Seizure Disorders
A Pharmacological Approach to Treatment

Seizure Disorders
A Pharmacological Approach
to Treatment

B. J. Wilder, M.D.
Chief, Neurology Service
Veterans Administration Medical Center
and Professor of Neurology and Neuroscience
University of Florida College of Medicine
Gainesville, Florida

J. Bruni, M.D., F.R.C.P. (C)
Assistant Professor
Department of Medicine (Neurology) and
Department of Pharmacology
University of Toronto
and Staff Neurologist
Wellesley Hospital
Toronto, Ontario, Canada

Contributing Author

R. J. Perchalski, M.S.
Research Chemist
Veterans Administration Medical Center
Gainesville, Florida

Raven Press ■ New York

Raven Press, 1140 Avenue of the Americas, New York, New York 10036

Made in the United States of America

Great care has been taken to maintain the accuracy of the information contained
in the volume. However, Raven Press cannot be held responsible for errors or for
any consequences arising from the use of the information contained herein.

Library of Congress Cataloging in Publication Data

Wilder, B. J. (Buna, Joe), 1929–

Seizure disorders.

Includes index.
1. Epilepsy—Chemotherapy. 2. Convulsions—
Chemotherapy. 3. Anticonvulsants. I. Bruni,
J. (Joseph) II. Title. [DNLM: 1. Anti-
convulsants. 2. Epilepsy—Drug Therapy.
AQ 85 W673s]
RC374.C48W54   616.8'45   80–5248
ISBN 0-89004–539–9   AACR2

To the neurology residents and postdoctoral fellows who have trained at the Veterans Administration Medical Center and the University of Florida College of Medicine, Gainesville, Florida.

Preface

The technological advances in antiepileptic drug monitoring of the past 20 years have richly enhanced our understanding of seizure disorders, mechanisms of action of antiepileptic drugs, and the pharmacology and pharmacokinetics of these compounds. The availability of accurate and reliable quantitative analysis of antiepileptic drugs in biological fluids and tissues has led to significant improvements in the treatment of epilepsy and related seizure disorders.

Before 1970, most physicians were taught to treat epilepsy by increasing the dosage of the drugs selected until the seizures subsided or toxicity appeared. Toxicity was generally described as interference with motor or cerebellar function, sedation, mental confusion, psychosis or marked behavioral aberration, or hematopoietic depression or other gross abnormalities of physiological function. The subject of saturation kinetics for the antiepileptic drugs was not appreciated. Chronic low-grade drug toxicity was only rarely suspected. Compliance could only be estimated from loss of seizure control (noncompliance) or gross aberrations observed on the neurological examination (overcompliance). Drug interactions were poorly understood and could not be scientifically defined and documented.

Currently, the physician treating epilepsy is guided by the concentration of antiepileptic drugs in the blood. Knowing the relationship between this concentration and the dose administered is crucial to the effective use of these agents. The efficacy and toxic effects of the antiepileptic drugs can only be reliably assessed by their blood drug concentrations. Through quantitative analysis of these compounds, the physician can predict drug interactions, establish abnormal drug metabolism, identify noncompliant patients, and verify suspected subtle medication toxicity. Also, drug interactions are now better defined in terms of absorption, protein binding, biotransformation, physiological potentiation, and elimination.

This volume synthesizes the important clinical information and scientific data on the pharmacological and physiological aspects of the antiepileptic drugs that are relevant to the proper medical management of convulsive disorders. It brings together comprehensively and concisely the pertinent information on the chemistry, mechanisms of action, pharmacokinetics, clinical use, drug interactions, and toxicity of the major and important minor antiepileptic drugs. Also presented is the current international classification of epileptic seizures, integrated with older, more descriptive classifications. The pharmacological principles of the antiepileptic drugs, which govern their effective use, are reviewed. The treatment of the various seizure types, including febrile convulsions, status epilepticus, neonatal seizures, alcohol withdrawal convulsions, and infantile spasms, is well delineated. Further, the theoretical basis of antiepileptic drug monitoring and the relationship of plasma drug concentrations to seizure control or drug toxicity are considered. The toxic effects of acute and long-term antiepileptic drug therapy are also discussed. The inclusion of a detailed description of the various techniques for the quantitative analysis of antiepileptic drugs should provide a practical understanding of the procedures that are so important to the recent therapeutic advances.

In the preparation of this work, we have drawn on our experience formerly as family practice physicians and now as neurologists and epileptologists, who have long been involved as clinicians in the management of epileptic patients and as researchers in the field of epilepsy and antiepileptic drugs. We hope that both the physician treating seizure disorders and the student of epilepsy will accept this volume not only as a guide to therapy but also as the pharmacological basis for developing a personal expertise in approaching the problems of a challenging disorder. The extensive reference list should serve as a good source of information on the treatment of seizure disorders and should be helpful in further research efforts on the pharmacology of antiepileptic drugs.

B. J. Wilder
J. Bruni

Acknowledgments

We express our appreciation to the administrative and medical personnel of the Veterans Administration Medical Center at Gainesville for providing an atmosphere of interest in epilepsy research and quality medical care for patients with seizure disorders.

We would like to express our sincere appreciation to Ms. Millie Walden for her dedication and assistance in the writing of this book. We also thank the personnel of the Neurology Service for their assistance in the many clinical and pharmacological studies cited in this book.

We acknowledge the support of the Medical Research Service of the Veterans Administration and the Epilepsy Research Foundation of Florida, Inc.

Contents

---

*This chapter was written by R. J. Perchalski, M.S., Research Chemist, Veterans Administration Medical Center, Gainesville, Florida.

1

Classification of Epileptic Seizures

Epilepsy is one of the most common neurological disorders. Convulsive seizures may occur during or after many of the acquired diseases or disorders that affect the nervous system. Transient seizures may be caused by drug or alcohol intoxication or withdrawal or electrolyte imbalance. Seizures are often the most prominent sign of brain dysfunction caused by diseases or injuries of the brain. They may be only one of a wide variety of neurologic disturbances that indicate abnormalities of brain structure and function.

The word epilepsy comes from the Greek: a "phenomenon in which man appears to be seized by forces from without." Epilepsy was recognized as early as 2080 B.C. when laws and rules regarding the marriage of epileptic persons and the validity of their court testimony were laid down in the Code of Hammurabi.

Although Hippocrates considered epilepsy as a disease of the brain, it was Charles Le Pois in the early 17th century who first stated that all epilepsies are of brain origin. John Hughlings Jackson and William Gowers were the leaders in the modern understanding of epilepsy. Jackson introduced the concept of a discharging epileptic focus in 1870. He considered petit mal (absence seizures) and grand mal (generalized tonic-clonic seizures) to be manifestations of paroxysmal discharges beginning in a focus and spreading from a focus in the brain (Taylor, 1958). Gowers in 1885 modified this focal concept by classifying the epilepsies into those arising in a demonstrable area of the brain (partial seizures) and those occurring as an expression of a condition of the brain which is not evidenced by a demonstrable structural lesion (primary generalized seizures) (Gowers, 1885).

INCIDENCE

The incidence of epilepsy (number of new cases of epilepsy occurring within a given population within a given period of time) has been variously reported to range

1

from 0.11% to 0.7%. The Epilepsy Foundation of America (1975) reports an incidence rate of approximately 4%, with a prevalence rate (number of epileptic patients in a population at a specific time) of 2% of the population in the United States. The highest incidence of epilepsy occurs among the age groups of <1 to 4 years. Of all new cases of seizure disorders, 77% occurs before the age of 20. The high incidence of epilepsy before age 5 (30% of the total) probably includes the incidence of febrile seizures that occur during the first 5 years of childhood.

DEFINITIONS AND DESCRIPTIONS

The term epilepsy implies chronicity or recurrence of seizures, with the primary defect originating in the brain. The term seizures can mean an epileptic attack or any convulsive or nonconvulsive episode resulting from a transient insult or intoxication of the central nervous system (CNS). The most remarkable clinical characteristic of epilepsy is the discontinuity of symptoms, with widely varying intervals between attacks. These intervals may be measured in minutes (as in the case of myoclonic spasms or absence attacks), hours, days, weeks, months, or even years. Epileptic seizures also vary widely in clinical presentation and duration. Thus a comprehensive and yet simple definition of epilepsy is not available.

Epilepsy is best referred to as a paroxysmal disorder of the brain. More than 100 years ago, John Hughlings Jackson described epilepsy as "an occasional and excessive disorderly discharge of nervous tissue." This conveys a concept of a neural irritative process or an abnormal state of nervous tissue discharge. Electrophysiological research during the past 40 years has strongly confirmed Jackson's original concept. Epilepsy is a symptom of brain dysfunction in which there is an occasional irritative or paroxysmal discharge of neurons, which is manifested as seizures. The seizures may be convulsive or nonconvulsive. The transient modifications in brain function that mark the seizure include alterations in or loss of consciousness or conscious contact, abnormal movements, and changes in sensation, emotion, visceral function, and behavior. Seizures derived from local abnormalities in the brain may be partial or focal in their extent. Other seizures are generalized from the start and involve widespread areas of the brain simultaneously. The concept of a paroxysmal discharge implies an abnormal increase in brain function in which whole populations of neurons are involved. The discharge can spread from focal abnormal areas into normal areas.

Epileptic activation can involve physiologically normal tissue by spreading directly from a contiguous area of the brain or by projecting and propagating paroxysms of abnormal discharge along neural pathways to distant neuronal centers. When epileptic discharge spreads from a focus to adjacent brain, the results of the successive and sequential epileptic activation of an increasing area of brain tissue are observable. One of the best examples of this is the focal motor seizure, which can be observed to spread from the hand to the face to the trunk and subsequently to the lower extremity before spreading to the opposite side of the body. The correlation for this is the spread of epileptiform activity from the motor-hand area to the face, trunk, and leg areas before projection to the opposite hemisphere to produce a secondarily generalized tonic-clonic seizure.

TERMINOLOGY*

The terminology of epilepsy has evolved over many years as scientific knowledge has increased. The word epilepsy itself has many meanings; even today some would restrict its use to the supposedly idiopathic or primary disorder of generalized seizures without evidence of focal onset. The term grand mal describes the major generalized convulsion, which is characterized by loss of consciousness followed by a sequence of tonic and clonic convulsive activity melding into a state of postseizure depression. Grand mal seizures are now known as generalized tonic-clonic seizures. The term petit mal, formerly used to describe absence attacks, which occur primarily in children and are associated with an electroencephalogram (EEG) pattern of 3 per sec spike and wave discharge, has given way to the new terminology of absence seizures. Automatisms, psychic seizures, limbic seizures, and psychomotor attacks are older terms that implicate temporal lobe or limbic system localization; they are now known as complex partial seizures.

The term aura is used to indicate a warning of an oncoming seizure. Indeed, from anatomic and physiological standpoints, the aura represents the seizure onset and may be the most important part of the seizure; the symptoms and signs of the seizure may reflect the function of the part of the brain in which it originates. The aura may entirely represent a simple partial seizure, which is recognized by current classification.

Premonitory or prodromal symptoms are less clearly defined, and little physiological or biochemical information is available as to their exact meaning. However, patients and observers of patients can sometimes predict when seizures will commence. Mothers may report that children become irritable, dull, or withdrawn; patients may have headaches, malaise, and sensations of impending doom hours before the seizure occurs.

In the past, seizures were named on the basis of precipitating factors. These types of seizures are rare. The most common, which occurs in patients who are sensitive to light, often can be precipitated with photic stimulation; it is known as photic epilepsy. Similar seizures may be induced by viewing television, riding under trees in bright sunlight, or other visual stimuli. Musicogenic epilepsy is the term for seizures precipitated by music or particular sounds. Rarely, seizures may be precipitated by reading or by attempting to solve arithmetic problems. These types of attacks have been called reading epilepsy and *epilepsia arithmatica*. If a patient runs during a seizure, he may be described as having cursive epilepsy; if he laughs, he may be said to have gelastic seizures.

---

*Taken from the Report of the Commission on Classification and Terminology of the International League Against Epilepsy, 1980.

CLASSIFICATION OF EPILEPTIC SEIZURES

The contemporary classification of epileptic seizures has considered several aspects of the disorder. The first is the clinical expression of the seizure, that is, the events observed during the attack and the symptoms experienced by the patient. The second relates to the anatomic and physiological substrates of the seizure, based on the nature of the attack and on knowledge of brain function, the latter being reinforced by the EEG. Other considerations—etiological, pathological, and age factors—may be relevant to the seizure state and may incorporate knowledge of genetic inheritance or acquired disease.

Historically, epilepsy has been described as being either idiopathic or symptomatic. The term idiopathic implies that the cause of the epilepsy is unknown, and that the seizure is its only sign or symptom. The implication of the term symptomatic is that the cause is discoverable in terms of changes in the brain, usually of an acquired nature. In the broadest sense, all epilepsy is symptomatic. The genetic traits that may predispose some individuals to seizures, whether their causes are known or unknown, is the actual disease and is also that which is transmitted. A genetic inheritance appears to be particularly important in the generalized seizure disorders. However, the incorporation of genetic implications at our present state of understanding does not help in forming a basis of seizure classification. Epilepsy is best classified primarily by the nature of the seizure itself and secondarily by the inferred anatomic, physiological, and pathological correlates (Schmidt and Wilder, 1968).

An accurate seizure classification is important for the evaluation of possible etiological factors and subsequent therapy. Unanimity of seizure terminology is also important for the purpose of communication. It should be stressed that what is referred to here is a classification of epileptic seizures and not of the epilepsies (Merlis, 1970).

Although a completely satisfactory seizure classification is not available, the Classification of Epileptic Seizures of the International League Against Epilepsy is the most widely accepted (Gastaut, 1970). It is based on clinical features, electroencephalographic features, anatomic substrate, etiology, and age. Since the classification was introduced, however, only the clinical seizure type and ictal and interictal EEG features have been emphasized. The main feature of this classification is the distinction between seizures that are generalized from the beginning and those that are partial or focal at the onset and become generalized secondarily. The classification categorizes epileptic seizures as partial, generalized, unilateral, and unclassified, as summarized below.

I.   Partial seizures (seizures beginning locally)
   A.   Partial seizures with elementary symptomatology (generally without impairment of consciousness)
     1. With motor symptoms (includes Jacksonian seizures)
     2. With special sensory or somatosensory symptoms
     3. With autonomic symptoms
     4. Compound forms

    B. Partial seizures with complex symptomatology (generally with impairment of consciousness) (temporal lobe or psychomotor seizures)
   1. With impairment of consciousness only
   2. With cognitive symptomatology
   3. With affective symptomatology
   4. With "psychosensory" symptomatology
   5. With "psychomotor" symptomatology (automatisms)
   6. Compound forms
    C. Generalized seizures secondarily generalized
II. Generalized seizures (bilaterally symmetrical and without local onset)
    A. Absence (petit mal)
    B. Bilateral massive epileptic myoclonus
    C. Infantile spasms
    D. Clonic features
    E. Tonic seizures
    F. Tonic-clonic seizures (grand mal)
    G. Atonic seizures
    H. Akinetic seizures
III. Unilateral seizures (or predominantly)
IV. Unclassified epileptic seizures (due to incomplete data)

The Commission on Classification and Terminology of the International League Against Epilepsy has recently proposed a revision of the currently accepted International Classification of Epileptic Seizures (Gastaut, 1970). The development of more objective methods for the documentation of seizures, such as telemetered EEG monitoring with simultaneous videotape recording of the clinical attacks, has allowed further elaboration of the classification. The convention of describing epileptic seizures by clinical seizure type, electroencephalographic ictal and interictal expressions, anatomic substrate, etiology, and age has been changed. The proposed classification recommends that only the clinical seizure type and ictal and interictal electroencephalographic expressions of seizures be retained. Other factors, based on either historic or speculative information rather than on direct observation, have been omitted. The other major distinction of the proposed classification is the separation of partial seizures into simple and complex entities, depending on whether or not consciousness is disturbed. In the case of simple partial seizures, classification should be based on the initial manifestations, even though there may be further elaboration of simple partial events, for example, focal motor movements followed by adversion. In the case of complex partial seizures, the sequence is crucial. Even if the onset is a simple partial one, evolution to disturbance of consciousness makes it a complex partial seizure.

Thus a partial seizure is classified primarily on the basis of whether or not consciousness is impaired during the attack. When consciousness is not impaired, the seizure is considered a simple partial seizure; when impaired, it is classified as a complex partial seizure. Impairment of consciousness may be the first clinical sign of a complex partial seizure, or a simple partial seizure may evolve into a complex partial seizure. Impaired consciousness may be accompanied by aberrations of behavior (automatisms). A partial seizure, either simple or complex, may evolve into a generalized tonic-clonic seizure.

Simple partial seizures usually have unilateral hemispheric involvement and only rarely have bilateral involvement, whereas complex partial seizures usually have bilateral hemispheric involvement.

According to the proposed classification, all partial seizures can be classified as follows:

    I.   Simple partial seizures (consciousness not impaired)
        A.   With motor signs
            1. Focal motor without march
            2. Focal motor with march (Jacksonian)
            3. Versive (generally contraversive)
            4. Postural
            5. Phonatory (vocalization or arrest of speech)
        B.   With somatosensory or special-sensory symptoms (simple hallucinations, e.g., tingling, light flashes, buzzing)
            1. Somatosensory
            2. Visual
            3. Auditory
            4. Olfactory
            5. Gustatory
            6. Vertiginous
        C.   With autonomic symptoms or signs
        D.   With psychic symptoms (disturbance of higher cortical function)
            1. Dysphasic
            2. Dysmnesic (e.g., déjà vu)
            3. Cognitive (e.g., forced thinking)
            4. Affective (e.g., fear, anger)
            5. Illusions (e.g., macropsia)
            6. Structured hallucinations (e.g., music, scenes)
   II. Complex partial seizures (generally with impairment of consciousness; may sometimes begin with simple symptomatology)
        A.   Simple partial onset followed by impairment of consciousness
            1. With simple partial features (IA–ID) and impaired consciousness
            2. With automatisms
        B.   With impairment of consciousness at onset
            1. With impairment of consciousness only
            2. With automatisms
  III. Partial seizures evolving to generalized tonic-clonic (GTC) seizures (GTC with partial or focal onset)
        A.   Simple partial seizures (I) evolving to GTC
        B.   Complex partial seizures (II) evolving to GTC
        C.   Simple partial seizures evolving to complex partial seizures evolving to GTC

The proposed classification of generalized seizures is largely unchanged from the previous classification (see above), except that infantile spasms and akinetic seizures have been deferred to a classification of the epilepsies. The category of unilateral seizures has also been deferred to this classification.

The criteria upon which the newly proposed classification of epileptic seizures is based are defined as follows.

Simple and Complex Partial Seizures

Partial Seizures

With motor signs.

Any portion of the body may be involved in focal seizure activity, depending on the site of origin of the attack in the motor strip. Focal motor seizures may remain strictly focal or may spread to contiguous cortical areas, producing a sequential involvement of body parts in an epileptic "march." The seizure is then known as a Jacksonian seizure. Consciousness is usually preserved, but the discharge may spread to structures whose participation is likely to result in loss of consciousness and generalized convulsive movements. Other focal motor attacks may be adversive, with head turning to one side. Speech involvment is either in the form of speech arrest or occasionally vocalization. When aphasia occurs, it is transitory. Occasionally, a partial dysphasia is seen in the form of epileptic pallilalia, with involuntary repetition of a syllable or phrase. Automatic utterance occasionally occurs.

Following a focal motor seizure, there may be a localized paralysis in the previously involved region. This is known as Todd paralysis and may last from minutes to hours.

When focal seizure activity is continuous, it is known as *epilepsia partialis continua.*

With somatosensory or special sensory symptoms.

Somatosensory seizures arise from those areas of cortex subserving sensory function, principally the postcentral gyrus region. They are usually described as pins and needles or a feeling of numbness. Occasionally, a disorder of proprioception with loss of spatial perception occurs. Like motor seizures, somatosensory seizures also may march and spread at any time to become complex partial or generalized tonic-clonic seizures. Special sensory seizures include visual seizures varying in complexity (depending on whether the primary or association areas are involved) with images varying from flashing lights to well-formed visual hallucinatory phenomena, including persons or scenes. Like visual seizures, auditory seizures may also run the gamut from crude auditory sensation to such highly integrated functions as music. Olfactory sensations, usually in the form of unpleasant odors, may occur.

With autonomic symptoms.

Vomiting, pallor, flushing, sweating, piloerection, pupil dilatation, borborygmi, and incontinence may occur as simple partial seizures.

With psychic symptoms (disturbance of higher cerebral function).

These usually occur with impairment of consciousness (i.e., complex partial seizures). Dysphasia was referred to above. Dysmnesic symptoms include a distorted memory experience, such as a distortion of the time sense, a dreamy state, a flashback, a sensation as if a naïve experience had been experienced before, known as *déjà vu*, or as if a previously experienced sensation had not been experienced, known as *jamais vu*. When this refers to auditory experiences, these are known as *déjà entendu* or *jamais entendu*.

Cognitive disturbances, such as forced thinking in which the mind is riveted upon an obtrusive thought, memory, or melody, may be experienced. Occasionally, as a form of forced thinking, the patient may experience a rapid recollection of episodes from his past life, known as panoramic vision.

Affective symptomatology is a sensation of extreme pleasure or displeasure, as well as fear and intense depression with feelings of unworthiness and rejection. Unlike those of psychiatrically induced depression, these symptoms tend to come in attacks lasting a few minutes. Anger or rage is occasionally experienced; but unlike temper tantrums, epileptic anger is apparently unprovoked and abates rapidly. Fear or terror is the most frequent symptom, sudden in onset, usually unprovoked, and may lead to running away. Often associated with the terror are objective signs of autonomic activity, including pupil dilatation, pallor, flushing, piloerection, palpitation, and hypertension.

Epileptic or gelastic seizure laughter, strictly speaking, should not be classified under affective symptoms because the laughter is usually hollow and without affect. Like other forms of pathological laughter, it is often unassociated with true mirth.

Illusions take the form of distorted perceptions in which objects may appear deformed. Polyoptic illusions, such as monocular diplopia, distortions of size, or macropsia or micropsia, and distortions of distance may occur. Similarly, distortions of sound, including microacusia and macroacusia, may be experienced. Depersonalization, as if the person were outside his body, may occur. Altered perception of size or weight of a limb may be noted.

Structured hallucinations may occur as manifestations or perceptions without a corresponding external stimulus and may affect somatosensory, visual, auditory, olfactory, or gustatory senses. If the seizure arises from the primary receptive area, the hallucination would tend to be rather primitive. In the case of vision, flashing lights may be seen. In the case of auditory perception, rushing noises may occur. With more complex seizures involving visual or auditory association areas with participation of mobilized memory traces, complex formed hallucinations occur and may take the form of scenery, persons, spoken sentences, or music. The character of these perceptions may be normal or deformed.

Seizures with Complex Symptomatology

Automatisms.

These may occur in both partial and generalized seizures. They are described here for convenience. In the *Dictionary of Epilepsy* (Gastaut, 1973), automatisms are described as "more or less coordinated adapted (eupractic or dyspractic) involuntary motor activity occurring during the state of clouding of conciousness either in the course of or after an epileptic seizure and usually followed by amnesia for the event. The automatism may be simply a continuation of an activity that was going on when the seizure occurred or, conversely, a new activity developed in association with the ictal impairment of consciousness. Usually, the activity is commonplace in nature, often provoked by the subject's environment or by his sensations during the seizure; exceptionally, fragmentary, primitive, infantile, or antisocial behavior is seen. From a symptomatologic point of view, the following are distinguished: (a) eating automatisms (chewing, swallowing), (b) automatisms of mimicry, expressing the subject's emotional state (usually of fear) during the seizure; (c) gestural automatisms, crude or elaborate, directed toward either the subject or his environment; (d) ambulatory automatisms; and (e) verbal automatisms.

Ictal epileptic automatisms usually represent the release of automatic behavior under the influence of clouding of consciousness that accompanies a generalized or partial epileptic seizure (confusional automatisms). They may occur in complex partial seizures as well as in absence seizures. Postictal epileptic automatisms may follow any severe epileptic seizure, especially a tonic-clonic one, and are usually associated with confusion.

Masticatory or oropharyngeal automatisms may arise from the amygdala or insula and opercular regions. They are occasionally seen in the generalized epilepsies, particularly absence seizures and do not help in localizing the automatisms. The same is true of salivatory, mimicry, and gestural automatisms. In the latter, fumbling of the clothes, scratching, and other complex motor activity may occur in both complex partial and absence seizures. Ictal speech automatisms are occasionally seen. Ambulatory seizures may occur either as prolonged automatisms of absence, particularly prolonged absence continuing, or of complex partial seizures. In the latter, a patient may occasionally continue to drive a car, although he may violate traffic light regulations.

Automatisms are a common feature of different types of epilepsy. While they do not lend themselves to simple anatomic interpretation, they have in common a discharge involving various areas of the limbic system without implication of any one specific area responsible for the symptom. Crude and elaborate automatisms occur in patients with absence as well as complex partial seizures. As such, they have no definite localizing value. Of greater significance is the precise descriptive history of the seizures, the age of the patient, and the presence or absence of an aura and of postictal behavior, including the presence or absence of confusion.

Drowsiness and somnolence.

These imply a sleep state from which the patient can be aroused to make appropriate motor and verbal responses. In stupor, the patient may make some spontaneous movement and can be aroused by painful or other vigorously applied stimuli to make avoidance movements. The patient, in confusion, makes inappropriate responses to his environment and is disoriented in regard to place, time, or person.

Aura.

A frequently used term in the description of epileptic seizures is aura. According to the *Dictionary of Epilepsy* (Gastaut, 1973), this term was introduced by Galen to describe the sensation of a breath of air felt by some subjects prior to the onset of a seizure. Others have referred to the aura as the portion of a seizure experienced before loss of consciousness. This loss of consciousness may be the result of secondary generalization of the seizure discharge or of alteration of consciousness imparted by the development of a complex partial seizure.

The aura is that portion of the seizure that occurs before consciousness is lost and for which memory is retained afterwards. As in simple partial seizures, the aura may be the entire seizure. Where consciousness is subsequently lost, the aura is the signal symptom of a complex partial seizure. An aura is a retrospective term described after the seizure is ended.

The most important distinction between simple and complex partial seizures is the presence or impairment of the fully conscious state. In the context of this classification, consciousness refers to the degree of awareness and/or responsiveness of the patient to externally applied stimuli. Responsiveness refers to the ability of the patient to carry out simple commands or willed movement. Awareness refers to the patient's contact with events during the period in question. A patient aware and unresponsive will be able to recount the events that occurred during an attack and his inability to respond by movement or speech.

Generalized Seizures

Absence Seizures

The hallmark of the absence attack is a sudden onset, interruption of ongoing activities, a blank stare, and possibly a brief upward rotation of the eyes. If the patient is speaking, his speech is interrupted; if walking, he stands transfixed; if eating, he stops the food on its way to his mouth. Usually, the patient will be unresponsive when spoken to. The attack lasts from a few seconds to half a minute and evaporates as rapidly as it commenced.

With impairment of consciousness only.

This describes absence simple, in which no other activities take place during the attack.

With mild clonic components.

The onset of the attack is indistinguishable from the above, but clonic movements may occur in the eyelids, at the corner of the mouth, or in other muscle groups. These may vary in severity from almost imperceptible movements to generalized myoclonic jerks. Objects held in the hand may be dropped.

With increase in postural tone.

During the attack, tonic muscular contraction may occur, leading to increase in muscle tone. This may affect the extensor or the flexor muscles symmetrically or asymmetrically. If the patient is standing, the head may be drawn backward, and the trunk may arch, possibly leading to retropulsion. The head may tonically draw to one side or the other.

With diminution of postural tone.

There may be a diminution in tone of muscles subserving posture as well as in the limbs, leading to drooping of the head, occasional slumping of the trunk, dropping of the arms, and relaxation of grip. Rarely, tone is sufficiently diminished to cause the person to fall.

With automatisms.

Purposeful or quasipurposeful movements occurring in the absence of awareness during an absence attack are frequent and may range from lip licking and swallowing to clothes fumbling or aimless walking. If spoken to, the patient may grunt or turn to the spoken voice; when touched or tickled, he may rub the site. Automatisms are quite elaborate and may consist of combinations of the above-described movements, or they might be so simple as to be missed by casual observation. Mixed forms of absence frequently occur.

Tonic-Clonic Seizures

The most frequently encountered of the generalized seizures are the generalized tonic-clonic seizures, often known as grand mal. Some patients experience a vague, ill-described warning, but the majority lose consciousness without any premonitory symptoms. There is a sudden, sharp tonic contraction of muscles. When this involves the respiratory muscles, there is a cry or moan, and the patient falls to the ground in the tonic state, occasionally sustaining an injury. He lies rigid on the ground; during this state, tonic contraction inhibits respiration, and cyanosis may occur. The tongue may be bitten, and urine may be passed involuntarily. This tonic stage then gives way to a clonic convulsive movement lasting for a variable period of time. During this stage, small gusts of respiration may occur between the convulsive movements; usually, however, the patient remains cyanotic, and saliva may froth from the mouth. At the end of this stage, deep inspiration occurs, and all the muscles relax, after which the patient remains unconscious for a variable period of time. He then frequently goes into a deep sleep and, upon awakening, feels quite well, apart from stiffness, soreness, and headaches. Grand mal convulsions may occur in childhood and in adult life; they are not as frequent as absence seizures but vary from one per day to one every 3 months and occasionally years.

Myoclonic Seizures

Myoclonic jerks (single or multiple).

Myoclonic jerks are sudden, short, shock-like contractions that may be generalized or confined to the face and trunk, to one or more extremities, or even to individual muscles or groups of muscles. Myoclonus may be rapidly repetitive or relatively isolated and occurs most frequently around the hours of going to sleep or awakening.

Clonic seizures.

As described by Gowers (1885):

> The muscle contractions become more shock-like in character and the state of clonic spasm is reached in which the limbs, head, face, and trunk are jerked with violence and through similar spasms of the muscles of the tongue and jaws, the former is often bitten. In becoming less frequent, the contractions do not become less strong, and the last jerks often are as violent as those which have preceded it. At last the spasm is at an end and the patient lies senseless and prostrate, sleeps heavily for a time and then can be aroused. Urine frequently, and feces occasionally, are passed during the fit.

Tonic Seizures

Again to quote Gowers (1885), a tonic seizure is:

> A rigid, violent muscular contraction, fixing the limbs in some strained position. There is usually deviation of the eyes and of the head toward one side, and this may amount to rotation involving the whole body and may actually cause the patient to turn around, even two or three times. The features are distorted; the color of the face, unchanged at first, rapidly becomes pale and then flushed and ultimately livid as the fixation of the chest by the spasms stops the movement of respiration. The eyes are open or closed; the conjunctiva is insensitive; the pupils dilate widely as cyanosis comes on. As the spasm continues, it commonly changes in its relative intensity in different parts, causing slight alterations in the position of the limbs.

Tonic axial seizures with extension of head, neck, and trunk may also occur.

Clonic-Tonic-Clonic Seizures

Clonic-tonic-clonic seizures usually commence with a clonic phase passing into a tonic phase, as described above. Occasionally a series of myoclonic jerks precedes the tonic phase, leading to a "clonic-tonic-clonic" seizure.

Atonic Seizures

A sudden diminution in muscle tone occurs, which may be fragmentary, leading to a head drop with slackening of the jaw, the drooping of a limb, or a loss of all muscle tone, in turn leading to a slumping to the ground. When these attacks are extremely brief, they are known as "drop attacks." If consciousness is lost, this loss is extremely brief. The sudden loss of postural tone in the head and trunk may lead to injury, particularly of the face, by projecting objects. In the case of more prolonged atonic attacks, the slumping may be progressive in a rhythmic, successive relaxation manner.

(So-called drop attacks may be seen in conditions other than epilepsy, such as brainstem ischemia and narcolepsy-cataplexy syndrome.)

UNCLASSIFIED EPILEPTIC SEIZURES

The unclassified epileptic seizures include all seizures that cannot be classified because of inadequate or incomplete data. This category includes some seizures which by their nature defy classification in the previously defined broad categories. Many seizures that occur in the infant (e.g., rhythmic eye movements, chewing, swimming movements, jittering, and apnea) are classified here until videotape confirmation and electroencephalographic characterization provide the data necessary for specific classification.

Epilepsia Partialis Continua

Epilepsia partialis continua under this name describes cases of simple partial seizures with focal motor signs without a march. These usually consist of clonic spasms, which remained confined to the part of the body in which they originated but which persist with little or no intermission for hours or days at a stretch. Consciousness is not impaired, but postictal weakness is frequently evident.

Postictal Paralysis

Postictal, or Todd, paralysis refers to the transient paralysis that may occur following some partial epileptic seizures with focal motor components or with somatosensory symptoms. It has been ascribed to neuronal exhortion due to the increased metabolic activity of the discharging focus; it may also be attributable to increased inhibition in the region of the focus, which may account for its appearance in nonmotor somatosensory seizures.

2

Pharmacological Principles of Medical Therapy

An understanding of certain pharmacological principles as they apply to anti-epileptic drugs is necessary in order to prescribe drug therapy for the maximum benefit of the patient with epilepsy. Important concepts of pharmacokinetics include drug bioavailability, distribution, metabolism, excretion, half-life, steady state, and drug interactions. By applying pharmacokinetic principles, the physician can make allowances for individual differences in absorption, distribution, protein binding, and elimination that may arise from multiple factors. These principles can be applied to describe the time course of drug concentrations as a function of dose and dosage interval. The basic pharmacological parameters of some antiepileptic drugs are shown in Table 2.1. Extensive reviews of drug kinetics are available (Fingl, 1972; Feldman, 1974; Greenblatt and Koch-Weser, 1975; Gibaldi and Levy, 1976; Hvidberg and Dam, 1976; Fingl, 1978).

PHYSICOCHEMICAL PROPERTIES

The passage of drugs across biological membranes is largely determined by the physicochemical properties of the drugs and cell membranes across which the drugs are transported in their passage through the body. Factors that determine the ability of a drug to cross biological membranes include molecular weight of the drug, its lipid and water solubility, degree of ionization and pH, protein binding, and the presence or absence of active transport mechanisms. An additional feature is the presence of a specialized blood-brain barrier.

Water solubility is important for drug dissolution and absorption in the gastrointestinal tract. Molecular size is important in the transport of drugs across membrane

15

TABLE 2.1. *Pharmacological parameters of commonly used antiepileptic drugs*

Drug	Absorption	Time to peak plasma level (hr)	Volume of distribution (liters/kg)	Half-life (hr)	Protein binding (%)
Phenytoin	Slow	8–12	0.5–0.8	10–40[a]	70–95
Phenobarbital	Moderate	2–3	0.7–1.0	50–150	40–60
Primidone	Slow to moderate	2–4	0.6–0.7	6–18	0–10
Carbamazepine	Slow to moderate	2–4	0.8–1.4	8–20	70–80
Ethosuximide	Rapid	3–7	0.6–0.7	20–60	0–10
Valproic acid	Rapid	1/2–2	0.15–0.42	8–12	90–95
Trimethadione	Rapid	1–3	0.6–0.8	16–20	0
Clonazepam	Rapid	1–3	2–3	22–33	40–50
Diazepam	Rapid	1–3	1–2	20–50	90–95
Methsuximide	Rapid	1–4	0.6–0.8	1–2[b]	0–10
Acetazolamide	Moderate	2–3	0.8–1.0	48–96	80–90

[a]Dose dependent.
[b]Rapidly metabolized.

pores. Large molecules, such as proteins, are unable to cross biological membranes; thus the degree of protein binding affects drug transport. The degree of protein binding is also an important consideration in the understanding of certain drug interactions. Modern analytic techniques for antiepileptic drug monitoring measure total (protein-bound plus unbound) drug concentration, but it is important to note that only the free, unbound drug is pharmacologically active and able to equilibrate between plasma and tissues.

Lipid solubility is the most important property, and the ability of a drug to cross biological membranes is in proportion to its lipid solubility (expressed as the partition coefficient of the drug between an aqueous buffer and an organic solvent). The degree of ionization influences lipid solubility, with un-ionized molecules generally being lipid soluble and readily transported across biological membranes. Ionized molecules are poorly lipid soluble and poorly diffusible. The degree of ionization of a drug is in turn dependent on its pK_a and the pH of the body fluids. Most antiepileptic drugs are weak bases or acids and exist as a mixture of ionized and un-ionized molecules. Changes in pH will change the degree of ionization and the ability of the drug to cross biological membranes.

Most antiepileptic drugs cross the membranes by passive diffusion, although some evidence suggests that valproic acid enters the central nervous system (CNS) by an active transport system (Frey and Loscher, 1978). The effect of ionization on passive diffusion can be shown with phenobarbital, which has a pK_a of 7.2 (the pH at which 50% of the drug is ionized and 50% is un-ionized). Alkalinization of the urine increases ionization of the drug, with a resultant increase in its renal excretion as passive diffusion across tubular cells back into the circulation is decreased. Table 2.2 shows the degree of ionization of organic acids of different pK_a in biological fluids of different pH. At pH 5, more of the organic acid is un-ionized and thus is more easily transported by passive diffusion than at pH 8.

TABLE 2.2. *Ionization of organic acids of different pK$_a$ in biological fluids of various pH*

pK$_a$	Percent un-ionized			
	pH 5	pH 6	pH 7	pH 8
8	99.9	99.0	91.0	50.0
7	99.0	91.0	50.0	9.0
6	91.0	50.0	9.0	1.0
5	50.0	9.0	1.0	0.1
4	9.0	1.0	0.1	0.01

The intramuscular administration of phenytoin illustrates the importance of pH effects. The pH of parenteral phenytoin is 12. If injected intramuscularly (pH of 7.4), the phenytoin precipitates, and absorption is poor and erratic (Wilensky and Lowden, 1973; Serrano and Wilder, 1974). The intramuscular administration of diazepam is also not recommended because of erratic and unpredictable absorption. Phenobarbital is well absorbed from intramuscular sites because of its lower pK$_a$ (Viswanathan et al., 1978).

PHYSIOLOGICAL CONSIDERATIONS

Kinetic variations in drug responses may come from differences in various physiological variables that involve hepatic, renal, gastrointestinal, and cardiac function. Pathological states in the function of any of these systems may result in abnormal drug kinetics (Prescott, 1975).

Hepatic failure may lead to a decrease in the rate of metabolism of antiepileptic drugs, and only by monitoring their plasma level can dosage adjustments be made. Phenytoin, phenobarbital, primidone, ethosuximide, carbamazepine, valproic acid, and the benzodiazepines are all significantly metabolized by the liver.

Chronic uremia influences both the hepatic metabolism of phenytoin and the renal excretion of its metabolites. Protein binding is reduced, and the biological half-life of phenytoin is decreased as a result of enhanced hepatic metabolism (Letteri et al., 1971; Odar-Cederlof and Borga, 1974; Gugler et al., 1975). Uremia decreases the protein binding of valproic acid (Gugler and Mueller, 1978; Bruni et al., 1980b), but the effects on valproic acid kinetics have not yet been established.

Gastrointestinal disease may cause disturbed absorption of drugs secondary to changes in gastrointestinal pH, rate of gastric emptying, the mucosal membrane, and mesenteric blood flow. Biliary tract disease may affect the enterohepatic circulation of drugs. Cardiac function can influence the rate of distribution of drugs, with resultant decreased elimination.

Of major importance in drug response is the relationship between age and drug sensitivity, and most drugs are more toxic in the newborn than in adults. Differences in sizes of body fluid compartments, protein binding, blood-brain barrier, and hepatic and renal functions must be considered. Phenytoin is poorly absorbed from the gastrointestinal tract in neonates (Painter et al., 1978) and should not be administered by this route. The differences in drug responses of pediatric patients have been reviewed (Jusko, 1972; Rane and Wilson, 1976).

DRUG ABSORPTION, DISTRIBUTION, AND ELIMINATION

Absorption

The general principles of the factors that can influence the absorption of antiepileptic drugs are discussed above. Changes in gastric pH may have a variable influence on drug absorption, since pH may influence gastric emptying, degree of drug ionization, solubility, and stability. The presence of food may retard absorption (e.g., phenytoin), increase absorption (e.g., carbamazepine), and retard the rate but not the extent of absorption (e.g., valproic acid). Plasma concentrations of drugs may be lower after oral than after intravenous administration.

The influence of formulation on drug bioavailability can be illustrated by phenytoin. Phenytoin suspension may be better absorbed than the capsule form, and the bioavailability of different brands of phenytoin may also vary (Pentikainen et al., 1975; Melikian et al., 1977; Arnold et al., 1978). The concurrent administration of a second drug theoretically may influence the bioavailability of a first drug by influencing gastric motility, gastric pH, splanchnic blood flow, or the formation of insoluble complexes.

The intramuscular administration of phenytoin and diazepam is not recommended for the reasons discussed above. If both oral and intravenous routes of administration are contraindicated, dosage regimens that allow for a delayed absorption from intramuscular administration have been proposed (Dam and Olesen, 1966; Wilder et al., 1974a; Perrier et al., 1976). Intravenous administration results in rapid, complete, and predictable bioavailability. The controlled intravenous administration of diazepam and phenytoin is the preferred route in status epilepticus (Lombroso, 1966; Wallis et al., 1968; Wilder et al., 1977).

Distribution

The kinetics of drug distribution may influence the time of onset, peak effect, magnitude, and duration of drug action. Drug distribution depends on regional blood flow, cardiac output, pH gradients, plasma protein binding, and permeability of cell membranes (Shand et al., 1975). It influences the amount of available drug in the CNS and the rate of drug elimination. The effects of plasma and tissue protein binding of drugs are important considerations in drug distribution (Jusko and Gretch, 1976; Gillette and Pang, 1977).

Metabolism

Most of the antiepileptic drugs are metabolized by the cytochrome P450 system in hepatic microsomes. Metabolism usually changes drugs into more polar and less biologically active compounds (e.g., phenytoin, phenobarbital, ethosuximide). Some metabolites, however, have significant anticonvulsive properties (e.g., the metabolites of primidone, carbamazepine, trimethadione, methsuximide, diazepam, and valproic acid). Hepatic metabolism may be inhibited or stimulated (Conney, 1967; Kuntzman, 1969; Anders, 1971; Richens and Woodford, 1976). Genetic factors may be responsible for differences in drug metabolism (Kutt, 1971; Vessell, 1972).

Theoretically, altered drug metabolism is predictable when the effects are a function of drug concentration and no active metabolites are formed. Increased drug elimination, reduced steady-state drug concentration, and decreased duration of drug action result from enhanced drug metabolism. Drug half-life and total drug action will be decreased. Drug interactions that may result from concurrent drug administration are discussed in Chapter 14. The liver is the most significant organ for antiepileptic drug metabolism; the lungs, kidneys, and gastrointestinal tract also contribute to a minor degree.

Excretion

The basic mechanisms for renal excretion of drugs are glomerular filtration and pH-dependent tubular secretion. Fifty to sixty percent of phenobarbital may be eliminated by the kidneys, and impaired renal function may lead to decreased excretion of unmetabolized phenobarbital. Excretion of phenytoin metabolites may also be decreased (Letteri et al., 1971; Gugler et al., 1975).

Drugs and metabolites may be partly excreted in bile by passive diffusion or active transport. Lipid-soluble drugs are reabsorbed in the small intestine, thus completing enterohepatic circulation. Excretion of drugs in breast milk and saliva contribute little to drug elimination. Sedation or hyperactivity, however, may occur in breast-fed babies of mothers receiving primidone or phenobarbital. Phenobarbital excretion in the saliva is pH dependent. The lungs are an important route for paraldehyde elimination.

PHARMACOKINETICS

Important concepts of pharmacokinetics are derived from the mathematical analysis of absorption, distribution, and elimination of drugs. The concepts of biological half-life, zero-order and first-order kinetics, volume of distribution, and clearance must be clearly understood for proper application to the clinical situation.

Biological Half-Life

The biological half-life of a drug is the time required for the drug concentration to decrease by 50% after absorption and distribution are complete. For most drugs, half-life is independent of route of administration, plasma concentration, and dosage. Knowledge of the biological half-life of a drug is important in determining the optimum dosage interval and the duration of pharmacological effect. For drugs metabolized by enzyme systems that can become saturated (zero-order kinetics, e.g., phenytoin), it is important that half-life determinations be made at concentrations that do not saturate metabolizing enzymes; otherwise, the biological half-life increases. Half-life is generally determined by administering a drug intravenously and measuring the time of its disappearance from plasma.

Knowledge of the half-life of antiepileptic drugs allows determination of an optimum dosage interval and the time required for a drug to reach a steady-state plasma concentration. (Steady state refers to a stable plasma drug concentration at a constant dose rate.) Drugs with long half-lives and lack of significant gastrointestinal effects from single large oral doses, such as phenytoin and phenobarbital, can be administered to adults in single daily doses. Drugs with shorter half-lives, such as valproic acid, should be administered in two or three divided doses to maintain therapeutic plasma concentrations over a 24-hr period. Mathematical analysis predicts that a minimum of five drug half-lives must pass before a steady-state plasma concentration is achieved. Thus the effectiveness of a drug at a given dose cannot be fairly evaluated until this time, and dosage adjustment must be delayed.

First-Order Kinetics

Most antiepileptic drugs are metabolized by first-order enzyme kinetics. In this type of reaction, the rate of metabolism varies directly with drug concentration. As drug concentration increases, metabolism increases proportionately, and the half-life remains constant. The plasma concentration of the drug also increases proportionately with increasing dose. Figure 2.1 shows the relationship between dose and plasma drug concentrations for drugs with first-order enzyme kinetics.

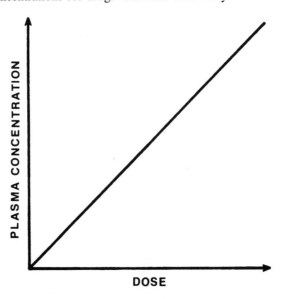

FIG. 2.1. Dose and plasma drug level relationship in first-order kinetics.

Zero-Order Kinetics

In zero-order kinetic reactions, the rate of metabolism reaches a maximum until enzyme saturation occurs; it then proceeds at a constant rate. The plasma drug concentration increases disproportionately with increasing dose, and the biological half-life increases with increasing dose. This relationship is shown in Fig. 2.2.

Zero-order kinetics are best demonstrated by phenytoin. With daily doses of phenytoin above 4 to 7 mg/kg, a small increase in the dose may result in a large increase in the plasma phenytoin concentration. The dose at which hepatic enzymes become saturated, however, varies among patients. With the knowledge that phenytoin may exhibit zero-order kinetics at high plasma concentrations, the physician should make only small dosage adjustments. Increasing the daily dose by 100 mg may lead to toxic plasma concentrations.

Volume of Distribution

The volume of distribution (V_d), expressed in liters per kilogram, describes the relationship between the amount of drug in the body and the plasma drug concentration. If a drug is confined to the blood stream, its V_d is equal to the blood volume. If a drug is highly bound to body tissue, the apparent V_d may be much greater than total body water. The degree of plasma protein binding also influences the apparent V_d. It is obvious that the plasma concentration of a drug is affected by dilution within the central compartment (in which the drug distributes rapidly), slower entry into the peripheral compartment, and rate of elimination from the body.

Single-Dose Administration

If a single oral dose of a drug is given, it can be predicted that it would be almost completely cleared from the body in five elimination half-lives. A single oral dose

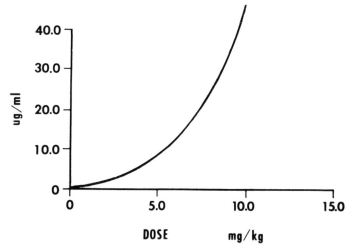

FIG. 2.2. Dose and plasma phenytoin level relationship in zero-order, or rate limited, kinetics.

of phenytoin would be almost completely eliminated in about 5 days. For a drug that follows first-order kinetics, it can also be predicted that unit doses given intravenously at half-life intervals will yield an initial plasma concentration after the first dose that will be half the peak value reached during chronic therapy. Steady-state plasma concentrations of the drug can be reached quickly if the initial dose is twice the maintenance dose administered at each half-life. This is the concept of "loading dose"; for phenytoin, a single dose of 12 to 14 mg/kg quickly yields therapeutic plasma concentrations.

Repetitive Doses and Dose Interval

In the chronic treatment of seizures, antiepileptic drugs are administered in repetitive doses. As mentioned above, with unit doses given at elimination half-life intervals, five half-lives are required to reach a steady-state plasma concentration. After a steady state is reached, plasma drug concentration varies with the dose and dosage interval. Administering the unit dose of drug at more frequent intervals decreases fluctuations of the mean steady-state concentration, but it does not change the rate at which the steady-state concentration is reached. Increasing the dose without changing the dosage interval increases the mean steady-state plasma concentration of the drug.

In practice, all antiepileptic drugs with elimination half-lives of 24 hr or longer can be administered once daily if no side effects (e.g., gastrointestinal) occur with single large doses. Children tolerate large doses poorly, and in them the drugs may have shorter half-lives. Even phenobarbital and phenytoin are administered to children in divided daily doses. In some adults, the drugs have shorter half-lives than usual and may require twice daily administration.

Drug Interactions

The administration of a second drug may alter the absorption, distribution, and elimination of a first drug. Important interactions of the antiepileptic drugs are presented in Chapter 14.

3

Medical Management of Seizure Disorders

The goal of medical management of seizure disorders is the prevention of seizures without medication toxicity. The physician must reach a seizure diagnosis and attempt to discover the etiology. The seizure diagnosis and therapeutic decisions are based largely on the patient's clinical history and electroencephalographic (EEG) record. The difficulty with this approach is that different seizure disorders may have similar clinical manifestations, and the EEG may not be definitive in some patients. For example, complex and atypical absence seizures may clinically resemble complex partial seizures, and the wrong therapy may be administered. Prolonged EEG recording techniques with simultaneous video recording of the seizure may help to assure that the seizure disorder is correctly diagnosed so that proper therapy may be instituted.

The availability of modern, noninvasive diagnostic techniques, such as computerized tomography (CT), increases the possibility of an etiological diagnosis, thereby allowing the prescription of specific therapy for some patients who were previously treated empirically. An etiological diagnosis cannot always be made. All patients with "idiopathic" seizure disorders should be reassessed periodically. This is especially true of patients with partial seizures, in those whose seizures become more difficult to manage without obvious cause, in cases of progressive EEG deterioration, and in patients in whom new neurological symptoms develop not attributable to antiepileptic drug toxicity. The ultimate diagnosis of a low grade astrocytoma or oligodendroglioma as the cause of a patient's idiopathic seizures is not rare.

A useful approach in the treatment of specific seizure disorders is presented in this chapter. (The pharmacological principles involved in the use of antiepileptic drugs are discussed in Chapter 2.) Although phenytoin and phenobarbital have been prescribed for more than 40 years, and many other antiepileptic drugs have had a long history of use, opinions differ about their effectiveness in the various seizure disorders. This may lead to multiple drug therapy.

With the application of plasma antiepileptic drug monitoring, polypharmacy can be reduced, and each drug can be used to optimum efficacy before another drug is added. Many patients can be successfully treated with one drug; only a few patients need more than two to achieve seizure control. When an additional drug is necessary, an attempt should be made to discontinue one or both of the previous drugs after achieving therapeutic plasma levels of the added drug. Thus the patient will experience fewer toxic drug reactions, and adverse drug interactions will be minimized. Table 3.1 divides the antiepileptic drugs and therapies into primary or major drugs and secondary or adjunctive drugs and therapies and gives the indication

TABLE 3.1. *Primary and secondary antiepileptic drugs and therapies*

Nonproprietary name	U.S. trade name	Daily dose (mg/kg)	Indications
Major drugs			
Phenytoin	Dilantin	4–7	Generalized convulsive seizures; partial seizures, simple and complex; status epilepticus
Carbamazepine	Tegretol	4–20	Same as for phenytoin
Phenobarbital	Luminal	1–5	Same as phenytoin (often used in combination with phenytoin); status epilepticus
Primidone	Mysoline	8–20	Same as for phenytoin
Ethosuximide	Zarontin	15–35	Absence seizures
Valproic acid	Depakene	10–60	Absence seizures, generalized tonic-clonic seizures; myoclonic seizures; adjunct in other seizure types
Secondary drugs and therapies			
Clonazepam	Clonopin	0.1–0.2	Absence seizures; myoclonus, akinetic attacks, infantile spasms
Trimethadione	Tridione	20–40	Absence seizures
Mephenytoin	Mesantoin	5–10	Same as for phenytoin
Methsuximide	Celontin	5–15	Same as for phenytoin
ACTH		40–60U	Infantile spasms
Chlordiazepoxide	Librium	1–6	Alcohol withdrawal seizures
Paraldehyde		0.1–0.2[a]	Alcohol withdrawal seizures; adjunct in status epilepticus
Diazepam	Valium	0.1–0.3[a]	Alcohol withdrawal seizures; status epilepticus, febrile seizures
Lorazepam	Ativan	0.05–0.15[a]	Status epilepticus
Acetazolamide	Diamox	10	Catamenial seizures
Ketogenic diet			Infantile spasms, Lennox-Gastaut syndrome, medically refractory seizures in infancy and childhood
Medium-chain-triglycerides diet			Same as for ketogenic diet.

[a]Single dose; total daily dose may depend on clinical situation.

for their use. The physician should be familiar with optimum dosage schedules, drug metabolism, absorption, distribution, elimination characteristics, half-lives, major toxic effects, and drug interactions peculiar to each agent (see Chapters 4 to 12). This knowledge should form the basis for treatment of the epileptic patient. Secondary drugs are often useful when primary drugs have resulted in allergic or idiosyncratic reactions, and they may be useful as adjuncts in combination with the major drugs.

Except in special circumstances or certain seizure types, antiepileptic drug therapy should be started with a single drug (see below). The physician should wait for the plasma drug level to reach a steady state before judging the efficacy of the drug. The dosage should then be adjusted to achieve optimum seizure control at a plasma drug level not exceeding the therapeutic range (see Table 3.2). Although unacceptable side effects do not often occur in the therapeutic range, the response may vary widely among patients. Thus therapeutic ranges are presented only as guidelines, and each patient's treatment must be individually determined. Usually, therapeutic plasma concentrations of an antiepileptic drug are associated with optimum seizure control. In some patients, however, seizure frequency and severity are reduced but not completely or satisfactorily controlled. When seizure control is unsatisfactory, a second drug should be considered. Certain drug combinations potentiate antiepileptic effects, and some combinations may also significantly potentiate toxicity.

The major exceptions for initiating therapy with a single drug are that the patient has (a) both absence and generalized tonic-clonic seizures, although in this case

TABLE 3.2. *Therapeutic plasma concentrations of the antiepileptic drugs*

Nonproprietary name	U.S. trade name	Normal range
Phenytoin	Dilantin	9–21 μg/ml
Phenobarbital	Luminal	20–50 μg/ml
Primidone	Mysoline	4–14 μg/ml
Ethosuximide	Zarontin	45–90 μg/ml
Carbamazepine	Tegretol	2–10 μg/ml
Clonazepam	Clonopin	40–100 ng/ml
Valproic acid	Depakene	40–100 μg/ml
Diazepam	Valium	200–500 ng/ml
Nitrazepam	Mogadon	40–90 ng/ml
Mephenytoin (measured as *N*-desmethylmephenytoin)	Mesantoin	12–25 μg/ml
Methsuximide (measured as *N*-desmethylmethsuximide)	Celontin	12–25 μg/ml
Mephobarbital (measured as phenobarbital)	Mebaral	20–50 μg/ml
Chorazepate (measured as *N*-desmethyldiazepam)	Tranxene	600–1,500 ng/ml
Trimethadione	Tridione	20–40 μg/ml
Dimethadione	Metabolite of tridione	700–1,400 μg/ml

treatment with valproic acid alone is often effective; (b) mixed seizure types; or (c) frequent or clustered tonic-clonic seizures or secondarily generalized partial seizures.

GENERALIZED TONIC-CLONIC AND SIMPLE PARTIAL SEIZURES

Phenytoin, carbamazepine, phenobarbital, and primidone are the most useful drugs for the treatment of generalized tonic-clonic and simple partial seizures. Valproic acid is also effective against generalized tonic-clonic seizures. Generalized tonic-clonic seizures can be controlled in 60 to 70% of patients; simple partial seizures can be controlled in a slightly smaller percentage of patients. Large, carefully controlled studies comparing the efficacy of the major drugs in the treatment of specific seizure types have not been performed.

The four major drugs may be used in the following order and combinations: (a) phenytoin or carbamazepine, (b) phenytoin plus carbamazepine, (c) phenytoin or carbamazepine plus phenobarbital, and (d) phenytoin or carbamazepine plus primidone. Valproic acid can be used in combination with any of the major drugs. However, interactions should be anticipated when this agent is used in combination with phenytoin and phenobarbital (see Chapters 7 and 14).

Initial therapy should consist of phenytoin or carbamazepine alone, since both drugs appear to be equally efficacious (Cereghino et al., 1974; Troupin et al., 1975; Simonsen et al., 1976; Shorvon et al., 1978; Kosteljanetz et al., 1979). Primidone is probably as potent as phenytoin or carbamazepine but often has disagreeable side effects, principally sedation, malaise, and personality alterations. We use primidone only rarely as a primary antiepileptic drug. Valproic acid may be used as the sole agent for the treatment of generalized tonic-clonic seizures if the patient also has absence seizures and/or myoclonic jerks. Phenytoin and phenobarbital or primidone in combination act synergistically. The combination of phenobarbital and primidone should be avoided because of potentiation of sedative side effects. A significant portion of primidone is converted metabolically to phenobarbital.

In children, carbamazepine may be preferred over phenytoin because of the frequent occurrence of hirsutism, acne, gingival hyperplasia, and interference with vitamin D and calcium metabolism associated with phenytoin therapy. Phenobarbital alone is often effective in children, although hyperactivity, excessive sedation, personality changes, and alterations in sleep patterns may occur.

There is little evidence that polypharmacy leads to better seizure control than monotherapy (Simonsen et al., 1976; Shorvon and Reynolds, 1977). When a second drug is added to the regimen, an attempt should be made to withdraw the first drug gradually if the addition of the second has effected seizure control. If seizures recur when the first drug is withdrawn, the patient should be maintained on therapeutic doses of both drugs. Valproic acid is often useful as adjunctive or sole therapy if the above regimens fail to effect satisfactory control. Thirty to fifty percent of refractory patients will have a satisfactory response to this agent (Simon and Penry, 1975; Pinder et al., 1977; Bruni and Wilder, 1979a).

The EEG may not be useful in determining drug efficacy in generalized tonic-clonic and simple partial seizures, and little correlation exists between clinical response and interictal EEG findings. The EEG may remain unchanged or show either an improvement or, rarely, deterioration following institution of treatment.

Unfavorable prognostic factors for generalized tonic-clonic and simple partial seizures include: (a) presence of an underlying structural lesion, (b) presence of seizures since infancy or childhood, (c) delay in the initiation of appropriate therapy, (d) presence of multiple seizure types (e.g., myoclonic, atonic, and generalized tonic-clonic), and (e) mental retardation.

COMPLEX PARTIAL SEIZURES

Although phenytoin, carbamazepine, and primidone are equally effective in the treatment of complex partial seizures, carbamazepine is the major drug. It may be used alone or in combination with either phenytoin or primidone, or both. Phenobarbital is occasionally used as a supplemental medication but may exacerbate the attacks. Significant seizure control can be achieved in more than 50% of patients with these three anticonvulsants alone or in combination. Secondarily generalized tonic-clonic seizures and associated automatisms are usually alleviated. Methsuximide may be of benefit in refractory cases, but development of tolerance to its antiepileptic effect may occur (Wilder and Buchanan, 1981). It may cause oversedation in combination with primidone or phenytoin.

We use the primary antiepileptic drugs in the same order and combination as outlined above for the treatment of generalized tonic-clonic and simple partial seizures. Primidone has been suggested as the preferred drug for the treatment of complex partial seizures, but no controlled study is available to prove its superiority. With the availability of carbamazepine in recent years, the use of primidone has declined.

Valproic acid may be helpful in 30 to 50% of patients when used as adjunctive therapy for complex partial seizures (Simon and Penry, 1975; Pinder et al., 1977; Bruni and Wilder, 1979a; Bruni et al., 1980a). It should be tried when other therapies have failed. Controlled studies are needed to compare its efficacy to that of the other antiepileptic drugs. We have observed significant improvement in more than one-third of medically refractory patients with complex partial seizures when valproic acid has been added to the regimen. When valproic acid is used in combination with phenytoin or phenobarbital, the potential for drug interactions should be anticipated (see Chapter 14).

Despite reports of the efficacy of the benzodiazepines in the treatment of tonic-clonic and partial seizures (Browne and Penry, 1973), these drugs have not gained popularity. Most of the reported studies were uncontrolled. Clonazepam has been reported to be better than placebo in a small controlled study of complex partial seizures (Birket-Smith et al., 1973) and slightly better than valproic acid when used as adjunctive therapy (Lance and Anthony, 1977). Acetazolamide may be useful as an adjunct in patients with premenstrual exacerbation of complex partial seizures.

ABSENCE SEIZURES

Ethosuximide and valproic acid are agents of first choice for the treatment of absence seizures. Drugs of second choice are listed in Table 3.3. Concomitant generalized tonic-clonic attacks are first treated according to the schedule outlined above, or therapy may be initiated with valproic acid. In the treatment of absence seizures alone, ethosuximide is the preferred drug because of lower cost, fewer side effects, more constant plasma drug levels, less frequent administration, and fewer drug interactions. Some patients may require combination therapy. The EEG is a good indicator of the efficacy of ethosuximide and valproic acid, since clinical response to these drugs is accompanied by normalization of the EEG (Villarreal et al., 1978).

In a study of 175 patients, ethosuximide was considered the most effective agent available at that time against absence seizures and myoclonus (Kiørboe et al., 1964). Eighty-seven of 110 children with absence seizures had more than a 50% reduction in seizures, compared with 16 of 23 adults. The drug was discontinued in nine patients because of side effects. Reports of early studies on the efficacy of ethosuximide are difficult to assess: most of these studies defined dissimilar populations, plasma ethosuximide levels were not monitored, and the number of concurrently administered drugs varied. Nevertheless, numerous reports confirm the efficacy of ethosuximide in the treatment of absence seizures (Livingston et al., 1962; O'Donohoe, 1964; Weinstein and Allen, 1966).

With the availability of plasma drug monitoring, a study involving 117 patients with absence seizures reported complete control of seizures in 53 patients (Sherwin et al., 1973). The majority of these patients had plasma ethosuximide concentrations greater than 40 μg/ml. A positive correlation was found between degree of seizure control and plasma level of ethosuximide.

In a group of 37 previously untreated patients, seizures were completely controlled in 19%, 90 to 100% controlled in 49%, and 50 to 100% controlled in 95% of patients (Browne et al., 1975). Plasma ethosuximide levels ranged from 40 to 100

TABLE 3.3. *Recommended drug therapy of absence seizures*

Drug or combination of drugs	Daily dose (mg/kg)
Ethosuximide	15–35
Valproic acid	10–60
Ethosuximide + valproic acid	
Ethosuximide + clonazepam	
Trimethadione (alone or in combination)	20–40
Paramethadione	20–40
Clonazepam[a]	0.1–0.2
Acetazolamide (as adjunct)	10

[a]Coadministration with valproic acid may cause seizure exacerbation.

μg/ml. Improved psychometric performance was observed in 17 patients, and side effects were minor.

With valproic acid therapy, a 75% reduction in absence seizures can be expected in two-thirds of patients with refractory simple and complex typical absences and in one-half of patients with refractory atypical absences (Simon and Penry, 1975; Pinder et al., 1977; Bruni and Wilder, 1979a; Bruni et al., 1980a). Failure of ethosuximide and valproic acid alone or in combination is an indication for the use of clonazepam or trimethadione.

Prior to the introduction of ethosuximide, trimethadione was the drug of choice for the treatment of absence seizures. Because of the high incidence of potentially serious side effects, however, it is now rarely used.

Clonazepam is indicated in medically refractory simple and complex absence and atypical absence seizures. Sedation is often a dose-limiting side effect. We use this drug only after failure with ethosuximide and valproic acid, or a combination of both.

INFANTILE SPASMS AND MYOCLONIC SEIZURES

The drug therapy of myoclonic seizures is difficult to evaluate because of differences in the study populations and the wide variety of conditions associated with the disorder. Myoclonus is a broad term for a number of disorders that have different causes and pathophysiological characteristics, numerous clinical and EEG manifestations, and various responses to therapy. Myers (1975) has listed more than 100 causes of myoclonus; it is not surprising that the response to any particular therapy may be variable.

The myoclonic epilepsies are more common in infancy and childhood. Their classification is complicated, but Jeavons (1977) has proposed a satisfactory scheme, which divides patients into six groups:

1. Infantile spasms (West syndrome, salaam spasms)
2. Myoclonic astatic epilepsy (Lennox-Gastaut syndrome, akinetic, petit mal, petit mal variant with myoclonic jerks)
3. Myoclonic absence (complex absence with myoclonus)
4. Myoclonic epilepsy of childhood (true myoclonic epilepsy)
5. Myoclonic epilepsy of adolescence (petit mal myoclonus, generalized epilepsy of adolescence with myoclonic jerks, bilateral massive epileptic myoclonus)
6. Photomyoclonic epilepsy (myoclonic epilepsy with photosensitivity).

There is no conclusive evidence that any of the antiepileptic drugs are effective in the treatment of infantile spasms; nitrazepam, currently unavailable in the United States, may be an exception (Volzke et al., 1967; Jan et al., 1971). In one review (Browne and Penry, 1973) were 19 reports of a favorable response to the benzodiazepines (usually nitrazepam), but most of the trials were uncontrolled. In a comparison of the efficacy of nitrazepam and diazepam in the treatment of myoclonic seizures, both drugs resulted in more than a 50% improvement in five of nine patients (Killian and Fromm, 1970). The efficacy of adrenocorticotropin (ACTH) and corticosteroids in the treatment of infantile spasms was first reported in 1958 (Sorel and Dusaucy-Bauloye, 1958) and has been reviewed by Sorel (1972) and Lacy and Penry (1976). ACTH or the corticosteroids, however, are of only short-term benefit in infantile spasms. The long-term prognosis is less satisfactory, and the incidence of mental deficiency, neurological deficits, and mortality is generally unchanged by treatment. Further discussion of ACTH and corticosteroids is given in Chapter 12.

Infantile spasms of undetermined etiology and normal development before their onset are favorable prognostic factors (Jeavons et al., 1973). The prognosis also depends on the patient's age at onset of spasms, mental state at time of presentation, and the presence of other types of seizures (Jeavons et al., 1973). Cortisone, hydrocortisone, dexamethasone, prednisone, and ACTH are equally effective in the treatment of infantile spasms (Lacy and Penry, 1976).

Clonazepam and valproic acid are sometimes of benefit in the treatment of infantile spasms and other myoclonic seizure disorders, but larger, controlled studies are needed (Dumermuth and Kovacs, 1973; Martin and Hirt, 1973; Vassella et al., 1973). From results of small studies, valproic acid appears to be highly effective in the treatment of myoclonic seizures (Simon and Penry, 1975; Jeavons et al., 1977; Pinder et al., 1977; Bruni and Wilder, 1979a; Bruni et al., 1980a). The Lennox-Gastaut syndrome is particularly difficult to treat, and multiple drug therapy is usually necessary for the management of these seizure types. The ketogenic diet and the medium-chain triglycerides diet may be effective in controlling seizures in the Lennox-Gastaut syndrome, as well as in other refractory seizure types of infancy and childhood (Livingston, 1972). In these diets, the daily ratio of fat to nonfat (carbohydrate and protein) is approximately 4:1. The urine should be tested daily for ketones, and supplementary calcium and multivitamins should be given (see Chapter 12). Other types of seizures occurring in conjunction with myoclonic seizures should be treated appropriately.

FEBRILE SEIZURES

Febrile seizures are convulsions occurring in infancy or childhood, usually between 3 months and 5 years of age, which are associated with fever but not with intracranial infection or other defined central nervous system (CNS) causes. Seizures associated with fever in children who have suffered a previous nonfebrile seizure should be excluded. Febrile seizures are to be distinguished from epilepsy (National Institutes of Health, 1980).

After a febrile seizure is terminated, efforts should be made to rule out a possible intracranial cause. In the uncomplicated febrile convulsion, however, complete blood cell count, measurement of blood levels of electrolytes, calcium, and glucose, skull X-rays, and CT scans of the brain are rarely useful. The role of the EEG in the evaluation of febrile seizures remains controversial; an abnormal EEG does not reliably predict the development of epilepsy in a patient with febrile convulsions.

Children who experience febrile seizures usually enjoy normal health following the episode, but they are at greater risk of impaired health than children who do not have febrile seizures. A second febrile seizure will occur in 40% of affected children, and 9% of these will experience recurrent febrile seizures. About 2 to 3% of children who have one or more uncomplicated febrile seizure will develop nonfebrile seizures or epilepsy. The risk of the subsequent development of epilepsy increases to as much as 13% if the child has any two of the following risk factors (Lennox-Buchthal, 1976; Nelson and Ellenberg, 1978; Fishman, 1979; National Institutes of Health, 1980): (a) a family history of epilepsy, (b) abnormal neurological examination prior to the febrile seizure, or (c) an atypical prolonged or focal seizure at the time of the febrile episode.

Intellectual impairment, hemiplegia, or death following febrile seizures is extremely rare (Wolf, 1979). Mesial temporal sclerosis and the subsequent development of complex partial seizures have been reported (Falconer, 1972). Findings from the NINCDS Perinatal Collaborative Research Project, however, do not support the development of these sequelae (Nelson and Ellenberg, 1978). Febrile convulsions rarely presage complex partial seizures or other types of epilepsy and are generally benign and self-limited.

In a study of 666 children with febrile seizures (Annegers et al., 1979), major risk factors for the development of epilepsy included preexisting mental retardation or cerebral palsy, atypical features of the febrile convulsions (e.g., focal seizures), and febrile seizures lasting 10 min or longer. The risk of developing epilepsy by age 20 was 2.5% for children without such complications and 17% for children with them. For all children, the risk was approximately 6%.

Prolonged febrile seizures can be terminated by slow intravenous infusion of diazepam (0.1 to 0.3 mg/kg). Intravenous phenobarbital in doses of 10 mg/kg given at a rate of 50 to 100 mg/min is also effective. Particular attention should be paid to cardiorespiratory depression.

The primary question faced by the treating physician is whether to prescribe prophylactic treatment in order to prevent recurrent febrile seizures or the subsequent development of nonfebrile seizures or epilepsy. The NINCDS Perinatal Collaborative Project, a study of 1,706 patients with febrile seizures followed to age 7 years, indicates that prophylaxis does not prevent the development of epilepsy (Nelson and Ellenberg, 1978). Thus the major goal of prophylaxis would be the prevention of additional febrile seizures, which does not seem justifiable except in patients who experience frequent febrile attacks. The question of whether the risks of long-term drug administration outweigh the benefits is still unanswered.

Phenobarbital is the drug most widely used prophylactically. The daily administration of doses that yield plasma levels of 15μg/ml will prevent the recurrence of febrile seizures. If the patient does not tolerate phenobarbital, primidone may be substituted.

Phenytoin is ineffective in febrile seizure therapy in children younger than 3 years of age but may be used for prophylaxis in older children if phenobarbital and primidone are not well tolerated (Melchior et al., 1971).

Experience with diazepam and valproic acid in the prophylaxis of febrile seizures is limited. Diazepam has been suggested as an alternative prophylaxis and could be administered at the onset of each febrile episode, rather than continuously (Knudsen and Vestermark, 1978; Dianese, 1979). Valproic acid is said to be equally as effective as phenobarbital (Cavazzuti, 1975), but a larger number of patients will have to be treated before the relative merits of each type of prophylaxis can be properly assessed.

In experimentally induced febrile convulsions, both phenobarbital and valproic acid have been found effective, but carbamazepine and clonazepam have not (Julien and Fowler, 1977).

The administration of phenobarbital in less than loading doses (10 to 15 mg/kg) or the use of antipyretics at the onset of a febrile illness will not prevent febrile convulsions (Camfield et al., 1980; National Institutes of Health, 1980).

Clinically, the potential risks of continuing prophylaxis are those predictable side effects, toxic manifestations, or idiosyncratic reactions that may be peculiar to the drug chosen. When phenobarbital is chosen, these reactions are generally hyperactivity, irritability and, less commonly, somnolence, sleep pattern disturbances with prolonged nocturnal awakening, and interference with higher cortical or cognitive function, such as defects in short-term memory formation, inattentiveness, decreased attention span, and defects in general comprehension (Faer et al., 1972; Heckmatt et al., 1976; Lennox-Buchthal, 1976; Wolf, 1977; Wolf et al., 1977; Bower, 1978; Freeman, 1978; Ounsted, 1978; Livingston et al., 1979; Camfield, 1980; National Institutes of Health, 1980). Side effects and toxic reactions of phenobarbital prophylaxis have been reported in up to 40% of infants and children. Experimentally in animals, prolonged treatment with phenobarbital has been shown to cause a decrease in brain weight and brain content of DNA, RNA, protein, and cholesterol (Schain and Watanabe, 1976; Diaz et al., 1977).

NEONATAL SEIZURES

Neonatal seizures occurring in the first month of life in less than 1% of infants are often the presenting manifestation of serious neurological disturbance. Because of immaturity of the CNS, seizure phenomena in newborns differ from those in older children and adults. Well-developed tonic-clonic seizures are rare. Seizures in premature infants may be difficult to recognize since they may resemble reflex activity or random movements.

Neonatal seizures generally have a poor prognosis because of associated etiological conditions. The incidence of permanent neurological sequelae is high. The earlier the onset of seizures after birth, the worse the prognosis in terms of both mortality and permanent sequelae. The cause of neonatal seizures can usually be determined in 75% of patients. Causative factors include infection, metabolic disorders, drug withdrawal, birth trauma, hypoxia, and congenital malformations (Lombroso, 1974; Volpe, 1977) (see Table 3.4).

Seizures caused by perinatal hypoxia, hypoglycemia, intracranial hemorrhage, and drug withdrawal most frequently begin in the first few days of life, whereas intracranial infections generally present later. Hypocalcemia and developmental defects may present with seizures both early and late. In both premature and full-term infants, perinatal hypoxia is the most common cause of seizures.

Since many etiological factors may be responsible, a careful prenatal and natal history is important, and a complete physical examination is mandatory. Laboratory evaluation should include examination of the cerebrospinal fluid for bacterial meningitis, as well as determination of blood glucose, serum electrolytes, and blood urea nitrogen. The EEG is generally of little use in establishing an etiological diagnosis. Skull X-rays and CT scans are of value in the evaluation of the infant who has suffered a birth injury.

Treatment of neonatal seizures is urgent because of the permanent brain injury that may result from repeated or prolonged seizures. Supportive measures to combat hypoxia and hypotension are essential, and acid-base disturbances must be corrected. Hydration, maintenance of body temperature, and avoidance of aspiration are required. Treatment is then directed primarily to the underlying etiological factor or factors. Therapy should be instituted quickly. After an airway is established and oral secretions removed, an intravenous line should be established. Based on the frequency of metabolic abnormalities as causative factors, 5 ml of 25% glucose should be administered intravenously. If seizures persist, the infant should receive 5 mg/kg of 5% calcium gluconate solution by slow intravenous injection during electrocardiographic monitoring. If seizures are still uncontrolled, magnesium sulfate in a 2% solution, 20 to 50 mg/kg, can be administered intravenously. The administration of 50 mg i.v. pyridoxine hydrochloride is indicated if the seizures

TABLE 3.4. *Etiological factors in neontal seizures*

Congenital malformations	Intracranial infection
Porencephaly	Bacterial
Microgyria	Viral
Hydrocephaly	Toxoplasmosis
Heterotopias	
Megalocephaly	Birth trauma (intracranial hemorrhage)
Others	
	Hypoxia
Metabolic causes	
Hypoglycemia	Drug withdrawal
↓ Sodium, calcium, magnesium	
↑ Sodium	
Aminoacidurias	
Pyridoxine deficiency or dependency	
Hyperbilirubinemia	

still persist. If seizures persist despite these specific therapies, antiepileptic drug therapy is required. Phenobarbital (10 to 20 mg/kg) may be administered intravenously and then continued orally (5 mg/kg/day in two divided doses) to maintain a therapeutic plasma concentration. Diazepam and phenytoin generally are not used. If phenobarbital fails, however, intravenous diazepam may be tried (Smith and Masotti, 1971). Diazepam should be used cautiously, in conjunction with phenobarbital, because of possible cardiorespiratory depression that may occur with doses as low as 0.3 mg/kg.

The treatment of neonatal seizures related to infection, drug withdrawal, and amino acid disturbances requires specific therapies directed to the underlying cause. If these measures fail, additional empirical antiepileptic drug therapy may be required.

DRUG AND ALCOHOL WITHDRAWAL SEIZURES

Seizures in the alcoholic patient may be caused by (a) an idiopathic seizure disorder, (b) toxic-metabolic states, such as electrolyte disturbance, hypoglycemia, or meningitis, (c) trauma, or (d) alcohol withdrawal.

Alcohol withdrawal seizures, or "rum fits," are generalized tonic-clonic seizures that occur during withdrawal of alcohol in patients who otherwise have no seizures and have normal EEGs. Focal features of the convulsion are indicative of additional factors such as trauma. Withdrawal seizures are more likely to occur 12 to 48 hr after cessation of drinking. They usually number one or two (Victor and Brausch, 1967), and status epilepticus is uncommon (Victor and Adams, 1953), occurring only in a small percentage of patients. Up to 40% of patients progress to delerium tremens.

It is important to exclude other causes of seizures before a patient is considered to have alcohol withdrawal seizures. Idiopathic generalized tonic-clonic seizures or partial seizures may be aggravated by alcohol (Victor and Brausch, 1967). Also, because the alcoholic patient is frequently exposed to craniocerebral trauma, post-traumatic seizures may often coexist with alcohol withdrawal seizures.

Various drugs have been used for the treatment of alcohol withdrawal (Sellers and Kalant, 1976), but the benzodiazepines are the most effective. Paraldehyde is also effective, but it has some undesirable side effects. If a history of seizures is obtained, the addition of phenytoin in therapeutic doses is indicated. In treating the alcoholic patient with liver disease, it is important to keep in mind that phenytoin metabolism may be reduced (Kutt et al., 1964). In addition, the free fraction of phenytoin may be increased because of hypoalbuminemia and the reduced ability of albumin to bind phenytoin (Hooper et al., 1974). Phenytoin need not be continued beyond the withdrawal period if the patient does not have a history of seizures unrelated to alcohol withdrawal.

For the prevention of withdrawal seizures, all the benzodiazepines are probably equally effective; however, chlordiazepoxide is used most frequently. Dosage varies from 100 to 1,000 mg daily (1 to 6 mg/kg), depending on the severity of the withdrawal reaction, and may be given orally or intravenously. Paraldehyde also can be used effectively in the treatment or prevention of these attacks. An initial dose of 0.1 to 0.2 ml/kg can be given parenterally or rectally in oil, and a dose of 0.1 ml/kg may be repeated every 2 to 4 hr for maintenance control (see Chapter 12). If status epilepticus or repeated withdrawal seizures occur, treatment should proceed as outlined below in the section on status epilepticus.

Experimentally, valproic acid has been found to prevent alcohol withdrawal seizures in animals (Hillbom, 1975; Noble et al., 1976; Goldstein, 1979), but no well-controlled clinical studies have compared its safety and efficacy to the benzodiazepines.

METABOLIC SEIZURES

The treatment of metabolic seizures should attempt to correct the underlying disturbance (e.g., uremia, sepsis, hypoglycemia, hypocalcemia, hyponatremia, hypomagnesemia). If an adequate response is not elicited, antiepileptic drug therapy is indicated. If the metabolic disturbance is correctable, the drug therapy may be subsequently discontinued.

STATUS EPILEPTICUS

Status epilepticus is a medical emergency and requires immediate treatment to prevent permanent brain damage or death. It is usually defined as a state of continuous seizure activity persisting for at least 30 min, or as a series of convulsions occurring without recovery of consciousness during the intervals between attacks. This definition is satisfactory for life-threatening convulsive status, but nonconvulsive status or epileptic fugue states also occur; and myoclonic status may be present without loss of consciousness.

Mortality and Morbidity

The death rate of patients with convulsive status epilepticus is between 6 and 12%. Treiman and Delgado-Escueta (1980) have reported an 8% mortality during the acute phase of status. Janz and Kautz (1964) and Oxbury and Whitty (1971) have reported similar mortality rates of 6.6 and 8.3%, respectively.

Clinical signs of brain injury are common sequelae of convulsive status. Neurological examination often reveals findings similar to the consequences of postanoxic, hypoglycemic, or Wernicke encephalopathy. Memory defects, confusion, difficulty in problem solving, apathy, and poor coordination are common sequelae of status epilepticus; for example, Engel et al. (1978) and Treiman and Delgado-Escueta (1980) have reported memory deficits following complex partial status.

Pathological changes in brains of children and adults dying during and shortly after status epilepticus reveal ischemic neuronal changes in the hippocampus, in layers 3, 5, and 6 of the cortex, and in the Purkinje cell layer of the cerebellum.

Ischemic neuronal changes are also found in the thalamus, basal ganglia, hypothalamus, and periaqueductal gray (Fowler, 1957; Urechia and Lichter, 1958; Scholtz, 1959; Karlov et al., 1974). These changes may result in part from the hypoxia associated with the convulsion, but there is ample evidence that continuous seizure discharge produces changes at the neuronal level. The metabolic activity necessary to sustain seizure activity outstrips available glucose, which results in metabolism of neuronal amino acids and proteins (Epstein and O'Connor, 1966; Meldrum and Brierly, 1973; Meldrum and Horton, 1973; Meldrum et al., 1973; Meldrum and Nilsson, 1976).

Children are more susceptible than adults to brain damage from status epilepticus. Focal convulsive status may produce local edema and local neuronal changes that may cause hemiparesis and asymmetrical ventricular enlargement. We have observed progressive hemiparesis in children who have experienced repeated prolonged focal motor seizures. Similar findings have been reported by others (Aicardi and Chevrie, 1970). Ventricular enlargement has been observed in 76% of patients after status epilepticus (Aicardi and Brarton, 1971). Brain weight in experimental animals is reduced following status epilepticus, presumably because of decreased protein synthesis and catabolism of amino acids (Wasterlain, 1972*a,b*; Wasterlain and Plum, 1973).

Classification

Status epilepticus comprises several different clinical entities, including both convulsive and nonconvulsive status, and may be classified as follows:

I.   Convulsive status epilepticus
  A. *Generalized tonic-clonic status* is a common and most serious form of convulsive status epilepticus. The incidence of neurological sequelae is high, and death can occur.
  B. *Secondary generalized tonic-clonic status* can develop from focal or partial status. It occurs most commonly as a complication of adversive, focal motor frontal lobe, or complex partial seizures.
  C. *Partial seizure status* usually occurs as focal motor seizures or sometimes adversive seizures with tonic head and eye deviation to the side of clonic seizure activity. Epilepsia partialis continua is a special form of focal motor status, which may continue for days or weeks with only brief periods of interruption. Consciousness is not necessarily lost during these attacks but is usually impaired. The EEG usually shows focal spike or spike and wave activity, but there is evidence that extrapyramidal centers are involved (Juul-Jensen and Denny-Brown, 1966).
  D. *Myoclonic status* occurs less frequently than other forms of convulsive status epilepticus. Consciousness may not be lost in the intervals between the massive muscle spasms, and the patient may be fully alert. This entity occurs in infantile spasms, progressive myoclonic epilepsy, postanoxic encephalopathy, and rarely in patients with generalized seizure disorders who have absence attacks, myoclonic jerks, and generalized tonic-clonic seizures.
  E. *Tonic seizure status* is manifested in prolonged bouts of tonic extensor spasms, and patients are unconscious during the interseizure intervals. These attacks occur

more commonly in infants and young children with infantile spasms and older children with Lennox-Gastaut syndrome.

II. *Nonconvulsive status or epileptic fugue states* usually require EEG confirmation for their differential diagnosis.

  A. *Absence status* is accompanied by an EEG pattern of 3 Hz generalized spike and wave or slow wave discharge. The activity is usually synchronous and symmetrical.

  B. *Atypical absence status* has EEG evidence of 1.5 to 4 Hz generalized slow or spike and wave activity.

  C. *Complex partial status* is usually accompanied by 6 to 15 Hz rhythmical activity over one or both temporal lobes and sometimes alternates between the two temporal regions. Automatisms may be present, and some patients may be in a stuporous or comatose state.

Causes

The causes of status epilepticus are varied. The incidence of generalized tonic-clonic status epilepticus is six times higher in patients with complex or simple partial seizures or "symptomatic epilepsy" than in patients with primary generalized or idiopathic epilepsy (Janz, 1961, 1964). Many patients with status epilepticus as their first manifestation of epilepsy have structural lesions. Head trauma, strokes, and tumors are common causes of status epilepticus. Infections, alcohol abuse, and antiepileptic drug manipulation or withdrawal are well-known causes of status epilepticus in epileptic patients (Hunter, 1959; Treiman and Delgado-Escueta, 1980). Status epilepticus can also be precipitated by electrolyte imbalance, hypoglycemia, febrile illnesses, and CNS infections. Diabetic ketoacidosis may precipitate status epilepticus in nonepileptic patients. Acute infarction of the brain and hypertensive encephalopathy can sometimes trigger status epilepticus.

Pathophysiological Changes

The physiological basis for the development of status epilepticus is unknown. A number of associated causes have been mentioned above, but the factors that lead from a single convulsion to status epilepticus are elusive. Treiman and Delgado-Escueta (1980) have discussed various hypotheses in their comprehensive yet concise report on this subject.

Status epilepticus leads to a number of physiological changes that must be considered and corrected when treatment is begun. A potentially serious and life-threatening situation, dependent on the length of the status epilepticus when the patient is first seen, is severe acidosis and profound loss of base reserve. Arterial pH determinations may reveal pH levels as low as 6.75. It is imperative immediately to determine arterial pH if the patient has been in status epilepticus for a prolonged period of time. Correction of the acidosis is equally as important as the administration of the appropriate anticonvulsant therapy.

A number of other pathophysiological changes may be found in the patient with status epilepticus (Table 3.5). The situation is dynamic; these changes depend on

TABLE 3.5. *Pathophysiological changes of status epilepticus*

Parameter	Early status (15–30 min)	Late status (> 30 min)
Pulse	Rapid	Weak and rapid
Blood pressure	Mildly to moderately hypertensive	Normal to hypotensive
Arterial oxygen tension	Decreased	Decreased
Arterial carbon dioxide tension	Elevated	Elevated
Bicarbonate	Decreased	Severely decreased
Glucose	Normal to elevated[a]	Decreased
Potassium	Elevated	Elevated
Sodium	Normal[b]	Normal to elevated[b]
pH	Depressed (7.0–7.2)	Depressed (6.7–7.1)
Lactic acid	Elevated	Elevated

[a]Hypoglycemia may rarely be a cause of status epilepticus.
[b]Hyponatremia may be a causative factor and should be corrected immediately.

the length of status, the amount of generalized tonic-clonic activity the patient has experienced, and the underlying cause, if it is discernible. Prolonged status epilepticus can lead to myoglobinuria and renal failure, hypercalcemia, intravascular coagulation, cardiac arrhythmias, and hyperpyrexia, in addition to the above pH and electrolyte changes.

Treatment

Treatment should be directed toward restoring normal physiological homeostasis and arresting seizure activity. Immediate attention should be given to respiration and airway patency. An oral airway should be inserted. If there is evidence of significant cyanosis, weak or shallow respirations, aspiration, or respiratory obstruction, then intubation, oxygen, and assisted ventilation should be instituted.

An intravenous line should be immediately established and maintained with normal or half-normal saline. If glucose is administered, it should be given in a separate intravenous injection. (Phenytoin, a major drug in the treatment of status, is soluble in normal saline but not in glucose solutions.) (Salem et al., 1980).

Blood samples should be obtained for a complete blood cell count and analysis for antiepileptic drugs, electrolytes, glucose, and blood urea nitrogen; 50 cc of 50% glucose should be administered prophylactically for possible hypoglycemia.

If status epilepticus has been in progress for 15 min or longer, arterial blood should be obtained for immediate analysis of pH, arterial oxygen tension, arterial carbon dioxide tension, and bicarbonate content. If the pH is 7.21 or less, 100 mEq bicarbonate should be administered. In addition to correcting acidosis, bicarbonate reduces hyperkalemia by driving potassium from the extracellular to the intracellular space.

Thiamine and pyridoxine should be routinely administered to all patients in status epilepticus to prevent possible Wernicke encephalopathy in the unknown alcoholic patient and to treat the rare case of vitamin B_6 dependency.

Physiological homeostasis and seizure termination can be accomplished simultaneously. The restoration of acid-base balance, physiological pH, and proper electrolyte balance depends on the use of 0.5% or normal saline and bicarbonate (depending on arterial pH). The antiepileptic drug selected may be mixed with the intravenous solution or administered separately, depending on the drug. The drugs effective in the treatment of status epilepticus are described below; their use in the order of choice for the various types of status epilepticus is summarized in Tables 3.6 to 3.8.

Phenytoin

Phenytoin is a drug of first choice in the treatment of generalized tonic-clonic, simple and complex partial, tonic, and myoclonic status epilepticus. Intravenous administration of 15 mg/kg at a rate of 50 mg/min stops the status episode within 20 min in 80% of patients (Wilder et al., 1977). Phenytoin can be mixed in normal saline in concentrations of 5 to 10 mg/ml without worry of precipitation (Salem et al., 1980). Theoretically, the addition of bicarbonate to the solution would further increase the solubility of phenytoin (the commercially available parenteral phenytoin is adjusted to a pH of 12 with sodium hydroxide).

Patients receiving a mean total intravenous injection of 9.2 mg/kg phenytoin (6.7 to 14.3 mg/kg) developed brain phenytoin concentrations of 16 μg/g by the end of the infusion (infusion rate, 70 mg/min). After 60 min, the level had reached a mean of 23 μg/g. During the hour following infusion, the plasma-to-brain ratio decreased from 1.8 to 0.5 (Wilder et al., 1977). Similar results have been observed in animals (Ramsay et al., 1979). Thus phenytoin penetrates the brain rapidly, and effectively terminates generalized tonic-clonic status epilepticus in the majority of patients.

Following intravenous infusion of 15 mg/kg phenytoin, plasma levels of the drug have remained in the therapeutic range for 12 hr (Salem et al., 1981; Wilder et al., 1977), and 18 mg/kg phenytoin have resulted in therapeutic plasma phenytoin levels for 24 hr (Cranford et al., 1978). These data are important, for they demonstrate that plasma phenytoin levels remain at a sufficient concentration to permit the institution of oral phenytoin in regular maintenance doses.

Intravenous phenytoin is a safe and effective method of terminating status epilepticus and has the additional advantage of not depressing the cardiorespiratory system or producing adverse neurological effects other than transient nystagmus. Hypotensive episodes and cardiac arrhythmias attributed to intravenous phenytoin (Cranford et al., 1978) result from excessively rapid administration of the drug. In 275 patients treated with intravenous phenytoin, we have observed only minor side effects of anxiety, vertigo, mild hypotension, and mild bradycardia.

Intravenous phenytoin, in addition to being an effective anticonvulsant, is an antiarrhythmic and has its greatest effect in cases of ventricular irritability. It decreases atrioventricular conduction and probably should not be given to patients with second or third degree heart block. Electrocardiographic monitoring is desirable but not necessary during intravenous phenytoin loading.

TABLE 3.6. *Pharmacological treatment regimens for primary and secondary generalized tonic-clonic status, simple partial status, epilepsia partialis continua, tonic status, and myoclonic status[a]*

Drug	Route of administration	Dose	Rate of administration (mg/min)	Time to action (min)	Remarks
A[b]					
1. Diazepam and phenytoin	i.v. concurrently	0.15–0.3 mg/kg 15 mg/kg	2 50	2–15	Maximum 10 mg diazepam; if seizures persist, follow with A2
2. Phenobarbital	i.v.	10–15 mg/kg	100	10–15	If seizures persist, follow with A3
3. Lidocaine	i.v.	4–5 mg/kg/hr		Variable	Continue for 1 to 3 days or follow with D if necessary
B					
1. Lorazepam	i.v.	0.05–0.15 mg/kg (usual dose 4–8 mg)	1	5–10	Follow with B2 or B3; if seizures persist, follow with A3 and D if necessary
2. Phenytoin	i.v.	15 mg/kg	50	15–20	
3. Phenytoin	Oral	5 mg/kg every 2 hr × 3			
C[c]					
1. Phenobarbital	i.v.	10–15 mg/kg	100	10–15	If seizures persist, follow with B2, A3, and D if necessary
D					
1. Pentobarbital or thiopental sodium	i.v.	Administered by anesthesiologist in intensive care unit			

[a]Start oral valproic acid after seizure terminates and continue oral phenytoin and/or phenobarbital if used to control status.
[b]Follow with daily maintenance dose of phenytoin (6 mg/kg).
[c]If successful, follow with daily maintenance dose of phenobarbital (3–4 mg/kg).

TABLE 3.7. Pharmacological treatment regimens for absence status

Drug	Route of administration	Dose	Rate of administration (mg/min)	Time to action (min)	Remarks
Diazepam or	i.v.	0.15–0.3 mg/kg (not to exceed 10 mg)	2	5–10	May be repeated 5 × in 24 hr
Lorazepam and	i.v.	0.05–0.15 mg/kg (usual dose 4–8 mg)	1	5–10	
Valproic acid or	oral	15 mg/kg/day (in three divided doses)			Increase dose (5 mg/kg) every 3 days to obtain trough blood level of 50–100 µg/ml
Ethosuximide	oral	20 mg/kg/day (in two divided doses)			Increase dose to obtain blood level of 50–100 µg/ml

TABLE 3.8. Pharmacological treatment regimens for complex partial status

Drug	Route of administration	Dose (mg/kg)	Rate of administration (mg/min)	Time to action (min)	Remarks
A					
Phenytoin	i.v.	15	50	15–20	Continue on daily maintenance dose of 6 mg/kg; if seizures persist, follow with B
B					
Phenobarbital	i.v.	10–15	100	10–15	Continue on daily maintenance dose of 3 mg/kg

Phenobarbital

Phenobarbital is highly effective for suppressing generalized tonic-clonic, simple and complex partial, and tonic seizures. The major drawback to its use in status epilepticus is that the large doses needed induce significant depression of consciousness and may depress the cardiorespiratory system.

Phenobarbital, when given in large intravenous doses, rapidly penetrates the CNS. In one study in experimental animals, it achieved a brain-to-plasma ratio of 3 within 1 to 15 min after infusion of 10 mg/kg (Ramsay et al., 1979). Brain phenobarbital concentrations reached 40 μg/g within minutes following the injection and then fell to 25 μg/g 1 hr later.

Phenobarbital should be given in an initial dose of 10 to 15 mg/kg at a rate of 100 mg/min. It is completely soluble in intravenous solutions. In patients who are refractory to phenytoin, it can be given immediately following a full loading dose of intravenous phenytoin without fear of potentiating CNS depression.

Phenobarbital should be used with extreme caution if diazepam has been used previously. It potentiates the cardiorespiratory depressant effects of diazepam, and both respiratory and cardiac arrest can occur without warning. The treating physician should be prepared to intubate the patient and provide assisted or controlled ventilation if phenobarbital is administered after diazepam.

Diazepam

Diazepam was first shown by Gastaut et al. (1965) to be extremely effective in stopping clinical seizure activity. The review by Browne and Penry (1973) found that 88% of patients treated with diazepam responded with cessation of seizures, but the seizures returned after 10 to 20 min in a high percentage of patients. Prensky et al. (1967) have reported that only nine of 20 patients were seizure free 2 hr after the administration of diazepam for status epilepticus. Recurrence of seizures after intravenous diazepam results from rapid redistribution of the drug from both the intravascular space and the brain. Ramsay et al. (1979) have observed that plasma diazepam levels fell from 600 to less than 150 ng/ml within 45 min after an intravenous infusion of 0.3 mg/kg diazepam in experimental animals. Concurrently, brain diazepam levels fell from 600 to less than 300 ng/g in the same period of time. Delgado-Escueta and Horan (1980) has shown that plasma diazepam levels must exceed 200 ng/ml to stop status epilepticus.

Diazepam, both clinically and experimentally, is an excellent drug for arresting seizures, but it does not prevent their recurrence. To effectively control status epilepticus, diazepam should be given concurrently with a major antiepileptic drug, such as phenytoin, that prevents the recurrence of seizures. Diazepam should be given initially in a dose of 0.15 to 0.3 mg/kg at a rate of 2 mg/min. It should be used with extreme caution if it is to be given concurrently with or following phenobarbital. Infants, young children, and the elderly are more susceptible to cardiorespiratory depression or arrest than older children and young adults.

We recommend the concurrent administration of 0.15 to 0.3 mg/kg (not to exceed 10 mg) diazepam and 15 mg/kg phenytoin as the most effective treatment for generalized tonic-clonic and simple partial status epilepticus. They can be given at a rate of 2 and 50 mg/min, respectively. The seizures promptly cease and do not recur in the majority of the patients (more than 90% in our experience).

Lidocaine

We use lidocaine in patients who have been refractory to the previously described regimens (see Chapter 12). It can be administered safely after other drugs have been given. Lidocaine should be injected at a rate of 4 mg/kg/hr and continued for several days to prevent recurrence of status epilepticus.

Electrocardiographic monitoring should be done, and widening of the QRS complex on the electrocardiogram should alert the physician to reduce the rate of, or discontinue, administration. Phenytoin therapy should be continued during lidocaine infusion to maintain plasma phenytoin levels in the therapeutic range.

Lorazepam

Lorazepam, a long-acting benzodiazepine (see Chapter 10), is marketed as an antianxiety agent, but is currently undergoing clinical testing for the treatment of status epilepticus. It has potent anticonvulsant properties; when given intravenously, it is extremely effective in terminating status epilepticus. The drug does not significantly depress the cardiorespiratory systems (Walker et al., 1979).

For generalized tonic-clonic or partial status, lorazepam should be given intravenously in doses of 0.05 to 0.15 mg/kg at a rate of 1 mg/min. Walker et al. (1979) have recommended 4 to 8 mg for the treatment of both generalized and partial status epilepticus. Seizures usually cease within 5 to 10 min, and their recurrence is not a problem because of the long half-life of the drug (about 12 hr). Treatment with lorazepam should be followed by the administration of a major antiepileptic drug, such as phenytoin, which should be given in a dose of 15 mg/kg, either orally in three doses of 5 mg/kg each every 2 hr (Wilder et al., 1973b) or intravenously at a rate of 50 mg/min (Salem et al., 1981).

Steroids

The use of steroids is indicated in refractory status epilepticus, in cases known to be associated with mass lesions (e.g., neoplasms), or in cases caused by such agents as acute head trauma, parasitic CNS involvement, infantile spasms, arteritis, or sickle cell disease. We recommend 1 to 2 mg/kg/i.v. prednisone. This should be repeated as necessary, depending on the cause of the status epilepticus.

General Anesthesia

The use of deep general anesthesia in the treatment of status epilepticus is rarely necessary. It may be required, however, when the above regimens fail. Thiopental sodium or pentobarbital are the agents of choice and should be administered by an anesthesiologist. The electrocardiogram is monitored; the patient is intubated, and oxygen is delivered with assisted or controlled ventilation. Monitoring of the EEG is essential to assure that seizure activity is completely suppressed.

Paraldehyde

Paraldehyde is of historic interest in the treatment of status epilepticus. It is an anticonvulsant agent and is effective in the treatment of status epilepticus. It is used only rarely now, as more effective agents, as described above, are available. The use of paraldehyde as an anticonvulsant is discussed in Chapter 12.

At the International Symposium on Status Epilepticus held in Santa Monica, California in November of 1980, Morrell reported that paraldehyde given intravenously in a 2% solution in association with phenytoin is extremely effective, having a low complication rate in terminating convulsive status epilepticus (F. Morrell, personal communication).

FAILURE OF MEDICAL THERAPY

Twenty to thirty percent of patients with chronic, recurring seizures are refractory to medical therapy. Lack of adequate seizure control may be indicative of factors other than medical intractability, including: (a) noncompliance, probably the most important single factor, (b) inadequate drug dosage, (c) improper drug or combination of drugs for the particular seizure disorder, (d) precipitating or aggravating factors (e.g., stressful situations, alcohol, sleep deprivation), (e) progressive neurological disease, (f) rarely, drug toxicity, and (g) drug interactions that may influence plasma antiepileptic drug concentrations.

The monitoring of plasma antiepileptic drug levels is helpful in determining compliance, kinetic drug interaction, and inadequate or excessive drug dosage. Toxicity is usually apparent from the presence of neurological signs. However, behavioral changes or psychological reactions may occur in the absence of overt signs of drug toxicity, such as ataxia and lethargy. Improper drugs or combinations of drugs may be recognized after reassessing the initial etiological and seizure diagnosis. Reevaluation with more intensive EEG monitoring may be required to distinguish complex absence seizures from absence-like complex partial seizures. A progressive neurological disease may be evident only after reevaluation. Physical and emotional stress are frequent causes of seizure exacerbation, and these triggering factors should be eliminated if possible. Sleep deprivation, emotional stress, excessive fatigue, alcohol, and irregular and improper dietary habits may cause recurrence of previously controlled seizures.

Occasionally, severely refractory patients must be hospitalized for withdrawal of all medications except a single major drug specific for the particular seizure type. Optimum plasma levels of the drug should be obtained. The patient should be reevaluated and started on a second drug under controlled conditions.

TERMINATION OF DRUG THERAPY

When an epileptic patient has been successfully treated and is seizure free, the question of withdrawing medication invariably arises. Most physicians are wary of discontinuing antiepileptic medication because of the high incidence of seizure recurrence when all drugs are discontinued. Patients with documented epilepsy who have been seizure free for 5 years will experience a recurrence rate of 40% after drug withdrawal (Juul-Jensen, 1968). Almost half of the recurrences are seen soon after discontinuation of therapy (29% during the first year; 15%, 3%, 6%, and 3% in the 4 years thereafter).

We caution against medication withdrawal until patients have been seizure free for a minimum of 5 years. At that time, antiepileptic drugs may be discontinued one at a time, withdrawing the supposed least effective initially. The dosage is decreased slowly over a period of 6 to 8 weeks until the drug is completely withdrawn. If the patient remains seizure free for 1 month, the second drug is discontinued in a similar fashion, and so on.

When drug withdrawal is instituted, the patient should not drive a motor vehicle. Close contact with the patient's family should be maintained during this period. Stressful situations known to precipitate seizures should be avoided; if seizures recur, therapy should be restarted. If medication has been completely withdrawn, monotherapy should be restarted using the most appropriate drug for the particular seizure type.

4

Barbiturates: Phenobarbital, Mephobarbital, and Metharbital

Barbiturates are hypnotic sedative compounds that act as general depressants of the nervous system and skeletal, smooth, and cardiac muscles. They inhibit mitochondrial respiration, oxygen utilization, and certain enzyme systems in various tissues. These effects occur over a wide range of concentrations. The concentration required for anticonvulsant action or even hypnotic sedative effect, however, rarely produces effects outside the central nervous system (CNS). The higher anesthetic concentrations may produce transient reversible depression of other organ systems. Severe, acute barbiturate intoxication produces serious and direct effects on the cardiovascular and respiratory systems.

Three barbiturates are marketed as antiepileptic drugs: mephobarbital (Mebaral®), metharbital (Gemonil®), and phenobarbital (Luminal®). (Primidone, a deoxybarbiturate analog of phenobarbital, is described in Chapter 8.) All are derived from barbital, the first synthetic hypnotic barbiturate, which was made by substituting the hydrogen at the 5C position of barbituric acid with ethyl groups.

Barbital   Metharbital

Mephobarbital   Phenobarbital

All the commercially available hypnotic barbiturates exhibit anticonvulsant activity at anesthetic doses and inhibit epileptic seizures or convulsions induced by strychnine, electroshock, tetanus, or pentylenetetrazol. The selective anticonvulsant action of phenobarbital, however, is not related to its sedative or anesthetic effects. Furthermore, anticonvulsant activity is not diminished by the concurrent administration of drugs that counteract sedation (e.g., amphetamines and methylphenidate).

CHEMISTRY

Barbituric acid was first produced in 1864 from the combination of malonic acid and urea. Approximately 2,500 barbiturate compounds have since been synthesized by replacing the hydrogen atoms at the 5C and 3N ring positions. Currently, about 25 compounds are licensed by the U.S. Food and Drug Administration as hypnotics, anesthetics, and anticonvulsants. Barbituric acid has no hypnotic properties or depressant effects on the CNS. Substitution of various carbon-containing moieties for the hydrogen atoms at the 1N, 3N, and 5C positions, however, yields compounds that have widely different effects, ranging from anesthetic hypnotics to anticonvulsants and even convulsant compounds. Simple short-chain alkyl groups at the 5C position enhance sedative or hypnotic properties, whereas substitution of a phenyl group at this position confers special anticonvulsant properties against the tonic spasms of tonic-clonic seizures. Such substitution at the 3N and 5C positions also markedly alters the pK_a or ionization constants and lipid/water partition ratios and affects lipid solubility and drug distribution. The acid strength of the barbiturates depends on tautomerization of the 2C position from the keto (I) to the enol (II) form, which allows dissociation to occur:

I   II

Barbital

Barbital (5,5-diethylbarbituric acid; molecular weight, 184.20) is a long-acting sedative with little anticonvulsant activity at therapeutic doses. It is largely un-ionized at physiological pH and thus readily crosses biological membranes. It is eliminated solely by renal excretion at a very slow rate. The rate of clearance can be increased by alkalinization of the urine.

Metharbital

Metharbital (5,5-diethyl-3-methylbarbituric acid; molecular weight, 198.22) is easily absorbed, readily crosses biological membranes, and is rapidly metabolized to barbital. The anticonvulsant effect is minimal in comparison with the hypnotic action of the metabolite barbital.

Mephobarbital

Mephobarbital (5-ethyl-3-methyl-5-phenylbarbituric acid; molecular weight, 246.26) is similar to metharbital except for the substitution of a phenyl group for the ethyl radical at the 5C position. It is identical to phenobarbital except for the methyl group at the 3N position. The lipid/water partition ratio is increased from 3 to 100 by methylation of the nitrogen (Table 4.1). Largely un-ionized at physiological pH, the drug is rapidly absorbed, distributed, and metabolized to phenobarbital.

Phenobarbital

Substitution of the phenyl radical for the ethyl group at the 5C position markedly changes the activity of the parent drug, barbital. The resulting compound, phenobarbital, was introduced in 1912 by Hauptmann (1912). Phenobarbital (5-ethyl-5-phenylbarbituric acid; molecular weight, 232.23) has become one of the most widely used antiepileptic drugs. It remains one of the four major drugs used in the treatment

TABLE 4.1. *The pK_a, lipid/water partition ratio, and half-life of some barbiturates*

Proprietary name	Nonproprietary name	pK_a	Lipid/water partition ratio	Half-life (hr)
Luminal	Phenobarbital	7.3	3	60–90
Mebaral	Mephobarbital	7.8	100	< 1
Gemonil	Metharbital	8.1	50	< 1
Mysoline	Primidone[a]	—	—	8
	Barbital	7.9	1	48
Seconal	Secobarbital	7.9	52	6
Brevital	Methohexital	8.4	1,000	< < < 1

[a]Neutral deoxybarbiturate.

of generalized tonic-clonic and partial seizures. It is effective in the prevention and treatment of febrile seizures, alcohol and drug withdrawal seizures, and status epilepticus. Phenobarbital is considered to be a safe drug, but certain subtle and potentially harmful effects associated with its long-term administration should be considered. These toxic effects are discussed below and in Chapter 15.

Because metharbital is metabolized to barbital and is of low anticonvulsant potency, and mephobarbital is rapidly metabolized to phenobarbital, the following discussions concentrate on phenobarbital.

MECHANISM OF ACTION

Phenobarbital is effective against generalized tonic-clonic and simple partial seizures but not absence seizures (Schmidt and Wilder, 1968; Buchthal and Lennox-Buchthal, 1972a; Aird and Woodbury, 1974). In this spectrum of activity, it is similar to phenytoin, primidone, carbamazepine, and perhaps valproic acid; in other respects it is different from these agents. In contrast to phenytoin and to a lesser extent carbamazepine, phenobarbital does not block posttetanic potentiation (PTP), nor does it elevate brain levels of gamma-aminobutyric acid (GABA) or block absence seizure activity. Unlike primidone, it is only minimally effective against complex partial seizures. Thus some of the antiepileptic action of primidone, which is partly metabolized to phenobarbital and partly to phenylethylmalonamide, can be separated from phenobarbital.

The anticonvulsant activity of phenobarbital is not greatly different from the more rapid-acting hypnotic barbiturates; at therapeutic concentrations, however, the sedative effect is absent or only minimal. To a slight extent, phenobarbital can be distinguished from other barbiturates, such as pentobarbital, by its more selective action on motor cortex, seizure threshold of electrically induced focal seizures, suppression of afterdischarge in isolated cortex, suppression of penicillin-induced spikes, and picrotoxin-induced firing in tissue culture (Keller and Fulton, 1931; Aston and Domino, 1961; Vasquez et al., 1975; Oliver et al., 1977; Macdonald and Barker, 1978). The possible mechanism for this is discussed below. Phenobarbital is also more effective than phenytoin in the above experimental situations. It significantly raises the seizure threshold to maximal electroshock and subcutaneous pentylenetetrazol (Porter and Penry, 1980). Also, in subanesthetic doses, phenobarbital shortens the duration and raises the threshold of normal brain structures to electrically induced afterdischarge (Aston and Domino, 1961). Phenobarbital suppresses the discharges of epileptic foci in experimental animals and humans (Morrell et al., 1959; Mares et al., 1977). It inhibits the kindling process more effectively than any of the other antiepileptic drugs (Wada, 1977). This may be of importance in seizure prevention, for kindling may proceed by mechanisms similar to those of the development of primary and secondary epileptic foci in humans (Wilder, 1981).

Phenobarbital possesses no unique neuropharmacological action that alone would account for its anticonvulsant activity. However, some of its effects on the CNS are undoubtedly pertinent to its role as an antiepileptic drug. It acts on the mesencephalic reticular formation to induce widespread 20 to 30 Hz fast activity in cortical and subcortical areas. Aston and Domino (1961) showed that pentobarbital equally raised the afterdischarge threshold in the reticular activating system of the mesencephalic reticular formation and the cortex. Phenobarbital raised the cortical threshold more than that of the reticular formation, and phenytoin raised the threshold only in the cortex. These findings are consistent with the relative hypnotic and antiepileptic effects of these drugs, with pentobarbital having the greatest and phenytoin having almost no sedative effect. It would not be surprising if the induction of fast cortical EEG rhythms might be antiepileptic. The work on biofeedback has shown the greatest antiepileptic response in those patients conditioned to fast frequency EEG rhythms (Sterman and Friar, 1972; Sterman, 1977).

Phenobarbital has been shown to depress postsynaptic potentials and physiological excitations (Barker, 1975) and to interact with GABA to enhance inhibition and prolong hyperpolarization (Scholfield, 1978). Macdonald and Barker (1979) compared the effects of anticonvulsant and anesthetic barbiturates on postsynaptic action potentials in cultured mammalian neurons. They found that all barbiturates augmented responses to GABA and suppressed glutamic acid activation. The anesthetic barbiturates were more potent in augmenting the GABA response and reversing the GABA antagonists picrotoxin and penicillin. These responses are mediated by changes in membrane conductance. High concentrations of phenobarbital block Ca^{2+} entry into nerve terminals (Sohn and Ferrendelli, 1976), which would decrease transmitter release and postsynaptic excitation. Phenobarbital depresses postsynaptic potentials in sympathetic ganglia (Nicoll and Iwamoto, 1978), enhances presynaptic inhibition in the spinal cord and cuneate nucleus, and increases recurrent collateral inhibition in the hippocampus (Polc and Haefely, 1976; Wolf and Haas, 1977).

Hypnotic doses of phenobarbital depress brain oxygen consumption and increase high-energy phosphate compounds. It is generally accepted that high concentrations of ATP and NADH inhibit glycolysis. Thus high concentrations of glycogen found in phenobarbital-induced anesthesia can be attributed to decreased breakdown of glycogen rather than to increased synthesis. The slower brain energy metabolism observed after the administration of barbiturates is secondary to a reduction in neuronal activity resulting from some of the pharmacological and physiological effects of phenobarbital described above. This depression in brain oxygen consumption and energy metabolism does not exert any anticonvulsant effect. However, a phenobarbital-induced decrease in energy metabolism might be of value in the treatment of the posttraumatic or anoxic state (Maynert and Kusek, 1980).

All the barbiturates suppress brain electrical activity and generalized as well as focal epileptic discharge. Of the barbiturates, phenobarbital alone selectively suppresses epileptic activity without inducing a significant hypnotic effect. Prichard (1980a,b) has proposed that this may be attributable to the lower pKa of phenobarbital (pKa 7.3), which is close to the normal physiological pH of 7.4. At a pH of 7.3, the dissociation constant of phenobarbital is such that the unchanged (unionized) form of the drug is in sufficiently high concentrations for membrane penetration. Local acidosis resulting from seizure discharge, however, would favor a further shift of phenobarbital to the un-ionized form and tend to concentrate phenobarbital at the site of epileptic activity and spare other portions of the brain not involved in the seizure discharge. This might also account for the rapid return to consciousness following the use of phenobarbital in the treatment of status epilepticus. With the control of status, the brain pH would shift from an acidic state to the normal pH, with a concomitant shift of the active un-ionized phenobarbital to the inactive ionized state.

Although a precise mechanism of action for phenobarbital is unknown, many of the mechanisms discussed are plausible. A general decrease in postsynaptic activity and an overall decrease in electrical potential generation is central to the anticonvulsant effectiveness of the drug.

PHARMACOKINETICS

The pK_a of 7.3 and lipid solubility largely determine the absorption, distribution, metabolism, and elimination of the barbiturates. Table 4.1 shows the pK_a, lipid/water partition ratio, and half-lives of the three anticonvulsant barbiturates, as well as some hypnotic barbiturates (Prichard, 1980a).

Absorption

Phenobarbital, because of its pK_a of 7.3 and (lipid/water partition ratio of 3.0), is readily absorbed at the normal physiological pH. The drug is predominantly in the un-ionized state in the stomach and to a lesser degree in the intestinal tract. After oral ingestion, phenobarbital is absorbed fairly rapidly through the gastric and intestinal mucosa and achieves peak plasma levels within 2 to 3 hr (Viswanathan et al., 1978).

Distribution and Protein Binding

In the plasma, the drug is approximately 40 to 50% un-ionized. Reversible plasma protein binding of approximately 40% occurs in the albumin fraction (Mark, 1971). Thus this lipid-soluble agent freely diffuses across capillary membranes and is widely distributed to all tissues. The volume of distribution is calculated to be 1. Because some phospholipid and CNS protein binding occurs, phenobarbital tends to be in higher concentrations in the brain than in the plasma (Domek et al., 1960, Houghton et al., 1975; Ramsay et al., 1979). As would be expected, the cerebrospinal fluid concentration is equal to that of an ultrafiltrate of plasma (McAuliffe et al., 1977). Salivary levels are roughly equal to those of the plasma-free fraction. However, salivary pH must be known for accurate correlation with plasma levels of unbound phenobarbital (Schmidt and Kupferberg, 1975). Nishihari et al. (1979), correcting for pH, found a high correlation between salivary and free plasma phenobarbital levels. Phenobarbital has a relatively low affinity for proteins and phospholipids (Goldberg, 1980a), whereas phenytoin, carbamazepine, and valproic acid have a high affinity and consequently are highly protein bound.

TABLE 4.2. *Major uses of phenobarbital alone or in combination therapy[a]*

Seizure types	Dosage
Generalized tonic-clonic seizures	1.5–5 mg/kg/day
Partial seizures (focal)	1.5–5 mg/kg/day
Myoclonus	1.5–5 mg/kg/day
Febrile seizures	1.5–5 mg/kg/day chronically for prevention after second febrile convulsion
Drug or alcohol withdrawal seizures[b]	8–15 mg/kg i.v. initially; repeat as necessary to prevent seizures
Status epilepticus	8–15 mg/kg i.v.; repeat 5 mg/kg as necessary every 2–6 hr (monitor vital signs closely)

[a]Combination therapy; phenobarbital + phenytoin; phenobarbital + carbamazepine; phenobarbital + valproic acid (be wary of interaction); phenobarbital + acetazolamide; phenobarbital + phenytoin + carbamazepine.
[b]Drug withdrawal seizures may sometimes require prodigious quantities of the drug over 7 to 30 days.

Buchthal and Lennox-Buchthal (1972*a*) have collected extensive data on seizure control and plasma phenobarbital levels and suggest a therapeutic range of 15 to 30 μg/ml. Many clinical laboratories report the normal therapeutic range to be 15 to 50 μg/ml. Regardless of a so-called normal range, the physician should be wary of any unusual behavioral or personality changes in the patient taking phenobarbital.

Although phenobarbital is the most commonly used drug for the treatment and prevention of febrile seizures in infants and young children, a paradoxical hyperactive syndrome sometimes occurs. Porter and Penry (1980) have recommended achieving a minimal plasma concentration of 15 μg/ml for the prevention of febrile seizures. Wolf (1977) has advocated that phenobarbital should be given chronically for the management and most effective prevention of febrile convulsions. When administered only at the time of febrile episodes, the drug is ineffective in preventing convulsions. We do not recommend chronic phenobarbital treatment of febrile seizures except under special circumstances (see Chapter 3).

Phenobarbital is commonly and effectively used in the treatment of drug or alcohol withdrawal convulsions. It is the drug of choice in treating withdrawal convulsions secondary to the abuse of moderate or rapid-acting barbiturates and other hypnotic drugs. The drug may be effective in suppressing the myoclonic phenomenon of epilepsy or other forms of myoclonus.

Phenobarbital given intravenously is an excellent agent for the treatment of status epilepticus. We recommend an initial dose of 8 to 15 mg/kg over a period of 10 to 15 min. Patients who have received a full dose of phenytoin (10 to 15mg/kg) and continue to have seizures can be given a full dose of phenobarbital (8 to 15 mg/kg) without potentiation of side effects. Intravenous phenobarbital should be used with great caution following the intravenous administration of diazepam. Marked potentiation of cardiorespiratory depression may occur.

Phenobarbital may be effective when used in combination with phenytoin or carbamazepine in the treatment of generalized tonic-clonic or partial seizures. Little or no potentiation of sedative side effects is noted. When phenobarbital is discontinued, it should be withdrawn slowly over a period of 3 weeks to 3 months. Withdrawal seizures may occur if the drug is stopped abruptly.

Phenobarbital may be administered by oral, intravenous, intramuscular, or rectal routes. For chronic oral use, it can be best given in single daily doses of 2 to 5 mg/kg. Steady-state plasma levels will be achieved 20 to 30 days after initiation of therapy. The desired therapeutic range is approximately 20 to 40 µg/ml (Higher doses in the milligram per kilogram range, are usually required in children to achieve this range). We usually recommend giving the dose in the evening to avoid the sometimes transient occurrence of somnolence due to peaking of plasma levels 1 to 3 hr after drug ingestion. In general, a marked degree of tolerance to the mild hypnotic effects of the drug eventually develops (Butler, 1978).

Intramuscular administration of phenobarbital is followed by complete absorption and peak plasma levels that roughly parallel those achieved after oral administration (Viswanathan et al., 1978). Little pain is experienced after intramuscular injection. A mild local anesthetic effect may occur if the drug is administered adjacent to peripheral nerves because of a mild action similar to that of local anesthetics. Intravenous administration is safe if a rate of 100 mg/min is not exceeded. Ramsay et al. (1979) have shown that the drug rapidly penetrates the brain after intravenous injection (Fig. 4.2).

INTERACTIONS WITH OTHER DRUGS

Drug interactions that may occur when phenobarbital is administered with other physiologically active compounds are generally secondary to the enzyme induction described above. Certain situations require careful monitoring (Tables 4.3 and 4.4). Phenobarbital may result in decreasing plasma levels of bishydroxycoumarin, digitoxin, phenytoin, and other chronically administered drugs (see Chapter 14).

Physiological interactions may potentiate the effects of certain drugs in a synergistic or additive manner. The combination of phenobarbital and diazepam or clonazepam may lead to severe somnolence and even cardiorespiratory depression in the very old and the very young. The concurrent intravenous administration of phenobarbital and diazepam is definitely contraindicated because of potential cardiorespiratory depression and collapse. Phenobarbital and primidone should not be administered concurrently. About 15 to 20% of primidone is metabolized to phenobarbital, and additive effects and increasing plasma levels of phenobarbital are observed when the drugs are given together.

Some drug interactions occur because of competitive inhibition of metabolic enzyme systems. The result is increasing physiological effects and high plasma

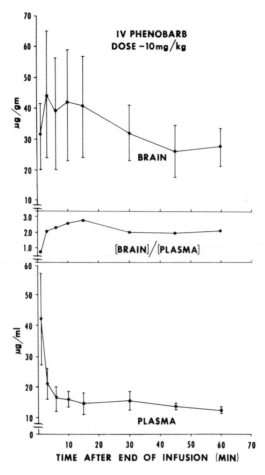

FIG. 4.2. Intravenous administration of phenobarbital in a therapeutic dose results in rapid penetration of the brain. Note that the brain/plasma ratio increases during the hour following administration.

drug levels. Valproic acid significantly interferes with the metabolism of phenobarbital. The addition of valproic acid to the regimen of a patient receiving phenobarbital may require a 30 to 50% reduction in phenobarbital dosage to maintain steady-state phenobarbital levels (Wilder et al., 1978). Phenobarbital inhibits the metabolism of the active metabolite of methsuximide, *N*-desmethylmethsuximide. Likewise, the metabolism of phenobarbital is inhibited, and levels may increase by 30 to 40% when methsuximide is added to the regimen of a patient who is receiving phenobarbital (Rambeck, 1979). These drugs compete for the same hepatic metabolizing enzymes.

TABLE 4.3. *Phenobarbital interactions with other drugs*

Decreases levels of
  Phenytoin
  Bishydroxycoumarin
  Digitoxin
Increases levels of
  N-Desmethylmethsuximide (methsuximide
    metabolite)
Potentiation of effect
  Diazepam
  Clonazepam
  Methsuximide
Addition of effects
  Phenobarbital metabolized from primidone
Phenobarbital levels increased by
  Valproic acid
  Methsuximide

TABLE 4.4. *Phenobarbital interactions with other drugs*

Drug	Effect
Alcohol	Decreased sedation with chronic alcohol abuse; increased sedation with acute intoxication
Steroids	Decreased steroid effect
Quinidine	Decreased quinidine effect
Tricyclic antidepressants	Decreased antidepressant effect
Bishydroxycoumarin	Decreased anticoagulant effect
Digitoxin	Decreased digitoxin effect
Phenothiazines	Decreased phenothiazine effect
Doxycycline	Decreased doxycycline effect
Rifampin	Decreased phenobarbital effect
Methsuximide	Increased phenobarbital effect
Valproic acid	Decreased valproic acid effect

TOXICITY

The major toxic or side effects of phenobarbital are related to its hypnotic properties. In general, patients tolerate plasma levels of 15 to 30 μ/ml without somnolence or excessive sedation. Phenobarbital is similar to other anticonvulsant drugs in that it may have deleterious effects on multiple organ systems. It is teratogenic in experimental animals and presumably in humans also.

A major concern should be the subtle toxic effects that frequently occur in patients on long-term therapy. Intellectual impairment often becomes obvious in retrospect when the drug is withdrawn. Barbiturate depression of cognitive function has been well described (Hutt et al., 1968). As many as 40% of children placed on phenobarbital experience unpleasant side effects. The most common are hyperactivity, irritability, and alterations in sleep patterns. Many elderly patients experience similar reactions. MacLeod et al. (1978) have carefully demonstrated impairment of immediate memory by phenobarbital at therapeutic plasma drug levels. The authors believe that such a defect in attentiveness might decrease a patient's ability to acquire new information. Camfield (1980) has shown that phenobarbital in the therapeutic range significantly decreases attention span and higher cognitive function in children receiving the drug to prevent febrile seizures. Such an effect on short-term memory is a problem of some importance, considering the number of school-age children who receive this drug. Experimental studies in animals are even more alarming in this regard. Schain and Watanabe (1976) have reported significant retardation of brain growth and maturation in developing rats maintained on phenobarbital. Others have reported similar effects of phenobarbital on the developing brain (Diaz and Schain, 1978; Wahlström and Nordberg, 1978; Yanai et al., 1979). Because of the potential adverse effects of phenobarbital on higher cortical function, patients should be treated with the lowest dose that effects seizure control.

5

Hydantoins: Phenytoin, Mephenytoin, and Ethotoin

Three hydantoin compounds, phenytoin (Dilantin®), mephenytoin (Mesantoin®), and ethotoin (Peganone®), have been marketed in the United States for the treatment of generalized tonic-clonic seizures, simple complex and partial seizures, and mixed types of convulsive attacks. These drugs are ineffective against and may exacerbate absence seizures.

The history of the experimental and clinical testing of phenytoin verifies the hypothesis that sedative and anticonvulsant actions may be unrelated. In the 1930s, phenobarbital was well established as an effective drug for the treatment of convulsive disorders, although its anticonvulsant effect was sometimes overshadowed by its sedative action. Late in the decade, Putman and Merritt (1937; Merritt and Putnam, 1938a) began a study designed to find an antiepileptic drug devoid of sedative effects. They soon reported on the anticonvulsant properties of phenyl derivatives in animal studies, and then recommended phenytoin for clinical trials. Clinical trials of phenytoin demonstrated its superiority over phenobarbital and its lack of significant hypnotic properties (Merritt and Putman, 1938b). Phenytoin has subsequently become the most widely used drug in the world for the treatment of generalized tonic-clonic and simple and complex partial seizures.

Mephenytoin, a derivative or analog of phenytoin, was first tested and introduced by Loscalzo (1945). It has a broader spectrum of activity against experimentally induced seizures than phenytoin, including effectiveness against pentylenetetrazol-induced convulsions. Its anticonvulsant usefulness, however, is limited by potent hypnotic effects and other potentially serious toxic reactions.

Ethotoin, introduced by Schwade and colleagues (1956), also has a broad spectrum of activity against experimentally induced convulsions, but its clinical use is limited by its low anticonvulsant potency and hypnotic properties. Ethotoin is now rarely used.

These drugs are five-membered ring structures synthesized from derivatives of phenol and urea.

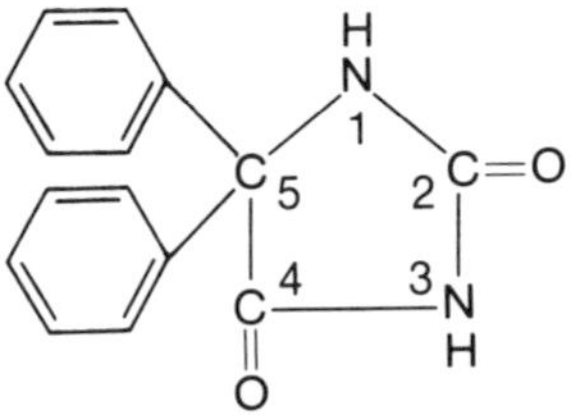

Phenytoin

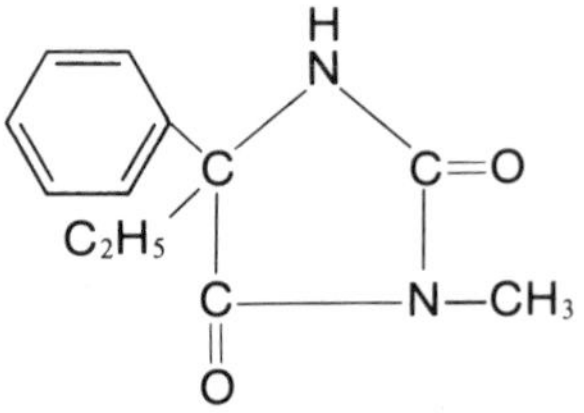

Mephenytoin

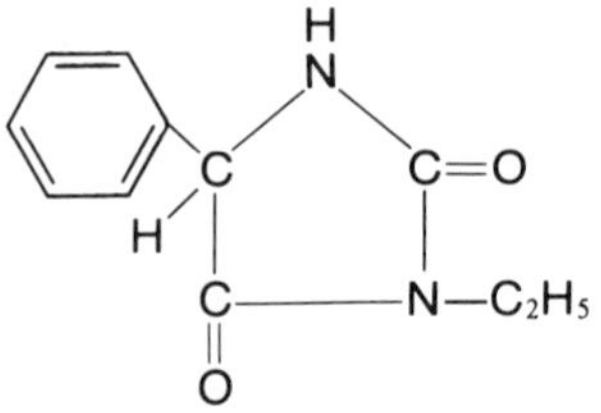

Ethotoin

CHEMISTRY

Phenytoin

Phenytoin (5,5-diphenylhydantoin) is a weak organic acid with a pK_a of 8.3 and molecular weight of 252.26. The aqueous solubility at pH 7.5 is 21.9 µg/ml and in plasma at 37°C is 75 µg/ml. Were it not for protein binding, the drug would theoretically precipitate in the blood (Glazko, 1972). Phenytoin behaves like an acid, ionizing from the keto to the enol form, as described for phenobarbital (Chapter 4). At physiological pH, the drug is almost completely in the un-ionized form and is free to cross biological membranes. Phenytoin is highly lipid soluble and penetrates the brain rapidly following intravenous injection (Ramsay et al., 1979; Wilder et al., 1977; Goldberg and Toderoff, 1976, 1978). The two phenyl radicals confer special anticonvulsant properties, and the absence of alkyl groups reduces hypnotic effects.

Mephenytoin

Mephenytoin (5-ethyl-3-methyl-5-phenylhydantoin), with *N*-methylation at position 3 in the nucleus and substitution of an ethyl group for a phenyl group at position 5, is a hydantoin homolog of the barbiturate mephobarbital. The presence of the alkyl groups at the 3 and 5 positions predicts potent hypnotic properties, and the phenyl group predicts anticonvulsant properties (see Chapter 4). Mephenytoin has a molecular weight of 218.25. It is insoluble in water but is lipid soluble and readily crosses membranes, as it is un-ionized at physiological pH.

Ethotoin

Ethotoin (3-ethyl-5-phenylhydantoin) differs from phenytoin by the addition of an ethyl group in position 3 and the deletion of one phenyl group from position 5 in the nucleus. This manipulation of the hydantoin ring reduces anticonvulsant potency and increases hypnotic effects.

MECHANISM OF ACTION

Phenytoin

Phenytoin is perhaps the most effective antiepileptic drug for preventing the development of generalized tonic-clonic seizures and the spread of seizure activity from an epileptic focus. It suppresses the paroxysmal electrical activity that characterizes the focal epileptic lesion. One of its major anticonvulsant actions is the blocking of posttetanic potentiation (PTP), which refers to the augmentation of the postsynaptic compound action potentials elicited by repetitive presynaptic stimulation. This physiological phenomenon of PTP is an important mechanism in the development of high frequency trains of impulses in excitatory brain circuits. Also, the spread of this activity to adjacent neurons and propagation to distant neuronal aggregates results in uncontrolled spread of excitation to the whole brain, leading to a maximal tonic-clonic seizure. The facilitation of synaptic transmission that occurs during PTP may be attributed to a number of factors that increase neuronal excitability, including (a) increased calcium-dependent neurotransmitter release, (b) partial depolarization of the postsynaptic membrane, (c) decreased transmitter degradation, and (d) increase in excitatory nucleotides. The anticonvulsant effect of phenytoin in blocking PTP or suppressing focal paroxysmal discharge cannot be ascribed to any single mechanism of action but rather to a multiplicity of effects that basically affect or change the effect of synaptic transmission: (a) ionic (Na^+, K^+, Cl^-) fluxes associated with depolarization, repolarization, and membrane stability, (b) calcium (Ca^{2+}) uptake in presynaptic terminals and Ca^{2+} energy metabolism, (c) the N^+-K^+ adenosine triphosphatase-dependent ionic membrane pump, (d) cyclic nucleotide build-up, (e) Ca^{2+}-dependent synaptic protein phosphorylation and transmitter release, and (f) cerebellar stimulation.

The specific actions of phenytoin that suppress PTP, local seizure spread from a focus, and interictal paroxysmal epileptiform activity are incompletely known but have been examined in a number of recent reviews (Ayala and Johnston, 1980; Delgado-Escueta and Horan, 1980; DeLorenzo, 1980; DeWeer, 1980; Ferrendelli, 1980; Laxer et al., 1980; Pincus et al., 1980; Woodbury, 1980*a,b,d*).

The major effects exerted by phenytoin on depolarized or partially depolarized neurons in the epileptic brain occur without significantly affecting the normal metabolic or physiological activity of the central nervous system (CNS). Antiepileptic action occurs at a therapeutic concentration that does not significantly alter normal physiological function.

A major pharmacological effect of phenytoin is exerted on active ionic fluxes associated with depolarization, repolarization, and hyperpolarization. This is clearly evidenced by its actions on ionic movements in blocking the membrane channels through which Na^+ moves from outside to inside the neuron during the depolarization process (DeWeer, 1980).

Ionic movement of K^+ from the intracellular to the extracellular space in the repolarization process may be facilitated by phenytoin (Schwartz and Vogel, 1977). The removal of excess extracellular K^+ by glial cells is also enhanced by phenytoin (Heinemann and Lux, 1973). Extracellular to intracellular movement of Cl^- may be stimulated by phenytoin. These ionic shifts result in hyperpolarization of the membrane (Ayala et al., 1977).

Phenytoin blocks not only the inward movement of Na^+ elicited by stimulation but passive or resting inward fluxes of the ion as well (DeWeer, 1980). The net effect of blocking Na^+ movement through sodium channels and the possible facilitation of K^+ and Cl^- fluxes would be to decrease neuronal excitability and to stabilize membrane potential toward the normal or hyperpolarized state.

The action of phenytoin on the uptake of Ca^{2+} by neuronal membranes and presynaptic terminals was noted in early experiments by Toman (1952). Phenytoin decreases membrane permeability to Ca^{2+}, resulting indirectly in the inhibition of a number of Ca^{2+}-dependent mechanisms. One of the most important in terms of synaptic transmission is Ca^{2+}-dependent neurotransmitter release. Thus phenytoin indirectly decreases transmitter release from presynaptic terminals by inhibiting the presynaptic terminal uptake of Ca^{2+}.

The effect of phenytoin on other Ca^{2+}-dependent mechanisms may be paramount to many actions of this drug that are unrelated to the CNS. According to Woodbury (1980a), therapeutic concentrations of phenytoin inhibit many glandular functions, including: (a) insulin release from pancreatic islet cells, (b) norepinephrine secretion by the adrenal medulla, (c) pancreatic glucagon release, (d) vasopressin and oxytocin release from the neurohypophysis, (e) thyrotropin and adrenocorticotropin release from the adenohypophysis, (f) salivary secretion, (g) calcitonin release, and (h) general glandular secretory activity.

The cyclic nucleotides adenosine monophosphate (cAMP) and guanosine monophosphate (cGMP), found in both the presynaptic and postsynaptic membranes, are biologically active compounds in the CNS which are elevated in epileptic foci and are thought to enhance seizure discharge. When transmitter substance is released into the synaptic cleft, adenosine triphosphate (ATP) is catalyzed in both presynaptic and postsynaptic membranes by adenyl cyclase to cAMP. This activates protein kinases, which in turn induce phosphorylation of special proteins in the membrane structures, resulting in alterations in ion permeability and increased excitability in the postsynaptic membrane (Iverson, 1979). In the presynaptic membrane, phosphorylation of synaptic vesicle protein occurs, resulting in the further enhancement of transmitter release. The phosphorylation of vesicle protein and the release of transmitter substances are Ca^{2+} dependent and thereby blocked by phenytoin (Ferrendelli and Kinscherf, 1977; DeLorenzo, 1980).

Phenytoin in physiological concentrations significantly reduces cerebellar content of cGMP in the resting state and cAMP and cGMP accumulation in cortex, striatum, thalamus, brainstem, and cerebellum after electrical stimulation. Both these cyclic nucleotides cause excitatory changes, and their suppression by phenytoin may be pertinent to seizure control. Ferrendelli (1980) has suggested that the phenytoin-induced depletion of cGMP in cerebellum may be due to decreased afferent input to Purkinje cells or to enhanced cerebellar inhibitory activity. Laxer et al. (1980) have concluded that the cerebellar cortex is indispensable for the maximal anticonvulsant action of phenytoin. Iverson (1979) has reported that phenytoin enhances Purkinje cell discharge and depresses basal nuclei discharge. These changes in cerebellar firing patterns have been associated with a reduction in seizures (Laxer et al., 1980). Similar findings of other investigators implicate phenytoin in an effect on the cerebellum in the control of cortical convulsive activity (Halpern and Julien, 1972; Strain et al., 1978; Puro and Woodward, 1973).

Neuronal membrane stability and extracellular-intracellular ionic equilibrium is maintained in the resting or basal state and reestablished after depolarization by the $(Na^+-K^+-ATPase)$-dependent ionic membrane pump. A major action of phenytoin is the stimulation of the ionic pump following depolarization of unstable neurons in epileptic foci or after convulsive seizures. Phenytoin reverses the ionic changes induced by seizures or paroxysmal epileptiform activity. The membrane pump is actively stimulated by phenytoin to extrude Na^+ and Ca^{2+} from the intracellular compartment and to move K^+ back into the intracellular space or into glial cells, which reduces extracellular K^+ and allows redistribution back into neurons (Festoff and Appel, 1968; Delgado-Escueta and Horan, 1980; Woodbury, 1980a). This action decreases neuronal excitability by restoration and stabilization of neuronal membrane potential.

Delgado-Escueta and Horan (1980) have summarized the anticonvulsant action of phenytoin as follows:
A. Inhibition of seizure spread
   1. Stimulation of the (N^+-K^+) pump
   2. Blockade of passive Na^+ influx
   3. Blockade of Ca^{2+} influx
   4. Enhancement of chloride-mediated inhibitory postsynaptic potentials (IPSPs)
   5. Inhibition of protein phosphorylation and neurotransmitter release
   6. Interaction with phospholipids, with secondary effects on membrane-bound enzymes
      (The latter two mechanisms would incorporate the suppression of cAMP and cGMP accumulation.)
B. Suppression of the epileptic focus
   1. Stimulation of the (Na^+-K^+) pump
   2. Enhancement of the inhibitory surround via stimulation of chloride-mediated IPSPs
   3. Interaction with phospholipids, with an effect on membrane-bound enzymes

Mephenytoin

Mephenytoin antagonizes pentylenetetrazol and raises the threshold to electro-shock seizures. In these actions, it simulates the activity of the anticonvulsant barbiturates. It also resembles phenytoin in that it blocks PTP in experimental animals. Thus it is effective in preventing the tonic phase of generalized tonic-clonic seizures (Butler, 1953). It prevents the hyperexcitability resulting from hypocalcemia and decreases Na^+ membrane transport and intracellular Na^+.

PHARMACOKINETICS

Phenytoin

Absorption

Phenytoin is administered orally as a sodium salt or as the acid. The salt is in a macrocrystalline form, and the acid is microcrystalline. Both are reliably absorbed from the stomach and intestinal tract. Critical factors influencing absorption are particle size and the incipient used in the formulation (Richens, 1979). Phenytoin is erratically and incompletely absorbed when administered in an amorphous form.

Following the administration of single dose, peak plasma levels can be expected to occur within 3 to 8 hr. The absorption of phenytoin varies significantly with the formulation used, and this variation can dramatically alter the time of peak plasma level. Of the current formulations on the market, the Parke-Davis brand appears to be one of the slowest and most evenly absorbed. When the drug is administered chronically in a single daily dose, the plasma levels slowly rise and peak after 8 to 12 hr (Wilder et al., 1972).

Intramuscular administration of phenytoin Na^+ results in crystallization, and absorption into the bloodstream is extended over a period of several days (Wilder and Ramsay, 1976). Muscle necrosis also occurs at the site of injection (Serrano et al., 1973).

Protein Binding

Phenytoin is approximately 90% bound to the albumin fraction of plasma proteins (Wilder et al., 1972; Richens, 1979; Goldberg, 1980*b*). Phenytoin concentrations in saliva and cerebrospinal fluid (CSF) accurately reflect the free fraction of the drug in plasma (Wilder et al., 1972; Schmidt and Kupferberg, 1975). Phenytoin may displace hormones and other drugs from binding sites, and thyroxine levels may be artificially low because of phenytoin displacement (see Chapter 15). Goldberg and Todoroff (1976, 1978) have demonstrated phenytoin binding to brain lipids, which may account for the high brain-to-tissue ratio demonstrated clinically (Wilder et al., 1977; Goldberg and Crandall, 1978). Subcutaneous fat does not bind phenytoin.

Distribution

Following intravenous infusion, phenytoin is widely distributed to all tissues; its volume of distribution is 0.6 liters/kg. In experimental and clinical studies, Ramsay et al. (1979) and Wilder et al. (1977) have demonstrated brain-to-plasma ratios of 1.8 to > 2 at 1 hr after infusion of approximately 10 to 13 mg/kg (Fig. 5.1). Phenytoin is also concentrated in liver, kidney, and salivary glands.

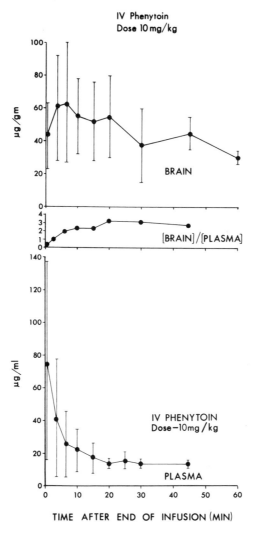

FIG. 5.1. Intravenous phenytoin in therapeutic doses administered at a rate of 50 to 100 mg/min results in rapid entry into the cortex. The brain/plasma ratio increases within minutes after infusion and remains high as phenytoin is bound to brain lipids.

Metabolism

Phenytoin metabolism occurs in the liver. The major metabolic pathway is by parahydroxylation and to a lesser extent metahydroxylation of one of the phenyl rings. The resulting 5-(*p*-hydroxyphenyl)-5-phenylhydantoin (*p*-HPPH) is conjugated with glucuronic acid and excreted as a glucuronide. Much smaller quantities of phenytoin are metabolized to diphenylhydantoic acid, a dihydrodiol, and a catechol from an epoxide intermediary (Chang and Glazko, 1972).

The most important aspect of phenytoin metabolism is that it is rate limited, and the enzyme system involved is saturable within the therapeutic range of plasma concentrations. This fact may have grave consequences if ignored. Small increases in dose may result in dramatic increases in plasma levels. In many patients, the earliest manifestations of phenytoin toxicity are subtle changes in behavior and alterations in higher cortical function. Plasma phenytoin levels should be monitored within 2 to 3 weeks after dosage increases. The magnitude of plasma level increases that can occur following small increases in the daily dose is shown in Chapter 2 (Fig. 2.2). Because of the rate-limited metabolism of phenytoin, the elimination half-life may vary from 7 to 40 hr (Arnold and Gerber, 1970). The rate of metabolism is directly related to the plasma concentration in a given subject, (Levy, 1980). In adults, however, the half-life after oral administration averages 22 hr. Children between the ages of 6 months and 6 years have shorter biological half-lives than adults (Curless et al., 1975). Elderly patients may more slowly eliminate the drug than adolescents and adults. The elimination half-life after intravenous infusion is shorter than after oral dosing (Glazko et al., 1969).

Elimination

Phenytoin is eliminated in urine principally as its major metabolite *p*-HPPH, which is largely conjugated with glucuronic acid. Sixty to 80% of an ingested dose of phenytoin can be accounted for in the urine as *p*-HPPH. An additional small amount ($< 5\%$) is excreted as unchanged phenytoin (Bochner et al., 1973). Because of protein binding and its pK_a of 8.3, phenytoin is found in low concentrations in the glomerular filtrate; this small amount is reabsorbed from the renal tubules. Three to 5% can be found in the feces as unabsorbed phenytoin or as a product of biliary excretion from the enterohepatic circulation.

Mephenytoin

Mephenytoin is readily absorbed from the gastrointestinal tract and reaches peak plasma levels 2 to 4 hr following oral administration. It is partly protein bound (20 to 50%) and fairly widely distributed. The presence of the phenyl group insures brain uptake. The brain-to-plasma ratio is not known; however, the CSF-to-plasma ratio is 0.5 to 0.8, which corresponds to the ratio of free drug to total drug in the plasma.

Mephenytoin is metabolized by the hepatic microsomal enzymes to 5-ethyl-5-phenylhydantoin (Nirvanol®) by demethylation. Many of the severe toxic reactions are attributed to this metabolic by-product. Nirvanol is hydroxylated and conjugated with glucuronic acid in the liver and excreted.

CLINICAL USE

Phenytoin

Phenytoin, the most effective drug for the treatment of convulsive disorders, is the treatment of choice in primary or secondary generalized tonic-clonic seizures. It is also indicated for the treatment of simple and complex partial seizures and mixed seizure types of infancy and childhood. It is ineffective against and may exacerbate absence seizures.

Intravenous phenytoin (15 mg/kg) in combination with small doses of diazepam (5 to 10 mg) is the treatment of choice for status epilepticus (see Chapter 3). It is also effective in terminating prolonged febrile convulsions and alcohol withdrawal seizures when given intravenously (10 to 15 mg/kg).

Phenytoin is customarily administered by the oral route. The drug is supplied in 100 mg capsules and 50 mg chewable tablets and as 125 mg/5 ml adult and 30 mg/ 5 ml pediatric suspensions. The capsules and tablets contain the sodium salt in a macroparticle form. The liquid suspensions contain phenytoin acid in a microsuspension, which is absorbed more rapidly than the macroparticle form.

Single-Drug Therapy

The usual daily dose is approximately 5 to 7 mg/kg, and therapy can be initiated at the full calculated daily dose. Steady-state plasma drug levels occur after 7 to 10 days. Plasma levels should be monitored so that appropriate dosage adjustments can be made. Phenytoin follows zero-order kinetics or rate-limited metabolism; thus small increases in daily dose may result in large increases in plasma levels (see above).

In acute seizure situations, a loading dose of phenytoin can be given by administering 13 to 15 mg/kg of the drug in three divided doses over a 4-hr period (Wilder et al., 1973b) or by an intravenous dose of 13 to 15 mg/kg (Salem et al., 1981). Record et al. (1979) proposed a slightly different method; they gave 19 mg/kg orally divided in two to four increments over a 3 to 21 hr period. This regimen achieves and maintains therapeutic plasma concentrations for 18 to 24 hr. If the intravenous route is chosen, the drug should be administered at a rate not to exceed 50 mg/min. Rapid administration can result in hypotension and asystole. The drug can be safely mixed without precipitation in 50 to 500 ml normal saline (Salem et al., 1981).

When therapeutic plasma antiepileptic drug levels are needed as rapidly as possible, intravenous phenytoin is the drug of choice. In contrast to phenobarbital, diazepam, or paraldehyde, phenytoin does not significantly alter neurological examination: cardiorespiratory function is not depressed, coma (if present) is not deepened, somnolence is not induced, and continued seizure protection is afforded by the long half-life (18 to 25 hr) of the drug.

Renal failure poses a problem that requires careful monitoring of both bound and unbound plasma levels of the drug. Free plasma levels can be obtained by measuring saliva concentrations.

Combination Therapy

The antiepileptic drugs most commonly used in combination therapy are phenytoin and phenobarbital. The anticonvulsant effects of the two drugs are additive in the experimental situation and appear to be so clinically (Leppik and Sherwin, 1977). This combination is recommended in generalized tonic-clonic and partial seizures that are refractory to single-drug therapy. When plasma levels of the drugs are in the therapeutic range, toxicity or side effects do not potentiate, and interactions between the two drugs are not significant.

The combination of phenytoin and carbamazepine may have increased anticonvulsant effectiveness. Interactions are rare, and potentiation of side effects or toxicity does not occur. Phenytoin and ethosuximide provide an effective combination for the treatment of concurrent absence and convulsive seizures. Interactions and potentiation of side effects or toxicity are extremely rare. Phenytoin and primidone appear to have additive anticonvulsant effects and are often effective in refractory complex partial seizures.

Phenytoin and valproic acid may be used in combination for the treatment of generalized seizures or simple and complex partial seizures. Although the anticonvulsant effects are not predictable, dramatic results occur commonly enough to warrant a trial in refractory patients. The combination of these two drugs may be particularly effective in patients with refractory generalized tonic-clonic and absence seizures with or without myoclonus. When this combination therapy is used, the drug interaction discussed below should be anticipated (also see Chapter 15).

The combination of phenytoin and methsuximide may show additive anticonvulsant activity in patients with refractory complex partial seizures with or without secondary generalization (Wilder and Buchanan, 1981). Drug interactions, as discussed below, may be avoided by careful monitoring of plasma drug levels.

The combined use of phenytoin and diazepam, except in the case of status epilepticus, does not offer additional anticonvulsant effectiveness, except when myoclonus accompanies generalized tonic-clonic seizures. Tunnicliff et al. (1979) have reported phenytoin competition for diazepam binding sites in animal cortex synaptosomal membranes.

Triple combination therapy with phenytoin and other agents may be more effective than the above therapies in selected situations. The various drug interactions that may occur should be kept in mind.

Mephenytoin

The spectrum of anticonvulsant activity of mephenytoin is similar to that of phenytoin. Although sedation and other toxic reactions may limit its usefulness, it should be considered as a substitute for phenytoin in cases of phenytoin allergy or when other undesirable reactions to chronic phenytoin therapy, such as gingival hyperplasia or hirsutism, are present.

Mephenytoin is supplied as 100 mg scored tablets. The usual daily dose is 5 to 10 mg/kg, given in divided doses. The therapeutic plasma level ranges from 9 to 15 μg/ml.

Mephenytoin may be used in combination with other antiepileptic drugs, but potentiation of sedative effects can be anticipated when it is used in combination with the barbiturates, primidone, or methsuximide.

INTERACTIONS WITH OTHER DRUGS

Phenytoin

Phenytoin interacts with a number of drugs presently used in medical practice. These interactions are comprehensively reviewed by Richens (1977*a*), Eadie and Tyrer (1980), and in Chapter 15. The mechanisms of these pharmacokinetic interactions involve drug absorption, protein binding, metabolism, enzyme induction or inhibition, and elimination. The most predictable interactions involve alterations in phenytoin metabolism.

Some of the drugs that increase plasma phenytoin concentrations are shown in Table 5.1. Disulfiram (Antabuse®), which is widely used in alcohol rehabilitation programs, is an enzyme inhibitor. It causes significant elevation of plasma phenytoin concentrations, depending on the steady-state level of phenytoin when therapy is started (Labram, 1975). Isoniazid, a commonly used antituberculosis agent, is also an enzyme inhibitor. Elevation of phenytoin levels is less predictable than with disulfiram, and the extent of inhibition depends on the patient's acetylator phenotype. Slow acetylators develop isoniazid concentrations high enough to retard phenytoin metabolism (Brennan et al., 1970). Sulthiame (an antiepileptic drug not licensed in the United States), chloramphenicol (a broad spectrum antibiotic), and propoxyphene (an analgesic) have been reported to raise phenytoin levels but not predictably. The metabolite of methsuximide, *N*-desmethylmethsuximide, and phenytoin compete for metabolism. Both drugs undergo saturation kinetics at their higher therapeutic ranges; when methsuximide is added, therefore, phenytoin levels may significantly rise to the toxic range (Rambeck, 1979). Phenobarbital and primidone both induce metabolizing enzymes and in turn compete for these enzymes. These

TABLE 5.1. *Drugs that increase plasma phenytoin concentrations*

Anticoagulants (oral)	Phenobarbital
Chloramphenicol	Primidone
Disulfiram	Propoxyphene
Isoniazid	Sulthiame
Methsuximide	Tricyclic antidepressants

opposite effects are generally cancelling, and no significant change occurs in phenytoin levels.

Plasma phenytoin concentration or its half-life may be decreased by the drugs shown on Table 5.2. Sporadic heavy use of ethanol may significantly lower phenytoin levels in patients with normal liver function. Chronic heavy use of ethanol, depending on liver function, may result in either lowering or elevation of phenytoin levels (Kutt, 1975). The addition of valproic acid to phenytoin results in a predictable lowering of phenytoin levels in a majority of patients. This interaction is one of protein binding displacement of phenytoin by valproic acid, which results in more rapid metabolism of phenytoin. The reduction of phenytoin levels may not occur if preexisting phenytoin levels are elevated to the point of enzyme saturation (Bruni et al., 1979*b*).

Phenytoin may significantly induce enzymes that result in increased biotransformation of bihydroxycoumarin. A number of interactions involving phenytoin and hormones, vitamins, immunoglobulins, collagen, and other endogenous biological compounds have been reported (Table 5.3). Interactions involving benzodiazepines, carbamazepine, phenothiazines, tolbutamide, methylphenidate, acetylsalicylic acid, and other drugs and phenytoin have been observed, but these interactions are rare, insignificant, and unpredictable.

Mephenytoin

No drug interactions between mephenytoin and other drugs, aside from the potentiation of hypnotic effects of the barbiturates and succinimides, are known. Because mephenytoin is structurally similar to phenobarbital, mephobarbital, and phenytoin, similar interactions might be expected.

TABLE 5.2. *Drugs that decrease plasma phenytoin concentrations or half-life*

Alcohol	Phenylbutazone
Carbamazepine	Salicylates (massive doses)
Folic acid	Valproic acid (transiently)

TABLE 5.3. *Drugs whose plasma concentrations are decreased by phenytoin*

Bihydroxycoumarin	Phenylbutazone
Contraceptive pill	Quinidine
Dexamethasone	Thyroxine
Digitoxin	Valproic acid
Doxycycline	Vitamin D
Metyrapone	

TOXICITY

Hydantoins induce toxic side effects in a number of organ systems. The effects on the CNS are usually transient and occur as a result of acute overdose, chronic mild overdosage, interactions with other drugs, or changes in the physiological state of the individual. Toxic effects generally can be correlated with the level of the drug in the blood.

The most prominent toxic effects are usually related to the particular drug used or to as yet unexplained involvement of a particular functional system of the brain. Mephenytoin and ethotoin tend to show hypnotic effects early, as blood levels exceed the therapeutic range. Phenytoin, even at high blood levels, causes relatively mild sedation.

Phenytoin has a predilection for causing dysfunction in: (a) higher cortical function (concentration, judgment, decision making), (b) behavior (ranging from inappropriate affect to changes in thought content), and (c) cerebellovestibular integration of motor activity (nystagmus, ataxia, incoordination, and disintegration of skilled activity). These alterations of normal function may begin to occur at the upper limits of the normal therapeutic range (18 to 20 µg/ml), or they may not appear until blood levels reach 1½ to 2 times the normal range (30 to 40 µg/ml). Higher blood levels of phenytoin (> 40 µg/ml) begin to cause dysfunction in the extrapyramidal motor system, the reticulocortical activating system, and the autonomic nervous system. Stupor and coma occur when phenytoin levels exceed 40 µg/ml.

Clinical manifestations of phenytoin intoxication depend largely on whether the high blood levels are reached slowly, as chronic toxicity, or rapidly, as in overdosage. Accidental or purposeful massive overdosage causes the rapid progression of all the above-mentioned effects. Wilder et al. (1973a) followed three children who accidentally ingested 75 to 300 mg/kg phenytoin. All were stuporous on admission to the intensive care unit of the hospital, and all had plasma phenytoin levels between 40 and 42 µg/ml. The levels continued to rise for 1 to 2 days before falling to less than 10 µg/ml over a period of 4 to 12 days. All the children recovered without demonstrable sequelae.

Death from massive phenytoin overdosage can be prevented by supportive measures in an intensive care unit. Because of its wide distribution and high degree of protein binding, phenytoin cannot be removed by exchange transformation, hemodialysis, or peritoneal dialysis (Schulte and Good, 1966; Tenckhoff et al., 1968).

Chronic toxicity develops over a period of time when the dose exceeds the metabolic rate of degradation. In this situation, clinical signs of toxicity may be subtle and go unrecognized for months or years. If nystagmus and ataxia are early signs of chronic phenytoin intoxication, the condition is easily recognized, and the drug can be temporarily discontinued and restarted at a lower dose. Recovery occurs uneventfully, and no permanent changes in function can be detected. When chronic phenytoin toxicity produces slowly progressive alterations in higher cortical function and behavior, the signs may go unrecognized. In such situations, inappropriate diagnoses of dementia, schizophreniform psychosis, personality disturbances, and mental retardation may be entertained. Blood phenytoin levels may range from 20 to 50 μg/ml in these cases, and signs of cerebellovestibular dysfunction may not be obvious. The physician should be particularly alert for changes in behavior or higher cortical function in any patient who is receiving phenytoin. Blood phenytoin levels should be periodically monitored in most patients who receive the drug, even though seizure control has been effected. Particular care should be given to children, who rapidly develop from childhood to adolescence. The changes in endogenous hormone secretion that occur at this stage of maturation retard the rate of metabolism of phenytoin. Toxicity can occur in this situation even though the patient remains on the same daily dose.

Phenytoin and other hydantoins produce toxic effects in other organ systems. Such effects may be of an acute or a chronic nature and may be unrelated to high blood levels or overdosage of the drug. These reactions to anticonvulsant therapy are comprehensively covered in Chapter 15.

Mephenytoin

Mephenytoin may induce toxic side effects similar to those of phenytoin and phenobarbital. Sedation, ataxia, incoordination, and interference with higher cortical function occur with overdosage. More serious toxic reactions of mephenytoin include involvement of the hematopoietic system. Lymphadenopathy, agranulocytosis, pancytopenia, leukopenia, and aplastic anemia may occur with chronic administration. Temperature elevations and exfoliative dermatitis can occur. Periarteritis and lupus erythematosus occur with greater frequency than with phenytoin therapy. Unlike phenytoin, mephenytoin rarely induces gingival hyperplasia and hirsutism. Psychotic reactions and severe behavioral disturbances with the use of mephenytoin have been reported and may be caused by the metabolite Nirvanol®, which was marketed as a psychotropic agent in the 1920s and later withdrawn because of toxic effects.

6

Carbamazepine

Carbamazepine (Tegretol®) was developed by Geigy Laboratories in Europe in the 1950s. It was introduced in 1962 for the treatment of trigeminal neuralgia, for which it still remains the drug of choice (Blom, 1962). In 1963 its anticonvulsant properties were demonstrated in animals (Theobald and Kunz, 1963), and extensive clinical trials were started in Europe to determine its safety and efficacy in patients with seizure disorders. By 1968, sufficient evidence of safety and efficacy was available for approval of the drug in the United States for the treatment of trigeminal neuralgia. Additional testing on the efficacy of carbamazepine in epilepsy was carried out in this country in the early 1970s; it was approved for the treatment of adult seizure disorders in 1974. Although its approval was retarded by rare reports of potential hematological toxicity, extensive clinical use has shown this to be a rare reaction. Carbamazepine has not been approved for the treatment of seizure disorders in children. It is useful in the treatment of simple and complex partial and generalized convulsive seizures but is not effective in the treatment of absence seizures.

CHEMISTRY

Carbamazepine [5-carbamoyl-5H-dibenz(b,f)azepine, or 5H-dibenz (b,f)azepine-5-carboximide] is chemically related to the tricyclic antidepressants. It is an iminostilbene derivative with a molecular weight of 236.3. It is poorly soluble in water but readily soluble in propylene glycol, ethanol, and acetone.

MECHANISM OF ACTION

The precise mechanism of action of carbamazepine is unknown. Depression of synaptic transmission in the spinal trigeminal nucleus of the cat similar to that obtained with phenytoin has been observed (Fromm and Killian, 1967). Additional studies have shown depression of transmission in the nucleus ventralis anterior of the thalamus at blood levels of carbamazepine lower than those required to depress reticular formation, amygdala, hippocampus, hypothalamus, and pallidum (Holm et al., 1970). Depression in this thalamic nucleus may be significant because it has been implicated in the generalization and spread of seizure discharge (Holm et al., 1970; Kusske et al., 1972). At plasma carbamazepine concentrations above the therapeutic range, some depression of posttetanic potentiation similar to the action of phenytoin, but to a lesser degree, is observed (Krupp, 1969). Unlike phenytoin, which shows specific inhibition of sodium conductance at therapeutic levels, carbamazepine has an effect on ionic membrane conductances only at concentrations far higher than the highest therapeutic levels achieved in humans (Lipicky et al., 1972; Schauf et al., 1974).

The biochemical effects of carbamazepine are unknown. Like phenytoin, however, it inhibits ouabain-induced increases in cyclic AMP (Lewin and Bleck, 1977). A review of the mechanisms of action of carbamazepine has been published (Julien and Hollister, 1975).

PHARMACOKINETICS

Absorption

After oral administration of carbamazepine, absorption is slow, with peak plasma levels occurring within 6 to 24 hr. Plasma carbamazepine levels remained relatively constant from 10 to 24 hr after a single oral dose of 400 mg to normal volunteers (Morselli, 1975). With long-term carbamazepine therapy, peak plasma levels may be observed as early as 2 to 3 hr after ingestion, and absorption may be even more rapid. Since carbamazepine is often administered concurrently with other antiepileptic drugs, which may alter its metabolism, peak plasma times are variable. Administration with meals leads to increased absorption of carbamazepine (Levy et al., 1976).

The generally poor absorption of carbamazepine may be related to its poor water solubility, and its increased absorption with meals may be related to improved solubilization by the secretion of gastric juice and bile. A study in neonates and children has demonstrated that carbamazepine is also slowly absorbed in this age group (Rey et al., 1979). The delay and absorption rate constants were quite variable, and the peak level times were shorter than in adults.

Distribution

The volume of distribution of carbamazepine in adults ranges from 0.8 to 1.4 liter/kg. Its large volume of distribution implies that carbamazepine is distributed throughout body water, and that it binds significantly to tissues. In neonates and children, the volume of distribution is 1.5 to 2 times greater than in healthy adult volunteers (Rey et al., 1979). The brain concentration of carbamazepine is equal to or as much as 1.5 times higher than the plasma concentration (Levy et al., 1976; Friis and Christiansen, 1978). Phenytoin does not seem to influence the brain-to-plasma ratio of carbamazepine (Friis et al., 1977), but the percentage of carbamazepine epoxide relative to carbamazepine in the brain increases with concurrent phenytoin therapy. The brain concentration of carbamazepine epoxide may be important; experimentally, the epoxide possesses anticonvulsant properties (Frigerio and Morselli, 1975).

In animal studies, carbamazepine crosses the placenta (Morselli, 1975). It has also been detected in the plasma of newborns whose mothers were receiving carbamazepine (Rane et al., 1975).

Protein Binding

At plasma concentrations achieved clinically, carbamazepine is 75 to 80% protein bound (DiSalle et al., 1974; Hooper et al., 1975; Kutt, 1978). Unlike the effect on protein binding of phenytoin, uremia does not appear to alter carbamazepine binding, but hepatic disease slightly lowers binding (Hooper et al., 1975). *In vitro* studies reveal that other antiepileptic drugs do not significantly displace carbamazepine (Rawlings et al., 1975).

Metabolism and Elimination

In humans, carbamazepine is almost completely metabolized to carbamazepine-10, 11-epoxide, which is pharmacologically active, and to carbamazepine-10,11-dihydroxide. Iminostilbene and small quantities of the parent drug are also excreted in the urine. The epoxide and dihydroxide are excreted as free compounds in the urine or are first conjugated with glucuronic acid. The metabolites of carbamazepine and the parent drug excreted in urine account for only a portion of the administered drug; further studies are required to fully determine the metabolic fate of carbamazepine.

The half-life of carbamazepine varies from 8 to 20 hr and is partly dependent on dose, age of the patient (shorter half-lives in children), presence of other anti-epileptic drugs that may stimulate its metabolism, and chronicity of treatment (Frigerio and Morselli, 1975; Morselli, 1975; Eichelbaum et al., 1976). The mean half-life in neonates and children is approximately 9 hr (Rey et al., 1979); the half-life of carbamazepine epoxide is 8 to 14 hr (DiSalle et al., 1974).

During long-term therapy with carbamazepine, epoxide concentrations are present in variable ratios to concentrations of the parent drug, with a range of 15 to 50% of the carbamazepine levels (Morselli, 1975). The metabolite appears to be present in higher concentrations in patients on combined antiepileptic drug therapy (Westenberg et al., 1978). This effect, in conjunction with lower plasma carbamazepine levels when the drug is administered with other antiepileptic drugs, is suggestive of enhanced carbamazepine metabolism. Relatively more of the metabolite seems to be produced in children, which may be attributable to enhanced hepatic metabolism (Pynnönnen et al., 1977).

CLINICAL USE

Carbamazepine, one of the major anticonvulsant drugs used in the treatment of simple and complex partial seizures, is also effective in the treatment of generalized tonic-clonic seizures and in the mixed seizure types of childhood. It is not effective in the treatment of absence seizures. It is often effective as a sole agent in the treatment of the above-mentioned seizure types but can be given in combination with any of the other antiepileptic drugs. Potentiation of side effects is not seen when blood levels of carbamazepine and the other drugs chosen are in the therapeutic range. Drug interactions may occur and are discussed below.

Carbamazepine is supplied as 200-mg scored tablets, which can be divided easily for initiation of therapy. Daily doses of 4 to 20 mg/kg carbamazepine are needed to achieve therapeutic plasma concentrations. The initial dose should be small (100 to 200 mg in two daily doses for adults) to prevent gastrointestinal and other unpleasant side effects. This dosage can be increased in daily increments of 200 mg every 3 to 5 days until seizure control is obtained or therapeutic plasma concentrations are achieved. Since carbamazepine has a short half-life, administration in two or three divided daily doses is recommended. Ingestion with meals may help relieve some of the initial nausea without decreasing absorption of the drug.

Extensive clinical studies in Europe and North America have confirmed the efficacy of carbamazepine in the treatment of partial seizures (simple and complex) and generalized tonic-clonic seizures in both children and adults. Carbamazepine was initially used as a secondary drug because of the early reports of hematological toxicity. This is a rare reaction, however; the toxicity of carbamazepine is probably no greater than that of the other antiepileptic drugs.

In 1974, a review of 250 articles on the use of carbamazepine concluded that carbamazepine was efficacious in the treatment of generalized tonic-clonic seizures and partial seizures, especially complex partial seizures. This review confirmed earlier reports that carbamazepine was equivalent in efficacy to phenytoin and phenobarbital (Bird et al., 1966). Double-blind studies comparing phenytoin and carbamazepine have reported similar conclusions (Cereghino et al., 1975; Parsonage, 1975; Troupin et al., 1975; Simonsen et al., 1976; Dodrill and Troupin, 1977; Hassan and Parsonage, 1977; Troupin et al., 1977; Callaghan et al., 1978; Shorvon et al., 1978; Wilkus et al., 1978; Kosteljanetz et al., 1979). The psychotropic effects of carbamazepine were also evaluated, with phenytoin as reference (Dodrill and Troupin, 1977). Patients receiving carbamazepine made fewer errors on mental tasks requiring attention and problem solving. Some improvement in emotional status was also suggested. Treatment with carbamazepine has no consistent effect on the electroencephalogram (EEG) (Schneider, 1977).

With evidence of the efficacy and toxicity of carbamazepine, when compared with the other antiepileptic drugs, it becomes difficult to choose a primary drug for the treatment of generalized tonic-clonic and partial seizures. This decision is often based on the physician's experience with a particular drug. Carbamazepine may be preferred in children who often experience sedation with phenobarbital and primidone and gingival hyperplasia, acne, and hirsutism with phenytoin. To help determine the drug of first choice in the treatment of partial and generalized tonic-clonic seizures, a 5-year Veterans Administration cooperative study is under way.

INTERACTIONS WITH OTHER DRUGS

During chronic administration, carbamazepine causes autoinduction of its metabolism, with a resultant decrease in the half-life. Its interaction with other drugs is shown in Table 6.1. Hepatic enzyme induction can reduce the effect of phenytoin (Hansen et al., 1971; Cereghino et al., 1973) and oral anticoagulants (Hansen et al., 1971). The significance of this interaction is that the sudden withdrawal of carbamazepine in a patient on chronic anticoagulant and carbamazepine therapy may cause a serious bleeding diathesis. The administration of other hepatic enzyme-

TABLE 6.1. *Carbamazepine interactions with other drugs*

Drug	Effect
Phenytoin	Decreased phenytoin effect
Doxycycline	Decreased doxycycline effect
Propoxyphene	Increased carbamazepine effect
Oral anticoagulants	Decreased anticoagulant effect

inducing drugs (e.g., phenobarbital, primidone, phenytoin) may enhance carbamazepine metabolism (Schneider, 1975). Carbamazepine may decrease the effect of the antibiotic doxycycline, and propoxyphene may increase the effect of carbamazepine. No interaction has been noted between carbamazepine and the other antiepileptic drugs except phenytoin (Hansen et al., 1971; Cereghino et al., 1973).

TOXICITY

The toxic effects of carbamazepine are similar to those of the other antiepileptic drugs diplopia, ataxia, blurred vision, drowsiness, gastrointestinal disturbances, and headache. These side effects are more common with plasma carbamazepine concentrations in the upper therapeutic range or higher; they are additive when carbamazepine is used concurrently with other antiepileptic drugs. Some tolerance develops to some of these side effects, and there is a marked interindividual variation in the severity of these symptoms and signs. Vertigo, psychosis, and tremor may be rarely observed. In a series of 255 patients, diplopia was present in 16%, drowsiness in 11%, blurred vision in 6%, and disturbances of balance and paresthesias in 3% (Livingston et al., 1974). Most of these adverse reactions are experienced in the first few weeks of therapy and often clear spontaneously without dosage adjustment.

Neurotoxic side effects most commonly require a reduction of dosage, although these are present in less than 5% of patients. As mentioned above, sedation is less common than with phenytoin. As is the case with other antiepileptic drugs, neurotoxicity may be more common in patients with underlying central nervous system structural disease. Age may be an important factor in hematological toxicity, and most cases of serious bone marrow suppression have been in older patients receiving carbamazepine for the treatment of trigeminal neuralgia (Pisciotta, 1975). The systemic and neurological side effects of carbamazepine have been reported by several investigators; their conclusions are essentially the same as those stated above (Killian and Fromm, 1968; Reynolds, 1975a).

A summary of hematological disorders associated with the use of carbamazepine showed 13 cases of aplastic anemia (Pisciotta, 1975). Of these, 10 patients died and three recovered. These patients had developed bone marrow depression after treatment for 3 weeks to 2 years. Carbamazepine was being used to treat trigeminal neuralgia in nine patients. The report concluded that carbamazepine could be implicated in only three patients. Regular hematological surveillance was recommended, especially during early therapy. It was also recommended that carbamazepine be discontinued if evidence of bone marrow suppression persists. A transient decrease in the white blood count is common at initiation of therapy but does not require withdrawal of the drug.

In our experience, serious hematological toxicity has not been encountered with the use of carbamazepine. In a double-blind, 6-month study (B.J. Wilder and J. Bruni, *unpublished data*), carbamazepine alone was as effective as phenytoin in the treatment of patients with previously untreated complex partial, simple partial, and generalized tonic-clonic seizures. No specific EEG effect was noted. Sedation was more commonly reported by patients receiving phenytoin, and diplopia was reported by 15% of patients with plasma carbamazepine concentrations below 8 μg/ml. Performance on motor tasks was better in the patients receiving carbamazepine than in those receiving phenytoin.

Other side effects of carbamazepine have been reported as isolated case reports or in a small number of patients. Because of its anticholinergic action, carbamazepine may rarely cause urinary frequency and retention. A cardiac rhythm depressant effect has been reported (Beerman and Edhag, 1978; Hamilton, 1978; Herzberg, 1978), and caution should be exercised in using carbamazepine in patients with cardiac arrhythmias or ischemic heart disease that may predispose to cardiac irregularities. An antidiuretic effect has been reported (Flegel and Cole, 1977; Perucca et al., 1978; Stephens et al., 1978); the mechanism is thought to be related to increased renal sensitivity to arginine, vasopressin, and resetting of osmoreceptors (Stephens et al., 1978). Water intoxication with hyponatremia may result. The manifestations include dizziness, headache, drowsiness, confusion, and nausea. These symptoms should not be attributed to direct drug toxicity. In a study of pediatric patients, significant changes in serum sodium or serum osmolality were not observed (Helin et al., 1977).

Transient elevations of hepatic enzymes may occasionally occur. Serious hepatotoxicity is rare, but fatal carbamazepine hepatitis has been reported (Zucker et al., 1977). Its incidence is unknown. The report suggested that hepatotoxicity may be related to the epoxide, since epoxides are known hepatotoxins. The rare hepatotoxicity, not unique to carbamazepine, has been reported with other antiepileptic drugs.

Skin rashes rarely occur in response to carbamazepine therapy. However, deposits of plasma proteins have been found in the skin during treatment with carbamazepine and phenytoin (Permin and Sestoft, 1977). The various dermatological reactions include sensitivity reactions, erythematous rashes, pruritic eruptions, urticaria, photosensitivity, pigmentary changes, neurodermatitis, exfoliative dermatitis, Stevens-Johnson syndrome, alopecia, erythema multiforme, erythema nodosum, and aggravation of lupus erythematosus. Carbamazepine, as well as phenytoin and phenobarbital, has been associated with increased sex hormone-binding globulin concentrations in both sexes (Barragry et al., 1978), but the significance of these changes in relation to impotence in male epileptic patients is uncertain.

The role of antiepileptic drugs in congenital malformations is uncertain; but all agents have been implicated (Bruni and Wilder, 1979b). No congenital malformation has definitely been linked with carbamazepine (Niebyl et al., 1979), but chromosome damage has been noted (Herha and Obe, 1977). Plasma carbamazepine levels should be monitored to avoid excessive concentrations. As mentioned above, carbamazepine crosses the placenta and enters the fetal circulation.

From the above considerations, carbamazepine should not be administered to patients with a history of hepatic disease or serious blood dyscrasia. It should not be administered concurrently with monoamine oxidase inhibitors, nor should it be used in patients with known sensitivity to any of the tricyclic compounds. Carba-mazepine should be used with caution in patients with cardiac irregularities or coronary artery disease.

The symptoms of acute overdosage of carbamazepine include drowsiness or coma, nausea, vomiting, restlessness, agitation, confusion, tremor, abnormal reflexes, mydriasis, nystagmus, flushing, cyanosis, and urinary retention. Hypo-tension or hypertension may result. The EEG may show generalized slowing. No specific antidote is available, and management is supportive.

7

Valproic Acid

Valproic acid (Depakene®), the newest antiepileptic drug, was approved for use in the United States in 1978. It was first synthesized by B. S. Barton in 1881, but its anticonvulsant properties were not discovered until 1963 by Meunier and colleagues (Meunier et al., 1963). While being used as a solvent in the screening of anticonvulsant compounds, valproic acid was found to protect the animals against pentylenetetrazol (PTZ) seizures. The first clinical trials, reported by Carraz and co-workers (1964), were followed by numerous clinical studies in Europe. Valproic acid has been approved for the treatment of seizures worldwide. It is marketed as valproic acid, sodium valproate, and magnesium valproate. In the United States, both the valproic acid formulation and its sodium salt are used. In addition to Depakene, a variety of other proprietary names are used internationally: Depakine, Epilim, Ergenyl, Labazene, and Atemperator.

In the Unites States, 100 patients were initially investigated in three separate studies at seven epilepsy centers. These studies, designed to evaluate the safety and efficacy of valproic acid, compared it with a placebo as sole or adjunctive therapy in absence seizures. Its efficacy in other seizure types has also been investigated, but well-controlled studies are still required to determine the proper place of this drug in the treatment of these other seizure types.

CHEMISTRY

Valproic acid (2-propylvaleric acid, 2 propylpentanoic acid, di-n-propylacetic acid) is a branched-chain carboxylic acid similar in structure to endogenous fatty acids. It differs from conventional antiepileptic drugs in that it is a much simpler molecule, lacking nitrogen and a ring moiety.

$$CH_3CH_2CH_2 \diagdown \atop CH_3CH_2CH_2 \diagup CH{-}C \diagup\diagdown {O \atop OH}$$

The compound has a molecular weight of 144, a pK_a of 4.95, and is highly water soluble. It is very soluble in organic solvents. Its molecular weight and pK_a influence its transport across biological membranes. Its water solubility and low molecular weight favor absorption, and its low pK_a (indicating that it is a strong carboxylic acid) theoretically retards transport, since at physiological pH it is more than 99% ionized. Whether an active process is involved in the absorption of valproic acid is unknown.

MECHANISM OF ACTION

The exact mechanism of action of valproic acid is unknown, but evidence supports an effect on the metabolism of gamma-aminobutyric acid (GABA). It was originally proposed that valproic acid causes competitive inhibition of GABA-transaminase in the GABA shunt (Godin et al., 1969) Fig. 7.1). This would result in increased brain levels of GABA, a major inhibitory neurotransmitter in supraspinal cord central nervous system (CNS) structures.

Simler et al. (1973) have found a correlation between increased whole-brain GABA levels and anticonvulsant effects on audiogenic seizures in genetically susceptible mice. Subsequent studies, however, have shown that brain and cerebellar GABA levels are increased only with concentrations of valproic acid unlikely to be achieved clinically (Sawaya et al., 1975; Anlezark et al., 1976). Harvey (1976) has proposed that valproic acid prevents the reuptake of GABA by glia and axonal terminals. Synaptic changes in GABA availability in synaptic regions may be more important than more global changes in GABA levels.

In doses experimentally effective against PTZ-induced seizures, valproic acid blocks the convulsant effects of bicuculline and picrotoxin, two GABA antagonists (Frey and Loescher, 1976). One group of investigators (Lust et al., 1976) has found

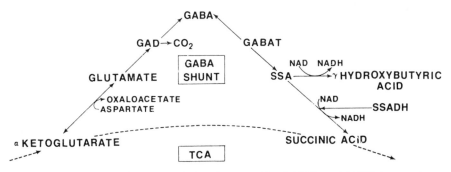

FIG. 7.1. Proposed valproic acid-induced competitive inhibition of GABA-transaminase (GABAT) and semialdehyde dehydrogenase (SSADH). TCA, tricarboxylic acid cycle.

both an increase in brain GABA content and a decrease in cyclic guanosine mon-ophosphate (cGMP), an inhibitory substance for cerebellar Purkinje cells. The investigators proposed that since Purkinje cells have an inhibitory output, their enhanced activity as a result of a decrease in inhibitory drive may be significant.

Some investigators have stressed the ability of valproic acid to inhibit the enzyme succinic semialdehyde dehydrogenase (SSADH), which normally converts GABA to succinate (Harvey et al., 1975; Sawaya et al., 1975; Anlezark et al., 1976). A decreased conversion of GABA to succinate might critically modify energy metab-olism, causing interaction with GABA-mediated synaptic inhibition.

There is some evidence that valproic acid augments GABA-mediated postsynaptic inhibition, suggesting that enhanced inhibition by GABA may explain its anticon-vulsant action (Macdonald and Bergey, 1978). Other findings suggest that the GABA hypothesis as previously outlined may be incorrect (Fowler et al., 1975; Emson, 1976; Whittle and Turner, 1978).

Electrophysiologically, valproic acid does not block an epileptic focus (Horton et al., 1977). The spread of seizure discharge is reduced, however, and fewer spike and wave discharges are observed on the electroencephalogram (EEG). Spike and wave activation by hyperventilation and photic stimulation is reduced (Jeavons et al., 1977; Harding et al., 1978; Bruni and Wilder, 1979a; Rowan et al., 1979; Bruni et al., 1980a). The 3/sec spike and wave pattern of absence seizures is blocked (Villarreal et al., 1978). Valproic acid has been found to influence thalamocortical excitability (Nowack et al., 1979) with a decrease in the average evoked response following stimulation of the ventrolateral thalamus at low frequencies. This decrease may be associated with effectiveness against absence seizures (Englander et al., 1977). Some of the anticonvulsant efficacy of valproic acid may result from re-stricting the ability of the thalamus to elaborate aberrant cortical activity into a generalized seizure.

At the membrane level, valproic acid causes a dose-related increase in potassium conductance with hyperpolarization of the resting membrane (Slater and Johnston, 1978). How this relates to GABA conductance is unknown.

PHARMACOKINETICS

Absorption

Valproic acid is rapidly and nearly completely absorbed. Peak plasma concen-trations are usually reached in 30 min to 2 hr, with bioavailability in the range of 80 to 90%. Administering the drug with meals slightly delays absorption, but the extent of absorption is unaltered (Meinardi et al., 1975). The relationship between daily dose and corresponding plasma concentrations is variable (Meijer and Hessing-Brand, 1973; Schobben and Van der Kleijn, 1974 a,b; Bruni et al., 1978a), al-though some workers have found it more constant than others (Ferrandes and Eymard, 1973; Loiseau et al., 1975; Klotz and Antonin, 1977). The causes for this pharmacokinetic variation may include differences in absorption or elimination.

The lack of such a constant relationship requires plasma concentration monitoring to determine when an adequate dose has been given.

Distribution

Both one-compartment models (Schobben and Van der Kleijn, 1974b; Klotz and Antonin, 1977; Bruni et al., 1978a) and two-compartment models (Gugler et al., 1977) have been used to describe the kinetics of valproic acid. Valproic acid is eliminated by linear kinetics, and enzyme saturation does not occur (Gugler et al., 1977; Klotz and Antonin, 1977). Valproic acid distributes mainly in the extracellular space (Klotz and Antonin, 1977), with an apparent volume of distribution of approximately 0.23 liter/kg (range, 0.15 to 0.42 liter/kg). Autoradiographic studies in mice have shown the drug to be present in high concentrations in blood and liver (Schobben and Van der Kleijn, 1974a,b). Two minutes after intraperitoneal administration, the drug was found in the gall bladder and subsequently in the intestinal tract. Large amounts of radioactive drug were also found in the kidney, urinary bladder, nasal cavity, and periosteum. The concentration in the cerebrum was approximately one-third that in blood.

Similar experiments in monkeys revealed that the drug easily crosses the placenta; there were no gross differences in concentration between mother and fetus (Schobben et al., 1977). In the cerebellum and occipital lobe, there was an uneven distribution between gray and white matter. In these distribution experiments, the contribution of rapidly formed metabolites is uncertain. A cerebrospinal fluid-to-serum ratio of 0.15 has been quoted (Meijer and Meinardi, 1976), and an active transport mechanism has been proposed for drug entry into the CNS. Less than 10% enters breast milk (Espir et al., 1976).

Protein Binding

Valproic acid is highly protein bound in the range of 90% or greater in the human (Jordan et al., 1976; Klotz and Antonin, 1977; Patsalos and Lascelles, 1977; Loscher, 1978; Patel and Levy, 1979; Fleitman et al., 1980). Species differences exist in the degree of protein binding, and the *in vitro* percentage of binding decreases with increasing temperature. The binding of valproic acid influences clearance of the drug, which is determined by restrictive and blood flow-independent elimination (Loscher, 1978). Other antiepileptic drugs do not influence valproic acid binding (Bruni et al., 1979a; Patel and Levy, 1979; Fleitman et al., 1980), but salicylate and phenylbutazone cause a decrease in binding. Uremia also reduces protein binding (Bruni et al., 1980c; Gugler and Mueller, 1978). Because valproic acid is highly protein bound, hemodialysis does not remove a significant amount from the circulation when the drug is present in therapeutic or toxic concentrations (Marbury et al., 1980).

Metabolism and Elimination

The plasma half-life of valproic acid is generally 8 to 12 hr, although in cases of overdosage, longer half-lives may be observed (Ferrandes and Eymard,

1973; Loiseau et al., 1975; Schobben et al., 1975; Espir et al., 1976; Richens et al., 1976; Bruni et al., 1978*a*). Owing to its short half-life, plasma concentrations fluctuate considerably. When determining plasma levels of the drug, sampling should be done at similar times in relation to dosing. It is uncertain if a diurnal circadian variation of plasma valproic acid levels occurs in humans as it does in the monkey (Lockard et al., 1977).

All metabolic degradation products of valproic acid in humans have not yet been identified. The elimination of valproic acid and its metabolites occurs principally in the urine, with minor amounts in the feces and expired air. Little unmetabolized drug is present in urine. Five metabolites were detected in rat urine, but their chemical structures were not determined (Eymard et al., 1971). Five metabolic products of valproic acid in rat urine and glucuronide conjugate of valproic acid were later identified (Kuhara and Matsumoto, 1974; Matsumoto et al., 1976). Metabolic pathways involving both β- and ω-oxidation were implicated in rats and later were found to be involved in the metabolism of valproic acid in humans (Gompertz et al., 1977).

Identification of valproic acid metabolites was made in the rat, mouse, dog, and human, and it was found that metabolic pathways may differ in different species (Jakobs and Loscher, 1978). β-Oxidation was found to be the preferred metabolic pathway in humans, with the formation of 3-hydroxy-2-propylpentanoic acid. The formation of 4-hydroxy-2-propylpentanoic acid resulted from involvement of the ω-oxidation pathway. A third metabolite of uncertain identity was also found. 5-hydroxy-2-propylpentanoic acid, suggested by some workers to be a metabolic product in humans (Ferrandes and Eymard, 1977), was found only in the serum of mice.

The full significance of the metabolites of valproic acid has not yet been determined. It is still not known whether some of the toxic effects of this drug are caused by the metabolites rather than the parent compound. Studies in our laboratory have shown that 3-hydroxy-2-propylpentanoic acid possesses anticonvulsant activity against PTZ-induced seizures.

CLINICAL USE

Valproic acid is a major antiepileptic drug for the treatment of absence, myoclonic, and primary generalized tonic-clonic seizures. It may be effective in complex partial seizures but is rarely effective against simple partial seizures. It may be used in combination with other antiepileptic drugs, but drug interactions and potentiation of side effects with barbiturates can be anticipated. These interactions and side effects are discussed below. Valproic acid is supplied as 250 mg capsules, and sodium valproate is supplied in a syrup at 250 mg/5 ml.

To prevent dose-related adverse effects, valproic acid therapy should be initiated gradually. The recommended initial daily dose is 10 to 15 mg/kg in three divided doses (250 mg three times a day). Increases at weekly intervals of 5 to 10 mg/kg/day can be made until seizures are controlled or side effects prevent further increases in dose. The maximum daily dose recommended by the manufacturer is 60 mg/kg/day. Rarely may higher doses be required to achieve optimum control, and plasma concentrations of up to 150 μg/ml may be required. The usual daily dose for adults is 1,500 to 2,000 mg. Administration with meals does not decrease bioavailability and often minimizes initial nausea. Because of its short half-life, valproic acid should not be administered once daily. Patients who cannot tolerate the doses required on the thrice daily dosage schedule may have to reduce individual doses and take the drug four times per day. This is necessary in rare situations when nausea and vomiting result from high peak concentrations within 30 min to 2 hr of valproic acid ingestion.

Valproic acid is currently approved by the U.S. Food and Drug Administration as sole and adjunctive therapy for absence seizures and as adjunctive therapy for other types of seizures when they occur in conjunction with absence seizures. Although valproic acid has a broad spectrum of antiepileptic activity, it is more effective in the generalized than in the partial epilepsies. It is particularly effective in patients who demonstrate 3/sec spike and wave discharges on the EEG.

The clinical efficacy of valproic acid has largely been studied in open trials as adjunctive therapy. The results of these trials have been summarized (Simon and Penry, 1975; Pinder et al., 1977; Bruni and Wilder, 1979a). Controlled trials have demonstrated the efficacy of valproic acid in the treatment of absence seizures (Meinardi, 1971; Suzuki et al., 1972; Gram et al., 1979). A 75% reduction in seizure frequency can be expected in about two-thirds of patients with simple and complex typical absence attacks and in 50% of patients with atypical absence seizures. We have treated approximately 80 patients with absence seizures that were refractory to other antiabsence seizure drugs (ethosuximide, clonazepam) and have observed similar results (Villarreal et al., 1978; Bruni et al., 1980a). For simple absence seizures, however, ethosuximide remains the drug of choice because of equal efficacy, a lower incidence of side effects, lower cost, less potential for drug interaction, and less frequent administration. Some patients may be optimally treated with either drug alone; others require combined therapy.

Valproic acid is the drug of choice in the treatment of myoclonic seizures associated with CNS degenerative disease (Jeavons et al., 1977; Villarreal et al., 1978; Bruni et al., 1980a). It has also been found useful in the treatment of postanoxic intention myoclonus (Carroll and Walsh, 1978; Fahn, 1978; Bruni et al., 1979d; Rollinson and Gilligan, 1979). We have not found it useful in the treatment of segmental spinal myoclonus, and its efficacy in nonepileptic myoclonus has not been determined.

In the treatment of generalized tonic-clonic seizures, the general experience is that approximately 50% of patients with seizures refractory to other drugs respond to valproic acid when it is added to previous therapy. Studies to determine the efficacy of valproic acid as sole therapy in generalized tonic-clonic seizures show the drug to be equally effective to phenytoin in recent onset primary generalized tonic-clonic seizures (B. J. Wilder and R. E. Ramsay, 1981, *unpublished data*). The efficacy of valproic acid in the treatment of simple and complex partial seizures has also been established in studies in which valproic acid was used as adjunctive therapy. Approximately 30 to 40% of patients can be expected to respond favorably.

The results of treatment of atonic or akinetic seizures with valproic acid show a 75% reduction in seizure frequency in 34% of patients (Pinder et al., 1977). In one study, valproic acid was as effective as primidone or phenobarbital in preventing febrile seizures (Cavazzuti, 1975). Infantile spasms and the Lennox-Gastaut syndrome do not respond as effectively to valproic acid as they do to the benzodiazepines (Pinder et al., 1977). Valproic acid has been used rarely in the treatment of refractory status epilepticus and has been reported to control it (Manhire and Espir, 1974; Barnes et al., 1976; Vayda et al., 1978).

In most patients with absence seizures, a positive correlation exists between clinical efficacy and improvement in the EEG, especially during chronic therapy (Villarreal et al., 1978; Bruni et al., 1980a). Some patients may have a good clinical response and poor EEG response, or vice versa. The effect of valproic acid on focal epileptiform discharges has not been fully established. In our experience, however, most focal EEG abnormalities remain unchanged despite good control of partial seizures.

Since valproic acid was first introduced, we have used it to treat nearly 250 patients, usually in combination with other antiepileptic drugs for the treatment of refractory absence attacks, generalized tonic-clonic seizures, myoclonic seizures, atonic attacks, and simple or complex partial seizures. We have been able to withdraw other medications in some patients with continued good seizure control. In others, the effects of valproic acid appear additive when used concurrently with other antiepileptic drugs. Because it has a broader spectrum of activity than most other antiepileptic drugs, it is rational to use valproic acid in the newly diagnosed epileptic patient who suffers from multiple types of seizures, such as absence and generalized tonic-clonic seizures. Previously, at least two drugs would have been used, one for each seizure type. If valproic acid alone does not result in satisfactory control, a second drug may be added.

Because valproic acid is believed to have a modifying effect on GABA metabolism, attempts have been made to use this drug in the treatment of some extrapyramidal movement disorders. The results have been variable. One report suggested that valproic acid may be useful in the treatment of tardive dyskinesia and other neuroleptic-related extrapyramidal signs (Linnoila et al., 1976). It has not been found to be of significant benefit in Huntington's chorea (Shouldon et al., 1976; Tan et al., 1976; Pearce et al., 1977; Symmington et al., 1978), and a recent study failed to demonstrate any efficacy in Parkinson's disease (Nutt et al., 1979).

INTERACTIONS WITH OTHER DRUGS

The interaction of valproic acid with other drugs is summarized in Table 7.1. The most commonly reported and significant interaction is an increase in plasma phenobarbital concentration when valproic acid is added to the regimen (Richens and Ahmad, 1975; Taburet et al., 1975; Vakil et al., 1976; Loiseau et al., 1978; Mesdjian et al., 1978; Wilder et al., 1978; Bruni et al., 1980b). We have found this to occur in more than 80% of patients. Unless the phenobarbital dosage is

TABLE 7.1. *Valproic acid interactions with other drugs*

Drug	Effect
Phenytoin	Transient decrease in total plasma phenytoin level, but phenytoin effect unchanged due to increase in free phenytoin; decreased valproic acid effect
Phenobarbital	Increased phenobarbital effect; decreased valproic acid effect
Primidone	Decreased valproic acid effect
Clonazepam	Precipitation of absence status
Salicylate	Increase in free valproic acid (decrease in protein binding)
Phenylbutazone	Increase in free valproic acid

decreased by 30 to 50%, excessive sedation may occur; this is caused by inhibition of phenobarbital metabolism by valproic acid. Valproic acid does not decrease pH-dependent renal phenobarbital excretion. Earlier findings of an increase in phenobarbital half-life after the coadministration of valproic acid are also compatible with inhibition of hepatic metabolism (Loiseau et al., 1978).

In patients receiving primidone, which is partly metabolized to phenobarbital, the derived phenobarbital concentration does not increase. The explanation for this is uncertain, but valproic acid may also inhibit the conversion of primidone to phenobarbital.

Pharmacokinetic interactions between valproic acid and phenytoin have also been observed (Vakil et al., 1976; Patsalos and Lascelles, 1977; Mattson et al., 1978; Wilder et al., 1978; Bruni et al., 1979*b*). The most common effect is a transient decrease in total plasma phenytoin concentration with an increase in the free fraction of phenytoin. This results from a displacement of phenytoin from protein binding sites, a transient increase in its hepatic metabolism, and increased excretion of the phenytoin metabolite, 5-(*p*-hydroxyphenyl)-5-phenylhydantoin. No increase in phenytoin dose is generally required; with a corresponding increase in the free fraction of phenytoin, the amount of unbound, pharmacologically active phenytoin is not decreased. After a variable period of weeks, valproic acid inhibits phenytoin metabolism, and total phenytoin levels increase again, generally to prevalproic acid concentrations. The free fraction of phenytoin remains elevated, and symptoms of phenytoin toxicity may be observed in some patients (Bruni et al., 1980*c*).

The addition of primidone, phenobarbital, phenytoin, or carbamazepine to the regimen of a patient already receiving valproic acid does not influence its protein binding, but lower valproic acid concentrations may result from induction of valproic acid metabolism. As mentioned above, *in vitro* experiments have demonstrated displacement of valproic acid by salicylate and phenylbutazone (Fleitman et al., 1980), but the clinical effects of these interactions are still undetermined.

Pharmacodynamic interaction between valproic acid and clonazepam has been shown (Jeavons et al., 1977). Nine of 12 patients had unwanted effects with this combination; drowsiness developed in four; and absence status developed in five. We have not observed this interaction in adults, but one child had absence seizure exacerbation with this combination of drugs. Most patients in whom intoxication developed with the coadministration of phenobarbital and valproic acid are affected by toxic phenobarbital levels, but some become encephalopathic without raised drug concentrations (Vrai, 1978). The two drugs may have some additive or synergistic effect in producing intoxication.

TOXICITY

There is usually a considerable delay between the introduction of a new drug and the full establishment of its toxicity. This should be kept in mind when a new drug is prescribed; such patients should be followed regularly. Even today, more than 40 years after the introduction of phenytoin, new adverse effects of the drug are still being documented. The side effects associated with valproic acid therapy have generally been mild; nausea, vomiting, abdominal cramps, diarrhea, and fatigue are the most common. In general, these occur transiently early in the course of therapy and often can be minimized by administering the drug with meals.

Drowsiness and sedation are most commonly seen in patients concurrently receiving phenobarbital, but they may occur with valproic acid alone if plasma concentrations of the drug are high. An encephalopathy may occur rarely in patients receiving both phenobarbital and valproic acid and usually can be attributed to high plasma concentrations of the former. High doses of valproic acid when initiating treatment may produce a transient encephalopathy accompanied by marked slowing of the EEG. Incoordination and ataxia are rare. Variable changes in appetite occur, but a significant number of patients have a weight gain unrelated to increased caloric intake. Mild and transient alopecia occasionally may occur. A postural and resting tremor develops in a few patients. This is correlated with high plasma concentrations of valproic acid.

The most serious, although uncommon, side effect of valproic acid is hepatotoxicity (Willmore et al., 1978; Suchy et al., 1979). Usually, hepatotoxic effects are manifested by transient hepatic enzyme elevations that return to normal values upon reduction of valproic acid dosage. Occasionally, valproic acid must be discontinued. Rare fatalities have been reported (Suchy et al., 1979). We have had to discontinue valproic acid therapy in two patients because of significant but reversible hepatotoxicity. A Reye-like syndrome producing an encephalopathy in children has also been reported (Young et al., 1980). We recommend regular monitoring of hepatic function during valproic acid therapy, especially early in therapy and when dosages are increased. Pancreatitis as a complication of valproic acid therapy has been reported (Camfield et al., 1979).

Abnormalities of laboratory tests associated with the use of valproic acid include mild thrombocytopenia (Sutor and Jesdinsky-Buscher, 1974; Winfield et al., 1976; Neophytides, 1979), false urinary tests for ketones and glucose, inhibition of the secondary phase of platelet aggregation (Richardson et al., 1976), hyperglycemia

(Jaeken et al., 1977; Wolf, 1978; Similä et al., 1979), prolonged bleeding times in the absence of thrombocytopenia (Barnes et al., 1976), decreased erythrocyte sedimentation rate (Nutt et al., 1978), and low fibrinogen levels (Dale et al., 1978). We have not found any of these abnormalities to be clinically significant. Platelet counts should be monitored during therapy.

Toxic effects from interactions with other antiepileptic drugs have been discussed above. Seizure exacerbation with the coadministration of clonazepam may occur, and it is wise to discontinue clonazepam therapy gradually if seizures increase. We have observed an exacerbation of complex partial seizures in two patients concurrently receiving valproic acid, carbamazepine, and phenytoin when plasma levels of these drugs were in the therapeutic range.

The effects of valproic acid on pregnancy are unknown. No human cogenital anomalies have thus far been attributed to valproic acid. In animals, valproic acid is teratogenic, causing dysmorphogenic effects that include cleft palate, fusion of vertebrae, renal agenesis, encephaloceles, ablepharia, and rib fusions (Whittle, 1976).

8

Primidone

Primidone (Mysoline®), a deoxybarbiturate, was first reported to be clinically effective as an anticonvulsant in 1952 by Handley and Stewart. It is one of the major antiepileptic drugs used for the treatment of simple and complex partial seizures and is ineffective against absence seizures and atonic and akinetic attacks. Infantile spasms and myoclonic seizures are generally refractory to the drug. Primidone is probably more effective than phenobarbital in the treatment of either primary or secondary generalized tonic-clonic seizures.

CHEMISTRY

Primidone [5-ethyldihydro-5-phenyl-4,6(1H,5H)-pyrimidinedione] is a nonpolar, neutral compound with a molecular weight of 218.25. It is sparingly soluble in water (< 1 mg/ml) and most organic solvents. The drug is structurally deoxy-phenobarbital.

MECHANISM OF ACTION

The mechanism of action of primidone is difficult to evaluate because the drug is readily metabolized to two active metabolites, phenobarbital and phenylethylmalonamide (PEMA). Experiments in animals, however, have shown that primidone alone raises the tonic-clonic seizure threshold to electrical stimulation (Bogue and Carrington, 1953; Gallagher et al., 1970). Baumel et al. (1973) have concluded that primidone possesses independent anticonvulsant activity that is more potent than that of phenobarbital in preventing maximal electroshock seizures. In other studies, Baumel et al. (1972) have demonstrated an anticonvulsant effect of PEMA at high doses and an anticonvulsant potentiating effect on phenobarbital at low doses.

PHARMACOKINETICS

Absorption

Primidone, being un-ionized, is readily absorbed from the stomach and intestinal tract, even though the lipid/water partition ratio is low (< 0.05). Peak plasma levels are reached 2 to 4 hr after drug ingestion but may occur within 30 min or as late as 8 hr.

Distribution and Protein Binding

The drug is minimally bound to plasma protein, as indicated by the cerebrospinal fluid-to-plasma ratio of 0.6 to 0.997 (Schottelius and Fincham, 1978) and the saliva-to-plasma ratio of 0.73 (McAuliffe et al., 1977). It is widely distributed in the tissues. Its volume of distribution is 0.6 liter/kg, which is similar to that of phenytoin. Houghton et al. (1975) have reported a brain-to-plasma ratio of 0.87 in humans.

Metabolism and Elimination

Within 24 hr of primidone ingestion, PEMA appears in the plasma; after 24 to 96 hr, phenobarbital can be measured (Gallagher et al., 1972). Primidone reaches a steady-state plasma level after 48 to 96 hr of three times per day dosing. The metabolism of primidone follows a linear or first-order kinetic profile.

The half-life of primidone in adults is approximately 7 to 9 hr, whereas those of PEMA and phenobarbital are 16 to 24 hr and 48 to 120 hr, respectively. Kauffman et al. (1977) have reported a similar half-life for children. They could account for 92% of the daily dose of primidone in the urine, 42% appearing as unchanged drug, 45% as PEMA, and 5% as phenobarbital. In studying metabolic disposition of primidone in adults, we have accounted for 12 to 15% of the daily dose of primidone as phenobarbital or its hydroxylated metabolite (B. J. Wilder, *unpublished data*). A daily dose of 750 to 1,000 mg primidone yields plasma phenobarbital levels equivalent to levels yielded by a daily phenobarbital dose of approximately 150 mg.

CLINICAL USE

Primidone is considered by some to be the drug of choice for the treatment of complex partial seizures when monotherapy is used (Aird and Woodbury, 1974).

Primidone usually should not be administered in combination with phenobarbital because therapeutic doses of primidone usually yield therapeutic levels of the metabolite phenobarbital. As noted above, however, it may be safely and effectively combined with other antiepileptic drugs. Primidone and phenytoin may be used together without potentiation of side effects, but the anticonvulsant effects are additive. Primidone also may be used in combination with carbamazepine. The combination of primidone and ethosuximide may be used to treat patients who have both absence seizures and generalized tonic-clonic, simple partial, or complex partial seizures. Primidone can be used in combination with valproic acid or methsuximide, but more careful clinical observation and frequent monitoring of plasma drug levels are required because of the possibility of drug interactions and potentiation of side effects.

Primidone is marketed in 50 and 250 mg scored tablets. The usual adult daily dose ranges from 500 to 1,000 mg, or 8 to 15 mg/kg. The usual childhood daily dose can be calculated from the recommended daily dose of 10 to 20 mg/kg.

Primidone should be started at a low dose in children, beginning at a rate of 25 mg (half a 50 mg tablet) to 50 mg administered twice daily. This dose then should be gradually increased by 50 mg/day at 5- to 7-day intervals until a daily dose of 10 to 20 mg/kg is reached or seizure control is achieved. Therepeutic steady-state plasma drug levels of 5 to 15 μg/ml should be reached within 2 to 4 days after the calculated maintenance dose is achieved.

Treatment of larger children and adults should begin with 50 to 125 mg (half a 250 mg tablet) administered twice daily. The dose then should be increased by 125 to 250 mg/day, as described above, until a daily dose of 10 to 20 mg/kg is reached.

Phenobarbital, a major metabolite of primidone, should reach steady-state levels of 15 to 35 μg/ml in 15 to 20 days after the calculated therapeutic dose has been attained. Because of the much longer half-life of phenobarbital, measurement of phenobarbital levels may provide a more accurate assessment of primidone therapy than plasma primidone levels. Some patients, however, may not readily convert primidone to phenobarbital. PEMA levels are not routinely reported by clinical laboratories, and therapeutic levels have not been established.

Most physicians prefer to give primidone in two or three divided daily doses. Blood samples for monitoring plasma drug levels should be drawn at least 6 hr after the last administered dose. In the case of primidone, this time of sampling gives a value slightly higher than the trough level. Phenobarbital levels fluctuate only slightly ($<$ 20%) when steady state has been achieved (15 to 20 days of constant daily doses).

Primidone treatment should be initiated with extreme caution. Doses larger than those recommended produce predictable side effects in many patients. Patients may complain of severe malaise, vertiginous sensations, lethargy, somnolence, headaches, nausea, vomiting, peculiar gustatory sensations, incoordination, and loss of balance. Many patients who are abruptly started on high doses of primidone thereafter may refuse to take the drug. Behavioral changes may be noted soon after the start of primidone therapy. Withdrawal of primidone should be accomplished over a minimum of 3 weeks, as rapid discontinuation may result in withdrawal seizures (Schmidt et al., 1978).

INTERACTIONS WITH OTHER DRUGS

When used in combination therapy, primidone acts synergistically with phenytoin or carbamazepine in the control of generalized tonic-clonic or complex partial seizures.

The concurrent administration of phenytoin and primidone does not alter the metabolic disposition of the drugs. Phenytoin has been reported to increase the conversion of primidone to phenobarbital (Ruf and Sauter, 1977; Schottelius and Fincham, 1978), but we have found such an effect to be negligible. We have observed, however, that when phenobarbital and primidone are given concurrently, phenobarbital levels are much higher than when primidone is given alone. The concurrent administration of phenobarbital and primidone thus does not inhibit the metabolic conversion of primidone to phenobarbital. Instead, the resulting plasma phenobarbital levels are additive.

TOXICITY

The toxic effects of primidone are discussed in Chapter 15. These are similar to those produced by the other 5- and 6-membered ring anticonvulsants. The toxic effects described in Chapter 4 on the barbiturate anticonvulsants also apply to primidone. Primidone may have a greater effect than phenobarbital on blood-forming tissue, lymphoid tissue, and autoimmune systems. In addition, the cleavage of the deoxybarbiturate ring at the 2C position produces a straight-chain compound (PEMA), which may be responsible for some of the adverse reactions noted at the commencement of therapy.

Acute primidone intoxication from overdosage results in general depression of the central nervous system and disequilibrium manifested by somnolence, lethargy, ataxia, nystagmus, dysarthria, nausea, and vomiting; deep coma and areflexia have been reported. These signs are primarily due to primidone rather than its major metabolite phenobarbital (Brillman et al., 1974). Chronic toxicity from excessively high maintenance doses produces lethargy and somnolence, which are attributable to the phenobarbital metabolite.

9

Succinimides: Ethosuximide, Methsuximide, and Phensuximide

The anticonvulsant succinimides ethosuximide, methsuximide, and phensuximide demonstrate the differential effects of substituting various chemical groups in a heterocyclic molecule on a variety of experimental and clinical seizure types. Methyl and ethyl groups at position 2C of the succinimide ring antagonize experimentally induced pentylenetetrazol (PTZ) seizures, whereas a phenyl group substituted at the 2C position antagonizes experimentally induced maximal electroshock (MES) seizures. Methylation of position 5N adds to the anti-PTZ effect and imparts additional hypnotic activity or sedative effects. Phenyl substitution at the 2C position and alkyl substitution at the 5N and 2C positions provide anticonvulsant activity against both PTZ- and MES-induced seizures (methsuximide).

Anti-PTZ activity predicts an effect against absence seizures, and anti-MES effect predicts activity against generalized tonic-clonic and simple or complex partial seizures. Succinimide itself, like barbituric acid, is not an anticonvulsant compound. The structures of ethosuximide, methsuximide, and phensuximide indicate that one should be effective against absence seizures and produce minimal hypnotic effects, and the other two should be effective against convulsive and absence seizure types and induce sedative side effects (Sherwin, 1978; Ferrendelli and Kupferberg, 1980).

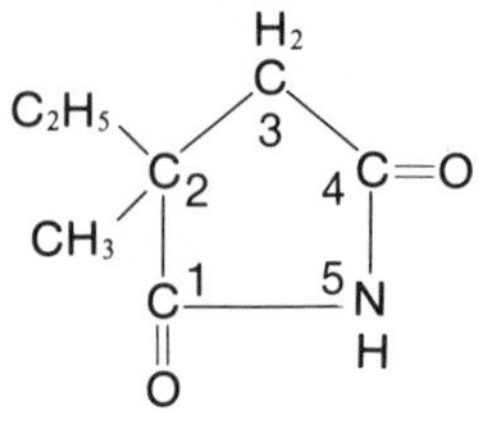

Ethosuximide

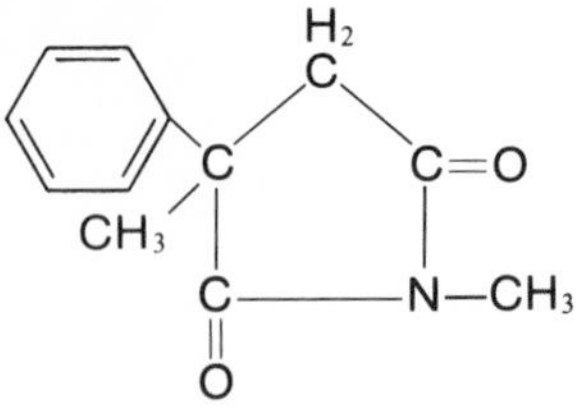

Methsuximide

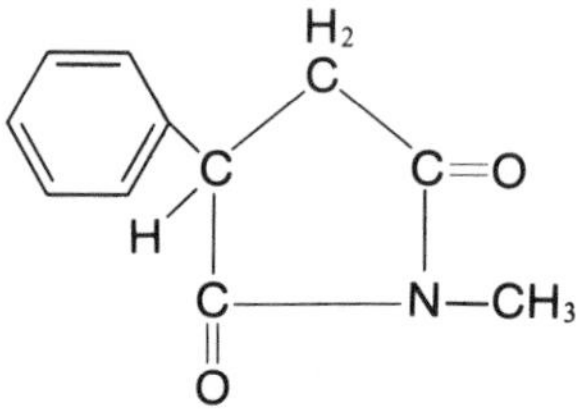

Phensuximide

ETHOSUXIMIDE

Ethosuximide (Zarontin®) was developed from a structure-activity research program designed to find a drug effective against absence seizures (Chen et al., 1951, 1963; Miller and Long, 1951, 1953*a,b*). The short-chain alkyl groups located at position 2C of the succinimide ring appear to be specific for seizures characterized by low frequency rhythmical spike and wave activity. Absence seizures are characterized by generalized 3/sec rhythmic spike and wave discharge. In addition, some clonic seizures have similar electrographic characteristics, and generalized tonic-clonic seizures are sometimes preceded by rhythmic spike and wave activity (Scholl and Schwab, 1971). Ethosuximide is the drug of choice in the treatment of simple and complex absence seizures and may rarely be effective in seizures with convulsive manifestations characterized by spike and wave or electroencephalographic (EEG) rhythmic slow wave abnormalities.

METHSUXIMIDE AND PHENSUXIMIDE

Methsuximide (Celontin®) and phensuximide (Milontin®) may prevent absence seizures and are effective against generalized tonic-clonic and simple or complex partial seizures. Phensuximide is substantially less effective than methsuximide for reasons discussed below. It is rarely used clinically and is of interest because of its structure and activity against experimentally induced PTZ and MES seizures.

CHEMISTRY

Ethosuximide

From its structure, ethosuximide (2-ethyl-2-methylsuccinimide) appears to be a weak acid, but the pK_a is unknown, and ionization does not occur in biological fluids or tissues. It is not lipophilic, which may account for its lack of anti-MES activity, and thus has no particular affinity for the brain or neuronal membranes. Its molecular weight is 141.17. It is much more water soluble than the other succinimides (190 mg/ml at 25° C).

Methsuximide and Phensuximide

Methsuximide and phensuximide are nonpolar, chemically neutral compounds. They are slightly lipophilic because of the phenyl group at the 2C position. Methsuximide (N,2-dimethyl-2-phenylsuccinimide) has a molecular weight of 203.23 and is water soluble (2.8 mg/ml at 25° C). Phensuximide (n-methyl-2-phenylsuccinimide) has a molecular weight of 189.21 and water solubility of 4.2 mg/ml at 25° C.

MECHANISM OF ACTION

Ethosuximide

The mechanism of action of ethosuximide is unknown. Since it is the drug of choice for absence seizures and has virtually no effect on generalized tonic-clonic and simple or complex partial seizures, its mechanisms of action may be different from the hydantoins, barbiturates, and carbamazepine. The antiabsence seizure effect may be due to mechanisms similar to those of the oxazolidinediones and valproic acid, which are also antiabsence seizure drugs, but a precise common mechanism of action is not apparent. Valproic acid is thought to act by elevating brain levels of gamma-aminobutyric acid (GABA). The oxazolidinediones are thought to act by changing intracellular and extracellular K^+ ratios, inducing an intracellular acidosis, or by altering GABA metabolism (see Chapters 7 and 11). Thus a common mechanism may be shared by these drugs if ethosuximide works to augment GABA activity by maintaining the continuity of anionic chloride channels.

The lack of its effect in generalized tonic-clonic and MES-induced seizures indicates that ethosuximide has little or no effect on membrane structure or function, in contrast to phenytoin and carbamazepine. The latter directly modify excitable membranes and ionic movements across these membranes that are associated with depolarization. This is further supported by the lack of effect of ethosuximide on calcium uptake in presynaptic terminals and cyclic nucleotide regulation (Sohn and Ferrendelli, 1977; Ferrendelli and Kupferberg, 1980).

Of additional interest is the action of ethosuximide in preventing the generalized spike and wave and absence-like seizures induced in animals by massive parenteral doses of penicillin (Prince and Farrell, 1969; Gloor and Testa, 1974; Guberman et al., 1975). Gloor and Testa (1974) have proposed that absence seizures involve epileptiform activity, which is reinforced and spread by low frequency repetitive discharges from the cerebral cortex to subcortical structures. Fromm and Kohli (1972) have shown that ethosuximide suppresses the activity of certain inhibitory pathways, a phenomenon not shared by drugs effective against tonic-clonic seizures.

Drugs effective against absence seizures have been shown to act on low frequency inhibitory pathways (Nowack et al., 1979). Ethosuximide also antagonizes the anticonvulsant action of picrotoxin, bicuculline, and electrical EEG convulsions induced by the anesthetic enflurane (Schettini and Wilder, 1974; Englander et al., 1977).

The drug has a number of effects on brain metabolism and enzyme function that seem to be unrelated to its antiabsence activity. Ethosuximide inhibits membrane (N^+-K^+)-ATPase (Gilbert and Wyllie, 1974). This is a paradoxical effect in terms of seizure inhibition and may be a factor in the exacerbation of seizures that sometimes occurs when a patient is placed on ethosuximide (Lorentz de Haas and Kuilman, 1964). The drug also depresses oxygen utilization by 20 to 30%. Cerebellar cyclic guanosine monophosphate (cGMP) is depressed, but cerebellar cyclic adenosine monophosphate (cAMP) is unaffected by ethosuximide. There is negligible effect on glutamic acid decarboxylase, monoamine oxidase, acetylcholinesterase, or arylsulfatase. Succinate dehydrogenase is increased by 20 to 30% (Leznicki and Dymecki, 1974; Ferrendelli and Kupferberg, 1980). Thus ethosuximide does not appear to affect systems that regulate GABA, acetylcholine, or catecholamine metabolism.

Although the effect of ethosuximide on chloride conductance has not been studied, Ferrendelli and Kupferberg (1980) have proposed that ethosuximide may increase chloride conductance either directly or indirectly through the augmented action of an inhibitory neurotransmitter, such as GABA, and by this process prevent seizures induced by the drugs that interfere with chloride conductance (e.g., PTZ, penicillin), as well as absence seizures (Macdonald and Barker, 1979).

Methsuximide and Phensuximide

No studies have precisely evaluated the effects of methsuximide or phensuximide on membranes or against rhythmic low frequency discharge. It might be presumed, however, that calcium uptake into presynaptic endings, transmitter release, sodium and potassium conductances, as well as chloride conductance might be affected.

PHARMACOKINETICS

Ethosuximide

Absorption

Ethosuximide, in both capsule and syrup forms, is readily and completely absorbed from the gastrointestinal tract. After a single dose, the drug can be detected in plasma within 1 hr, and maximal plasma levels can be measured after 3 to 5 hr. Plasma ethosuximide levels appear slightly sooner after administration of the syrup than after the capsules. There is a close correlation between the dose of ethosuximide and plasma level achieved. On constant daily dosing, steady-state plasma ethosuximide levels are reached after 10 to 15 days and remain constant over an extended period of therapy.

Because the drug is soluble in water and is chemically neutral, malabsorption should not occur in the absence of acute gastrointestinal problems. The failure to achieve adequate or therapeutic plasma levels after appropriate doses can usually be attributed to noncompliance or laboratory error in analysis (Buchanan et al., 1969, 1973, 1976; Browne et al., 1975).

Distribution and Protein Binding

The distribution of ethosuximide conforms to that of total body water and is evenly distributed, except for low concentrations in fatty tissue (Chang et al., 1972b). The volume of distribution is approximately 0.69 liter/kg in children and 0.62 liter/kg in adults (Buchanan et al., 1973). The drug is found in highest concentrations in the kidney because of excretion of free drug.

Protein binding is essentially absent, and the drug equilibrates in plasma, cerebrospinal fluid (CSF), and saliva (Sherwin, 1978). Placental transfer occurs, and unchanged ethosuximide is secreted in breast milk (Hill et al., 1973; Horning et al., 1973).

Metabolism and Elimination

Ethosuximide is extensively metabolized in the liver to four hydroxylated metabolites and to 2-acetyl-2-methylsuccinimide. The hydroxylated metabolites are largely conjugated with glucuronic acid and excreted in the urine as their glucuronides. The acetylmethyl metabolite is also excreted in the urine. Approximately 20% of ingested ethosuximide is excreted unchanged. The hydroxylated metabolites are inactive compounds, but the activity of the acetylmethylsuccinimide is unknown (Chang et al., 1972a; Horning et al., 1973).

Sherwin (1978) has reported the elimination half-life of ethosuximide, following cessation of chronic therapy, to be 18 to 72 hr (mean, 38.8 hr). Browne et al. (1975) have reported a similar half-life and noted that it did not vary between ages 5 and 15 years. Goulet et al. (1976) have reported much longer half-lives in adult volunteers; the half-life is long enough for the drug to be administered in a single daily dose.

Methsuximide and Phensuximide

Absorption

Both methsuximide and phensuximide are readily absorbed and achieve peak plasma levels within 2 to 4 hr.

Distribution and Protein Binding

Both drugs are fairly evenly distributed throughout the body, with higher concentrations in the brain and fat tissue than are found with ethosuximide (Glazko and Dill, 1972). Methsuximide and phensuximide are not protein bound and equilibrate with CSF and saliva (B. J. Wilder, *unpublished data*).

Metabolism

Methsuximide possesses considerably more anticonvulsant activity than phensuximide. The metabolic disposition of the two drugs is useful in understanding their differential potency. Methsuximide, which has a mean half-life of 1.4 hr, is rapidly metabolized by *N*-demethylation principally in the liver to 2-methyl-2-phenylsuccinimide. This metabolite, which has a mean half-life of 38 hr, achieves high steady-state plasma levels and exerts a major anticonvulsant effect. Phensuximide is rapidly metabolized to 2-phenylsuccinimide, which, like the parent drug, has a short half-life (mean, 7.8 hr). The desmethyl metabolite, however, is rapidly converted to 2-phenylsuccinamic acid, a compound that probably lacks antiepileptic activity (Strong et al., 1974; Kupferberg et al., 1977; Porter et al., 1979). The failure of phensuximide or its desmethyl metabolite to accumulate to the extent of the desmethylmethsuximide is probably the reason for its relative ineffectiveness. The short half-lives of the 5N methyl component of the parent drugs reduce their potency against absence seizures.

CLINICAL USE

Ethosuximide

Ethosuximide is one of the two major drugs used in the treatment of absence seizures; the other is valproic acid. It has no effect against generalized tonic-clonic or simple and complex partial seizures.

Ethosuximide is supplied as 250 mg capsules or as a syrup (250 mg/5 ml). It should be administered in single or multiple daily doses of 15 to 35 mg/kg. After 10 to 15 days of constant daily dosing, steady-state plasma levels should be achieved, and the dosage should be adjusted to bring plasma levels within the therapeutic range of 40 to 100 μg/ml. Sherwin and Robb (1972) have reported 40 μg/ml to be the lower limit and 120 μg/ml to be the upper limit of the therapeutic range. Browne et al. (1975) have reported that 79% of patients within a range of 41 to 99 μg/ml had a 75% or greater reduction in absence seizures. We have found some patients who did not respond until their plasma ethosuximide levels exceeded 125 μg/ml. The value of plasma level monitoring of this drug has been well established (Sherwin et al., 1973).

In predicting the relationship between dose and plasma ethosuximide level, one should be aware that the linear regression line of dose-to-plasma level is less in younger children than in older children and adults (Browne et al., 1975; Sherwin, 1978). This may be helpful in evaluating dosage adequacy and compliance. Complete control of absence seizures can be expected in 60% of patients who are carefully monitored and whose dose is adjusted to achieve optimum plasma levels. Sherwin (1978) has reported complete control in 74% of patients after 5 years of therapy. This time interval accounts for refinement of the regimen and the natural, spontaneous improvement that probably occurs.

Ethosuximide can be safely administered with the other major antiepileptic drugs. It is frequently administered in conjunction with phenytoin or carbamazepine to patients who have both absence and generalized tonic-clonic seizures. It also can be given in conjunction with primidone or phenobarbital to patients who have both absence and partial seizures. The combination of ethosuximide and valproic acid may be effective in patients with refractory absence seizures. Ethosuximide is usually not effective in myoclonus. If myoclonus is a prominent accompaniment of absence attacks, valproic acid should be substituted or administered concurrently.

Methsuximide and Phensuximide

Methsuximide is supplied as 150 and 300 mg capsules and is effective in the treatment of complex partial seizures (Cordoba and Strobos, 1956; Wilder and Buchanan, 1981), generalized tonic-clonic seizures, and absence attacks (Zimmerman and Burgemeister, 1954; Livingston and Pauli, 1957; French et al., 1958; Aird and Woodbury, 1974). The drug has a very short half-life and is rapidly metabolized to its major metabolite desmethylmethsuximide, which is principally responsible for the anticonvulsant activity of the drug (see above). Because of the long half-life of the metabolite, the drug can be administered in one or two daily doses of 5 to 15 mg/kg. Doses in this range result in plasma desmethylmethsuximide levels of 15 to 30 μg/ml. A therapeutic range of 10 to 25 μg/ml is desirable; higher levels produce sedative side effects. In the therapeutic range, the desmethyl metabolite follows first-order kinetics; as the plasma level increases, however, saturation or zero-order kinetics occurs, and serious toxicity can develop. Wilder and Buchanan (1981) have found the drug to be effective adjunctive therapy in the management of refractory complex partial seizures. Daily doses of 10 to 12 mg/kg produced plasma desmethylmethsuximide levels of 20 to 24 μg/ml. Marked seizure improvement occurred in 70% of the patients who were maintained on the drug.

Phensuximide has been reported to be effective in the treatment of absence seizures (Millichap, 1952), but it has a low order of efficacy and should only be used as an adjunctive drug in refractory cases of absence or generalized tonic-clonic seizures. It is supplied in 150 to 300 mg capsules. The recommended daily dose is 20 to 40 mg/kg.

INTERACTIONS WITH OTHER DRUGS

Ethosuximide

Ethosuximide does not significantly interact with the other major antiepileptic drugs or with other medicines (Smith et al., 1979a), but it may increase the lethargy and somnolence produced by barbiturates or the other succinimides.

Methsuximide and Phensuximide

Methsuximide interacts with the other antiepileptic drugs. Rambeck (1979) has reported that the concurrent administration of methsuximide and phenobarbital, primidone, or phenytoin results in significant plasma elevations of phenobarbital (as a metabolite of primidone) and phenytoin in these patients. The author attributed these elevations to competition by the drugs for common hydroxylating enzyme systems.

TOXICITY

Ethosuximide

Ethosuximide is generally well tolerated and produces few adverse reactions. Although there is a close correlation between dose and plasma level of ethosuximide, little correlation exists between side effects and dose or plasma level of the drug. In general, if a patient tolerates ethosuximide, the dose and plasma level can be increased to high levels without inducing adverse effects. We have treated patients whose plasma ethosuximide levels have exceeded 100 μg/ml for years with no noticeable side effects and no neurological signs of toxicity. This is in striking contrast to other antiepileptic drugs and to the other succinimides, of which the dose, plasma level, and adverse effects are definitely interrelated.

Transient side effects of nausea, fatigue, lethargy, dizziness, euphoria, photophobia, and anorexia may occur at the onset of therapy, but these usually disappear as treatment continues. Sometimes hiccups, behavioral changes, and dystonic movements are observed. Browne et al. (1975) have found no deterioration in psychometric performance following the institution of ethosuximide therapy. In contrast, performance improved and was attributed to the reduced frequency of clinical or EEG evidence of absence seizures. Leukopenia may occur shortly after the onset of therapy, but recovery of the white blood cell count usually occurs spontaneously or with the reduction of dosage. Generally, adverse reactions to ethosuximide are rare and of minor consequence. They usually clear with continued treatment but close monitoring is indicated.

Methsuximide and Phensuximide

The most common side effects of methsuximide are lethargy, somnolence, fatigue, and headaches; these are usually transient or dose related. Wilder and Buchanan (1981) have reported minor to major side effects of methsuximide in a few patients. Headaches, photophobia, and hiccups required withdrawal of the drug in three of 21 patients. In nine patients, complaints of somnolence and lethargy responded to reduction of dosage. Three patients experienced behavioral reactions that responded to reduction of dosage. Transient leukopenia has been reported, and other complaints and reactions similar to those for ethosuximide may occur. The presence of the phenyl group on the succinimide ring produces other toxic effects common to hydantoins and barbiturates.

10

Benzodiazepines: Diazepam, Clonazepam, Nitrazepam, Chlordiazepoxide, Clorazepate, and Lorazepam

The benzodiazepines were developed primarily as tranquilizers; they were subsequently shown to possess anticonvulsant properties to variable degrees. The two compounds that are used most in the treatment of seizures are diazepam (Valium®) and clonazepam (Clonopin®). Lorazepam (Ativan®) and nitrazepam (Mogadon®) are not licensed as antiepileptic drugs in the United States. Clorazepate (Tranxene®) has been approved as an antiepileptic drug for adjunctive therapy.

The first benzodiazepine was synthesized by Sternbach (1973) after he had initiated work in the 1930s on benzophenone structures. Testing of the new compound, called Rö 5-0690, was undertaken by Randall of Roche Laboratories in 1957. The chemical nature of this compound, originally named methaminodiazepoxide, was identified in 1958. The name was subsequently simplified to chlordiazepoxide (Librium®). Chemically, it is 2-methylamino-7-chloro-5-phenyl-3H-1,4-benzodiazepine-4-oxide, a seven-membered ring structure:

Extensive pharmacological studies carried out in the 1960s showed chlordiazepoxide to induce behavioral changes in animals. Further studies showed the drug to possess anticonvulsant properties against seizures induced by pentylenetetrazol (PTZ) and maximal electroshock (MES).

Additional benzodiazepines were subsequently synthesized. For example, diazepam was approved by the U.S. Food and Drug Administration in 1963. Nitrazepam was synthesized by substituting nitrogen for chloride at position 7. Clonazepam, a chlorinated derivative of nitrazepam that possesses a broad spectrum of anticonvulsant activity, was approved in 1976. Clorazepate was marketed in 1972 as a minor tranquilizer and in 1980 as an antiepileptic drug.

CHEMISTRY

The standard 1,4-benzodiazepine nucleus is shown in the following structure:

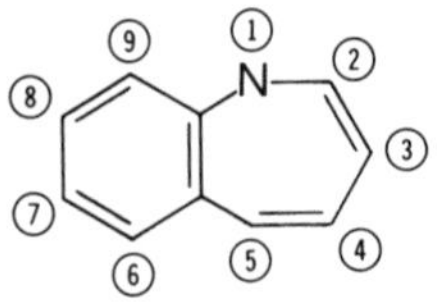

The basic structure of the benzodiazepines differs significantly from other classes of antiepileptic drugs. By manipulating the various substituents, various compounds with differing pharmacological potency were synthesized. The chemical structures of the benzodiazepines most commonly used in the treatment of seizure disorders are shown below:

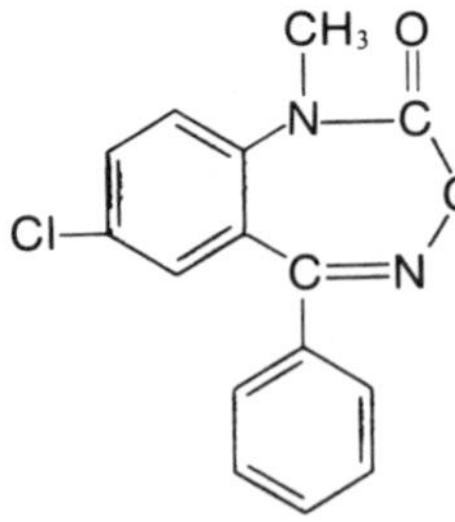

Diazepam 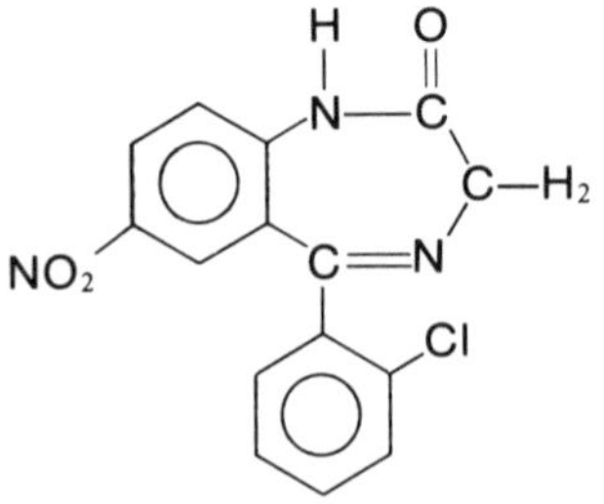   Clonazepam 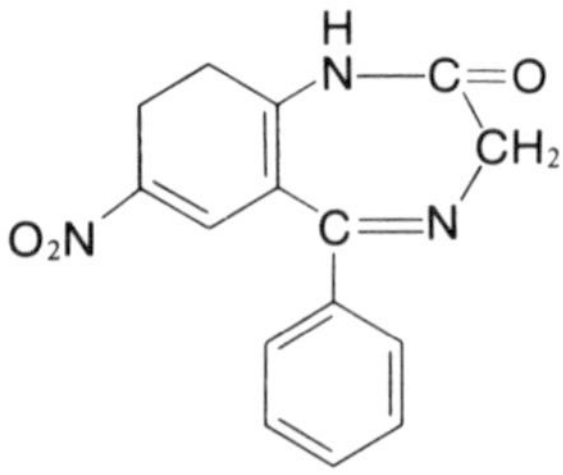   Nitrazepam

Diazepam (7-chloro-1,3-dihydro-1-methyl-5-phenyl-2H-1,4-benzodiazepine-2-one) has a molecular weight of 284.7. At physiological pH, it is poorly soluble in water but relatively lipid soluble. Parenteral diazepam is compounded with 40% propylene glycol, 10% ethyl alcohol, 5% sodium benzoate and benzoic acid as buffers, and 1.5% benzyl alcohol as preservative.

Clonazepam [5-(2-chlorophenyl)-1,3-dihydro-7-nitro-2H-1,4-benzodiazepine-2-one] is a light-yellow crystalline powder with a molecular weight of 315.7. It is available in the United States for oral administration only. Parenteral clonazepam has been used in other countries for the treatment of generalized tonic-clonic status epilepticus.

Nitrazepam (7-nitro-5-phenyl-3H-1,4-benzodiazepine-2[1H]-one is a yellowish crystalline compound. It is insoluble in water but soluble in alcohol. It is supplied in tablet form for oral use.

MECHANISM OF ACTION

Diazepam

Although the most striking anticonvulsant effect of diazepam is against PTZ-induced seizures, it also blocks seizures induced by picrotoxin, strychnine, and tetanus toxin. Electroshock seizure threshold is elevated, and extensor spasm secondary to MES is blocked. Diazepam blocks seizures after thalamic nuclear stimulation (Bancaud et al., 1972). Posttetanic potentiation is unaffected by the benzodiazepines (Swinyard and Castellion, 1966).

Electrophysiological studies have shown that the limbic system (hippocampus and amygdala), thalamus, and spinal cord are particularly sensitive to the action of the benzodiazepines (Schallek et al., 1972; Chou and Wang, 1977). GABAergic pathways are probably involved, and recurrent inhibition of hippocampal pyramidal neurons and cerebrocortical pyramidal cells is enhanced by diazepam (Zakusov et al., 1975; Raabe and Gumnit, 1977). Experimentally, diazepam has been found to augment cerebellar Purkinje cell discharge through an undetermined mechanism (Julien, 1972), but this effect has not been confirmed by other studies. A review of the subject supports the action of benzodiazepines on GABAergic synapses (Haefely, 1978). It is not known whether the main site of action is presynaptic or postsynaptic. It has been suggested that benzodiazepines enhance presynaptic inhibition in the spinal cord and dorsal column nuclei and postsynaptic inhibition in dorsal column nuclei, hippocampus, hypothalamus, cerebral cortex, and cerebellar cortex (Haefely, 1978). These all are examples of collateral and recurrent inhibition mediated by GABAergic neurons.

The cellular mechanisms responsible for the anticonvulsant effect of diazepam are unknown. The concept of specific benzodiazepine receptors has been advanced (Mohler and Okada, 1977). Diazepam binding is stereospecific, and the receptor is mainly located in the synaptic membrane fraction. The highest density of this receptor is in the cerebral cortex, followed by the hypothalamus and cerebellum. Competition for this receptor by the benzodiazepines closely parallels their pharmacological potency (Braestrup and Squires, 1978). Binding sites of the benzodiazepines have a neuronal localization and have not been demonstrated on astroglial cells. It has not been definitely demonstrated that benzodiazepine receptors are associated with gamma-aminobutyric acid (GABA) synapses, despite some evidence that GABAergic synapses are involved in benzodiazepine action. It has been shown that GABA can modulate the responsiveness of the benzodiazepine binding site (Tallman et al., 1978) and that GABAergic drugs lead to increased affinity of benzodiazepine binding sites (Gallagher et al., 1978).

Clonazepam

The pharmacological action of clonazepam is similar to that of other benzodiazepines. PTZ and electroshock convulsions are antagonized. Photic-induced seizures in baboons (*Papio papio*) are also blocked. In epileptic patients, the spike and wave discharges characteristic of absence seizures and the spike activity in focal cortical epileptic lesions are suppressed. Generalized abnormalities are more readily suppressed than focal abnormalities (Browne, 1978a). A decrease in local evoked potential amplitude and suppression of the spread of primary epileptiform discharges have been found (Guerrero-Figueroa et al., 1969a,b). Clonazepam is more potent than other benzodiazepines and other antiepileptic drugs against seizures in mice induced by parenterally administered local anesthetics, such as lidocaine or procaine (Pinder et al., 1976).

Neurochemically, clonazepam mimics the action of glycine, a spinal cord inhibitory neurotransmitter (Young et al., 1974); in addition, it increases serotonin concentration at synaptic regions (Jenner et al., 1975). It has been proposed that clonazepam-responsive myoclonus arises from a relative hypoactivity of the serotoninergic system (Chadwick et al., 1977a). It is uncertain whether a similar mechanism is responsible for the effect of clonazepam on other seizure types.

PHARMACOKINETICS

Diazepam

Absorption

Orally administered diazepam is rapidly and completely absorbed, with peak plasma concentrations occurring in 0.5 to 3 hr. Because absorption from intramuscular sites is slow and erratic (Baird and Hailey, 1972; Gamble et al., 1973), the drug should be administered orally or intravenously when possible. Studies on rectal administration showed good absorption (Agurell et al., 1975; Knudsen, 1977; Meberg et al., 1978). Oral administration with meals or antacids retards the absorption of diazepam (Greenblatt et al., 1978). This may depend on changes in gastric emptying and drug dissolution.

Protein Binding

Diazepam is strongly bound to plasma proteins in the range of 90 to 95% (Van der Kleijn et al., 1971). When other highly protein bound drugs are coadministered, the potential for interaction exists. In uremia, the protein binding of diazepam is decreased (Kober et al., 1979), but the overall clinical effect is uncertain. Drowsiness may be more common. Rarely, benzodiazepines cause a decrease in plasma phenytoin levels, but some data are conflicting (Houghton and Richens, 1975; Kutt, 1975).

Distribution

Diazepam has a large volume of distribution (1 to 2 liters/kg). The initial distribution pattern in brain primarily depends on blood flow, with highest concentrations occurring in the thalamus, hypophysis, mesencephalon, and cortical gray matter (Morselli et al., 1973). Diazepam concentrations at 5 and 30 min were uniform in gray and white matter. At later times, higher concentrations were absorbed in white matter-rich areas. Its metabolite N-desmethyldiazepam was found only after longer intervals, with higher concentrations in the lipid-rich white matter. Peripherally, diazepam and desmethyldiazepam had a strong tendency to accumulate in adipose tissue. The rapid rise of effective brain concentrations of diazepam has been confirmed, but it was also found that therapeutic brain concentrations are maintained for only a short time (Ramsay et al., 1979) (Fig. 10.1). This explains the phenomenon of recurrent seizures after initial intravenous administration of diazepam. Its short duration of action may be due to a redistribution phenomenon. Diazepam crosses the placenta and enters breast milk in small quantities.

Metabolism and Elimination

Orally administered diazepam has a biphasic decay curve with a phase I half-life of 2 to 10 hr and phase II half-life of 27 to 48 hr or longer (Browne and Penry, 1973). The initial half-life represents distribution of the drug, and the phase II half-life represents elimination. This biphasic elimination pattern is more marked after intravenous administration.

Repeated administration leads to accumulation of diazepam with steady-state plasma concentrations occurring in 4 to 10 days. Its major metabolite, N-desmethyldiazepam, begins to accumulate after several days, and it contributes to the anticonvulsant efficacy of diazepam. At steady-state levels, plasma concentrations of the metabolite are similar to concentrations of the parent drug (Zingales, 1973). The half-life of N-desmethyldiazepam is generally longer than the half-life of diazepam (Hillestad et al., 1974). Hydroxylation of N-desmethyldiazepam produces oxazepam, which is conjugated with glucuronide and excreted in the urine. Approximately 10% of an oral dose is excreted unchanged in the feces. Oxazepam is a physiologically active compound.

Hepatic disease may cause impaired elimination of the benzodiazepines with marked increases in the half-life (Klotz et al., 1977). The half-life may also be prolonged in elderly patients.

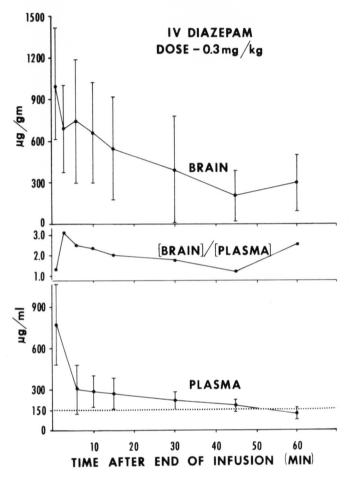

FIG. 10.1. Diazepam rapidly enters the brain following an intravenous infusion of 0.3 mg/kg. After 50 min, however, brain levels and plasma levels have fallen significantly, and the brain plasma ratio is only slightly greater than 1.

Clonazepam

Absorption

Clonazepam is rapidly absorbed from the gastrointestinal tract, being predominantly un-ionized at physiological pH. It readily crosses biological membranes. Maximal plasma concentrations usually occur in 1 to 3 hr but may be delayed as long as 10 hr. Bioavailability after oral administration is in the range of 80%.

Distribution and Protein Binding

The apparent volume of distribution of clonazepam is 2 to 3 liters/kg (Kaplan et al., 1974; Hvidberg and Sjö, 1975). The degree of protein binding is 40 to 50%

(Muller and Wollert, 1973). In laboratory animals, clonazepam crosses rapidly from blood to brain (Browne, 1978*b*). Successful treatment of tonic-clonic status epilepticus with intravenous clonazepam suggests that clonazepam enters the central nervous system quickly in humans. Because of its low protein binding, displacement interactions with other protein bound antiepileptics are not to be expected.

Metabolism and Elimination

Clonazepam is extensively metabolized, with less than 5% excreted unchanged in the urine (Muller and Wollert, 1973; Kaplan et al., 1974; Hvidberg and Sjö, 1975; Sjö et al., 1975). It is principally metabolized to 7-aminoclonazepam and to 7-acetaminoclonazepam. Hydroxylated derivatives, glucuronides, and sulfates are minor metabolites (Naestoft and Larsen, 1974; Pinder et al., 1976). Clonazepam metabolites lack significant antiepileptic properties.

The half-life of clonazepam is 22 to 33 hr, with a mean of 28.7 hr (Dreifuss et al., 1975), but this may be variable (Browne, 1978*a*). A constant dose-to-plasma concentration relationship has been reported (Dreifuss et al., 1975), but not all studies have confirmed this finding. No evidence of hepatic enzyme induction after chronic therapy is available. On the basis of half-life alone, clonazepam could be administered once daily; because large single doses are tolerated poorly, however, the drug requires administration in divided doses. Repeated administration leads to accumulation, with steady-state plasma concentrations occurring in 5 to 7 days. Its major metabolites begin to accumulate after several days and reach plasma concentrations similar to those of the parent drug.

The coadministration of other hepatic enzyme-inducing drugs may lead to enhanced metabolism of clonazepam (Huang et al., 1974; Nanda et al., 1977*a,b*). The effect of hepatic disease on clonazepam elimination has not been extensively studied.

CLINICAL USE

Diazepam

The major use of diazepam is in the initial treatment of status epilepticus. It has been reported to be effective in a wide variety of seizure types, but tolerance to its effects develops early in the course of treatment.

Diazepam is supplied for oral administration as 2, 5, and 10 mg tablets. As adjunctive therapy in the treatment of seizure disorders, daily doses of 0.25 to 0.75 mg/kg are usually required. Dose requirements vary widely, and responsiveness increases with hepatic disease and age. If used for chronic treatment of seizure disorders, which is rare, diazepam is usually given in two to four divided daily doses. When diazepam is administered intravenously for the treatment of status epilepticus, a total single dose of 0.1 to 0.2 mg/kg can be administered. If used alone, diazepam can be repeated every 30 to 60 min, with the total daily dosage not to exceed 100 mg. Extreme caution should be exercised in the use of intravenous diazepam. In order to prevent cardiorespiratory depression and hypotension, the rate of administration should not exceed 2 mg/min. Patients particularly at risk are those with preexisting cardiopulmonary disease and those receiving other medications that also cause cardiorespiratory depression.

The long-term treatment of seizure disorders with oral diazepam is generally unsatisfactory, despite reports of efficacy in uncontrolled trials. During chronic therapy, tolerance also develops and may contribute to decreased efficacy unless the dose is increased. In a review of the use of benzodiazepines for the treatment of epilepsy (Browne and Penry, 1973), it was concluded that the benzodiazepines suppress generalized EEG discharges and that they are effective in the treatment of absence, myoclonic, akinetic, photosensitive, and alcohol withdrawal seizures. Generalized tonic-clonic and partial seizures are less often controlled, and tonic-clonic seizures may be aggravated. The benzodiazepines were considered as helpful adjuncts in treating status epilepticus of all kinds, as well as eclamptic seizures.

In our experience, intravenous diazepam is useful in the initial treatment of tonic-clonic status epilepticus. Intravenous injection of diazepam may produce immediate seizure cessation (Lombroso, 1966; Parsonage, 1967; Prensky et al., 1967; McMorris and McWilliam, 1969; Nicol et al., 1969; Browne, 1978b; Duffy and Lombroso, 1978), but unless a major drug is also used, seizure activity resumes, requiring additional intravenous injections. We prefer an initial single injection of 5 to 10 mg diazepam coupled with simultaneously administered phenytoin, as described in Chapter 3. Browne and Penry (1973) have concluded that intravenous diazepam is particularly effective in absence status, somewhat less effective in tonic-clonic and psychomotor status, and least effective in infantile myoclonic status. Bilateral spike and wave activity is readily suppressed, but focal epileptiform activity is suppressed to a lesser degree.

Clonazepam

Although clonazepam is recommended for a wide variety of seizures, it should not be considered a major antiepileptic drug. It is supplied as 0.5, 1, and 2 mg tablets. The initial recommended daily dose for children is 0.01 to 0.03 mg/kg; the initial daily adult dose is 1.0 to 1.5 mg. Administration of clonazepam in divided daily doses minimizes the side effects. The dosage can be increased weekly by 0.25 mg/day in children and 0.5 mg/day in adults. Daily doses of 0.1 to 0.2 mg/kg usually produce optimum seizure control and therapeutic plasma concentrations of 20 to 80 ng/ml.

Clonazepam is presently approved for the treatment of typical and atypical absence seizures, myoclonic seizures, atonic seizures, and infantile spasms. It has been used successfully as adjunctive therapy for minor motor seizures, but the incidence of side effects was high (Nogen, 1978). Improvement has been noted in patients with myoclonic epilepsy, photosensitive epilepsy, atypical absence attacks, or fronto-temporal or generalized tonic-clonic seizures (Nanda et al., 1977b). Clonazepam as adjunctive therapy has also been found effective in patients with absence, generalized tonic-clonic, focal psychomotor, and mixed seizures, and myoclonic epilepsy, West syndrome, and Lennox-Gastaut syndrome (Lance and Anthony, 1977). In comparison with sodium valproate, clonazepam has been found equally effective in the control of absence and myoclonic seizures and less effective in the treatment of atonic and generalized tonic-clonic seizures, but it gave better results in partial epilepsies (Lance and Anthony, 1977). Both drugs significantly reduced the frequency of minor seizures, but clonazepam was less effective and had a high incidence of side effects (Shakir et al., 1979).

Despite these findings, definite indications are still lacking for the use of clonazepam, and most clinical trials have involved patients who were continued on their previous antiepileptic drugs when clonazepam was added (Pinder et al., 1976).

We do not use clonazepam as a primary antiepileptic drug. From general experience, however, it may be useful as adjunctive therapy in the seizure types named above. It can be stated, however, that clonazepam is a secondary antiepileptic drug that should be employed when other therapies are unsuccessful (Browne, 1978a). Controlled studies on the use of clonazepam as sole therapy are inadequate for a comparison of its efficacy with other antiepileptic drugs. A high incidence of adverse reactions and the development of tolerance are other factors that limit its usefulness. In the review by Browne and Penry (1973), for example, it was stated that clonazepam is extremely effective in the treatment of absence seizures, but these reactions make ethosuximide the preferred drug.

INTERACTIONS WITH OTHER DRUGS

The benzodiazepines interact with other psychotropic drugs at receptor sites, possibly resulting in excessive sedation. Interaction has been noted with tricyclic antidepressants, ethanol, phenothiazines, analgesics, antihistamines, and barbiturates. Hepatic metabolism is not induced by prolonged use of the benzodiazepines, but lower plasma phenytoin levels have been noted.

Clonazepam does not alter the steady-state plasma concentrations of other antiepileptic drugs, but the addition of phenobarbital or phenytoin may lower the plasma concentration of clonazepam (Hvidberg and Sjö, 1975; Nanda et al., 1977a). The mechanism is uncertain and may not be due to hepatic enzyme induction, since the levels of 7-aminoclonazepam were also decreased (Sjö et al., 1975). One study has suggested that the addition of carbamazepine results in decreased clonazepam levels (Lai et al., 1978).

A pharmacodynamic interaction between clonazepam and valproic acid has been noted (Jeavons et al., 1977). This combination of drugs in children may result in excessive sedation or precipitation of absence seizures. We have not observed this interaction in more than 15 adult patients. One child treated with valproic acid and clonazepam, however, did develop marked exacerbation of absence seizures, which became completely controlled when clonazepam was discontinued. Exacerbation of seizures has not been observed in adults. In children, a gradual decrease or discontinuation of clonazepam should be considered when valproic acid is added to their regimen.

TOXICITY

The common side effects of the benzodiazepines are extensions of their pharmacological activity: drowsiness and, rarely, coma. Hepatic, renal, and hematological toxicity are rare. Other unusual responses include nightmares, aggression, depression, delirium, and confusion. Intravenous diazepam may be associated with cardiorespiratory depression. Local phlebitis may occur with repeated injections. After prolonged therapy, psychological dependence may occur, and a withdrawal reaction may be observed if the drug is discontinued abruptly (de Bard, 1979).

The most common side effects of clonazepam therapy are drowsiness, ataxia, and behavioral changes (Pinder et al., 1976; Roussounis and de Rudolf, 1977; Browne, 1978a). Some tolerance to drowsiness and ataxia may develop during chronic administration. Behavioral changes in children include hyperactivity, poor concentration, irritability, aggression, and confusion. Uncommon side effects include hypersalivation, hypotonia, dizziness, dysarthria, anorexia, increased appetite, skin rashes, loss of libido, malaise, nausea, visual disturbances, weight gain, and thrombocytopenia (Masland, 1975; Veall and Hogarth, 1975). No definite correlation exists between the side effects and plasma clonazepam concentrations, although high concentrations are more likely to cause sedation and ataxia.

Increased frequency of seizures has occasionally been reported (Browne, 1978a), and absence seizures may be exacerbated when valproic acid is given concurrently with clonazepam. Intravenous administration of diazepam or nitrazepam has resulted in the development of tonic status epilepticus in patients with the Lennox-Gastaut syndrome (Tassinari et al., 1972).

The effect of clonazepam on the human fetus is unknown, but no dysmorphological effects have been noted in mice and rats. An increase in congenital abnormalities unrelated to dose has been observed in one species of rabbit (Pinder et al., 1976).

CLORAZEPATE

Clorazepate potassium (7-chloro-2,3-dihydro-2-oxo-5-phenyl-1H-1,4-benzodiazepine-3-carboxylic acid dipotassium salt) is an antiepileptic drug that may be useful as adjunctive therapy in refractory seizure disorders.

As a sedative, it offers no advantage over the other benzodiazepines. Clorazepate

It is apparent that the precise mechanisms of action of these drugs are unknown. Any drug that blocks repetitive transmission and raises seizure threshold should have anticonvulsant properties. It is difficult to explain why these drugs are effective in absence seizures and not in generalized tonic-clonic seizures.

TMO and its major metabolite DMO specifically antagonize the action of PTZ in a manner that suggests a common site of opposing action. The most prominent proposed mechanisms of pharmacological activity are (a) regulation of GABA metabolism, (b) blocking of extracellular potassium accumulation, (c) facilitation of presynaptic inhibition, (d) production of extracellular and perhaps intracellular acidosis, and (e) augmentation of GABA action on chloride conductance and inhibition.

PHARMACOKINETICS

Absorption

Both TMO and PMO are rapidly absorbed from the gastrointestinal tract, reaching peak plasma levels within 1 to 3 hr after ingestion.

Distribution and Protein Binding

TMO is distributed relatively equally in body water. Its volume of distribution is 0.6 to 0.8 liter/kg. Blood-to-tissue ratios of 0.61 to 0.94 suggest that the drug is not highly protein bound. The drug remains largely in the un-ionized state *in vivo* and moves freely from the extracellular to the intracellular compartment. Less than 10% unchanged TMO is excreted in the urine. The pharmacokinetic characteristics of PMO are similar.

Metabolism and Elimination

Both TMO and PMO are metabolized by the microsomal hepatic enzyme system (Chamberlain et al., 1965). The metabolism follows first-order kinetics within the therapeutic dose range. TMO (half-life, 3 hr) is rapidly demethylated to DMO, and PMO (half-life, 16 to 20 hr) is metabolized to demethylated PMO. These metabolites are active anticonvulsant agents, but DMO has been studied to a greater extent than demethylated PMO. They are present largely in the ionized state because of their pK_as of 6.13 and 5.9, respectively. Both compounds are eliminated in the urine slowly, with half-lives of 10 to 20 days. These metabolites are not distributed evenly because of ionization, pH gradients, and transport mechanisms. Their elimination can be increased, however, by alkalinization of the urine (Booker, 1972a; Withrow and Woodbury, 1972a–c).

CLINICAL USE

TMO and PMO are effective agents for the treatment of absence seizures. Because of their toxic side effects, however, they should be reserved for patients with refractory seizures that have not responded to ethosuximide or valproic acid. TMO and PMO are ineffective in the treatment of generalized tonic-clonic, partial, and myoclonic seizures, as well as in atypical absence or other seizure syndromes of childhood. These drugs sometimes precipitate generalized tonic-clonic attacks when therapy for absence seizures is started. If it is desirable to use TMO or PMO, the concomitant use of phenytoin, carbamazepine, or phenobarbital should be considered for the prevention of generalized tonic-clonic seizures.

Both TMO and PMO are administered orally in doses of 20 to 40 mg/kg daily. TMO is supplied in 300 mg capsules, 150 mg chewable tablets, and a solution containing 200 mg per teaspoon (40 mg/cc). PMO is supplied in 300 and 150 mg capsules and a solution containing 300 mg/ml. The initial dose should be approximately 10 to 15 mg/kg daily and slowly increased to a maintenance dose of 20 to 40 mg/kg. Clinical seizure control usually occurs when plasma DMO levels exceed 700 μg/ml and TMO levels reach 20 to 50 μg/ml. Steady-state DMO levels are achieved after 20 to 30 days of constant TMO dosage. DMO levels should be used to guide dosage after the steady-state level is reached; almost no fluctuation occurs because of the long half-life of DMO.

PMO levels and seizure control have not been studied. If PMO is used, however, demethylated PMO levels comparable to those of DMO should be achieved (Booker, 1972*b*).

INTERACTIONS WITH OTHER DRUGS

Because TMO and PMO are metabolized by demethylation, it is conceivable that any drugs that follow this metabolic pathway will interfere with their metabolism, and vice versa. Few studies have been done to investigate these potential interactions.

DMO exists predominantly in the ionized state at physiological pH. Large concentrations of the drug resulting from overdosage or from accumulation during chronic administration produce a metabolic acidosis because of displacement of bicarbonate. (Manfredi, 1963; Butler et al., 1966). Thus acid-base distortions produced by other drugs could affect the distribution and excretion of DMO (Withrow and Woodbury, 1972*c*).

TOXICITY

TMO, its metabolite DMO, and PMO are CNS depressants and in high doses produce sedation, ataxia, and incoordination. A most interesting CNS response is hemeralopia, or light blindness. Visual acuity is significantly affected when the patient goes from an area of low illumination to one of high illumination. The time for acuity adaptation is markedly prolonged, and the patient describes a phenomenon of transient snow blindness. The mechanism is thought to reside in the ganglion cell layer of the retina. Both light and color vision are affected (Sloan and Gilger, 1947).

Dermatological reactions of rash, erythema multiforme, and exfoliative dermatitis may occur early in the course of therapy and respond to drug withdrawal.

Depression of the bone marrow may be established before the peripheral blood count is altered. The earliest warning of pancytopenia may be a decrease in megakarocytes and platelets and a prolongation of clot retraction time.

Nephrosis may occur only after months of therapy. Renal disturbances are fortunately rare and respond to drug withdrawal. The rare occurrence of drug-related myasthenia has also been reported. These toxic reactions suggest an immune reaction. Caution should be exerted continually if these drugs are used (Gallagher, 1972).

TMO is highly teratogenic and should not be given to women contemplating pregnancy.

12

Other Drugs and Therapies

ACETAZOLAMIDE

Acetazolamide (Diamox®) is a carbonic anhydrase (CA) inhibitor that effectively abolishes the tonic extensor component of experimental maximal electroshock (MES) seizures. The main drawback to acetazolamide therapy is the early development of tolerance. Perhaps its most widespread use is in the adjunctive therapy of catamenial seizures. Acetazolamide and the CA inhibitors have been reviewed by Woodbury (1972, 1980c).

Chemistry

Acetazolamide (N-5-(aminosulfonyl)-1,3,4-thiadiazol-2-y-acetamide) inhibits the activity of the enzyme CA.

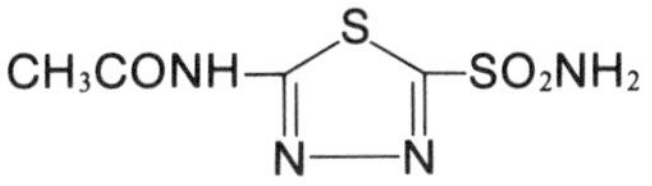

$$CH_3CONH-\overset{S}{\underset{N-N}{\big|}}-SO_2NH_2$$

It is a weak acid with a pK_a of 7.4 and exhibits a pH-dependent solubility in water.

Mechanism of Action

Acetazolamide acts through the inhibition of CA in the brain, which causes the accumulation of carbon dioxide, thereby inducing the anticonvulsant action. CA catalyzes the hydration and dehydration of carbon dioxide (Maren, 1967, Woodbury, 1980c). Carbon dioxide and acetazolamide have identical actions on the central nervous system (CNS). In addition to blocking CA in the brain, acetazolamide does the same in other tissues. Blocking CA in red blood cells causes greater carbon dioxide retention in the brain (Maren et al., 1954).

CA in the brain is localized in glial cells, astrocytes, and oligodendrocytes and their myelin products; it has not been found in neuronal cell bodies. The subcellular distribution of CA is in the cytosolic fraction, the membrane fraction, and in noncompact myelin (Tower and Young, 1973; Cammer et al., 1976; Sapirstein et al., 1978).

The anticonvulsant effect of the drug, as measured by the anti-MES effect (Millichap et al., 1955), correlates with the degree of inhibition of brain CA. Glial cells, in comparison with neurons, have a high bicarbonate concentration and a high pH. Blocking of the reaction $CO_2 + H_2O \rightleftharpoons H^+ + HCO_3^-$ in the glial cells by acetazolamide increases the pH and bicarbonate concentration in neurons and decreases them in glia. Glial cell CA plays a role in the transfer of H^+ and/or bicarbonate from neurons to glia. Interference with this transfer results in an increase of carbon dioxide in neurons sufficient to block the spread of seizure activity. Thus glia, in addition to maintaining potassium homeostasis in the brain interstitial fluid, regulates the acid-base balance, which is CA dependent (Schoffeniels et al., 1978; Woodbury, 1980c).

Acetazolamide may have a paradoxical effect in high doses (Woodbury and Kemp, 1977). In addition to inhibiting CA-dependent H^+ and bicarbonate transport, high doses of the drug inhibit CA-dependent anionic chloride and bicarbonate transport into glia and $[HCO_3]$-ATPase—which is necessary for anionic transport—thereby disrupting anionic and acid-base homeostasis in the brain. This may lead to increased neuronal excitability and seizures. Acetazolamide increases brain levels of gamma-aminobutyric acid (GABA), but increased carbon dioxide levels have also been shown to elevate brain GABA. The mechanism in the case of acetazolamide is probably secondary to its effect on CA, with subsequent increase in intracellular carbon dioxide (Woodbury, 1977).

Acetazolamide markedly alters choroid plexus function by its effect on CA. CA catalyzes the transport of chloride and bicarbonate from plasma into cerebrospinal fluid (CSF). The net effect of anticonvulsant doses of acetazolamide on the choroid plexus is to decrease CSF production by limiting chloride and bicarbonate transport across the plexus, which alters the acid-base balance in brain interstitial fluid (Woodbury, 1980c). Woodbury (1980c) has shown that the development of tolerance to acetazolamide is attributable to the induction of increased CA synthesis in glial cells and to glial proliferation. Experiments in both young and old animals suggest that the increased glial cell CA and glial proliferation that occurs with age may explain the reduced anticonvulsant effectiveness of acetazolamide in the elderly (Rauh and Gray, 1968).

Pharmacokinetics

Absorption

Acetazolamide, a weak acid, is un-ionized in the stomach, where absorption begins. Because of its poor solubility, however, absorption is completed in the upper intestinal tract. Peak plasma levels occur 2 to 3 hr after oral administration, and absorption appears to be complete after doses as high as 5 to 10 mg/kg (Maren et al., 1954).

Distribution and Protein Binding

Protein binding accounts for approximately 90% of the drug in plasma. The remaining free drug is available for diffusion into the tissue. This process is pH dependent, and acetazolamide is distributed throughout body water as the free drug in sufficient concentrations to inhibit CA. The greatest concentration of drug is found in red blood cells. Acetazolamide binds to CA; after 24 hr, almost all the drug distributed to various tissues is in a relatively stable CA-acetazolamide complex.

Acetazolamide slowly penetrates the brain and CSF, where the concentration is lower than in plasma. Although the brain contains a higher concentration than CSF, brain concentration depends on the concentration in CSF.

Metabolism and Elimination

Acetazolamide is not metabolized in the body, and all of an ingested dose can ultimately be accounted for in the urine. The CA-acetazolamide complex is relatively stable, so that the plasma half-life of the drug is approximately 2 to 4 days. Renal excretion occurs by both glomerular filtration and tubular secretion. Elevating the urinary pH will enhance excretion. Acetazolamide is also excreted in the bile and reabsorbed from the intestinal tract.

Clinical Use

Acetazolamide is effective in the treatment of absence, simple and complex partial, generalized tonic-clonic, and mixed types of seizures. However, tolerance develops after several weeks of continuous treatment. The drug may be particularly effective in some epileptic women who experience seizures or exacerbation of seizures during the menstrual or estral cycles (Poser, 1974). These patients often have mixed seizure types, including complex partial seizures. The mechanisms of this catamenial epilepsy are unknown. Water retention and electrolyte changes in the brain may reflect systemic alterations that occur during the menstrual cycle and have been implicated in the pathogenesis of the seizures (Millichap, 1969, 1974).

Seizure exacerbations may also occur during febrile illnesses, situations leading to water and electrolyte imbalance, and other temporary disorders. The transient use of acetazolamide in these situations avoids the development of tolerance to the drug and may give added protection above that of the chronically administered anticonvulsant agents. Acetazolamide is supplied in 250 and 500 mg scored tablets. The recommended daily dose is 10 mg/kg, administered in a single dose.

To treat seizure exacerbation before the commencement of menses, we recommend starting the drug 10 days before the expected onset and continuing it until the first day of the menstrual period. Because of its long half-life, acetazolamide reaches steady-state plasma levels approximately 5 to 7 days after the initial dose, and adequate levels continue for 3 to 5 days after the drug is discontinued. This regimen should be repeated monthly.

The use of acetazolamide should be considered if seizures are aggravated by pregnancy. Teratogenic effects of the drug have been described in animals, however, and the drug should not be administered during the first trimester. Because of the high degree of protein binding, relatively small quantities of the drug are secreted in breast milk.

Interactions With Other Drugs

Probenecid, which blocks renal tubular secretion of acids, decreases elimination of acetazolamide and prolongs its half-life. Absorption of other drugs from the gastrointestinal tract may be altered because of pH changes induced by blocking of intestinal mucosal CA. Amphetamine absorption is delayed, and salicylate absorption is increased (Schnell and Miya, 1970).

Many theoretical possibilities for drug interaction exist: (a) the drug inhibits CSF flow, (b) competes for plasma protein binding sites, (c) interferes with biliary secretion, and (d) may alter distribution of other drugs because of changes induced in pH and carbon dioxide and bicarbonate concentrations in various tissues (Woodbury, 1980c).

Toxicity

Few toxic reactions to acetazolamide, even in high doses, have been reported. Some patients complain of lethargy and paresthesias. Rare hypersensitivity reactions occur. Skin rashes, distension of the abdomen, and cyanosis have been noted. Teratogenic effects have been induced in experimental animals (Maren, 1971; Woodbury, 1980c).

CORTICOTROPIN AND CORTICOSTEROIDS

The anticonvulsant effect of steroids was reported by McQuarrie and colleagues (1942). Desoxycorticosterone acetate was shown to control seizures induced in epileptic patients given a water load and antidiuretic hormone. Since then, both adrenocorticotropic hormone (ACTH) and adrenocorticosteroid hormones have been used to improve the electroencephalogram (EEG) and reduce seizure frequency in epileptic children. Infantile spasms, generalized tonic-clonic seizures, refractory absence seizures, and atypical absence seizures have been favorably affected by these hormones (Miribel and Poirier, 1961; Schneider, 1961; Livingston, 1966). Massive infantile spasms often respond spectacularly to ACTH, but the effect frequently does not persist beyond cessation of treatment (Lacy and Penry, 1976). Complex and simple partial seizures usually do not respond to steroids, and little or no anticonvulsant effect can be expected in adult epileptic individuals. Because the beneficial effects of ACTH and adrenocortical steroids have been correlated with the relative maturation of the CNS, the value of these agents declines with the age of the patient. Exceptions to this are patients who are in an addisonian or postadre-nalectomy state. Corticosteroid therapy in these situations results in cessation of seizures and normalization of the EEG. Corticosteroids are sometimes useful in the treatment of selected cases of status epilepticus (see Chapter 3).

Chemistry

Corticotropin

Corticotropin, or ACTH, is a polypeptide consisting of 39 amino acid residues, the first being serine and the last phenylalanine, with a molecular weight of about 4,500. The loss of serine by hydrolytic cleavage results in biological inactivation; the loss of the terminal amino acid does not alter potency. Synthetic compounds have been prepared, but they offer no advantage over the naturally occurring pituitary ACTH.

Corticosteroids

The corticosteroids are synthesized from cholesterol by the adrenal cortex. They contain 21 carbon atoms arranged in four ring structures, as in cortisol:

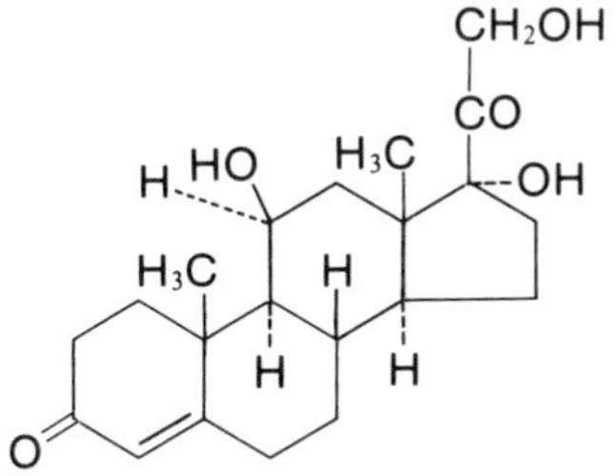

Adrenocorticosteroids are not stored to any extent in the adrenal gland. The rate of biosynthesis is in essence the rate of secretion and the subsequent concentration in plasma.

Mechanism of Action

Corticotropin

°The major action of ACTH is the stimulation of the synthesis of corticosteroids from the cortex of the adrenal gland. ACTH controls the target tissue (the adrenal cortex) by increasing the formation of adenosine 3':5'-cyclic phosphate (cAMP) in the cortical cells, which in turn increases the rate of synthesis of the steroid hormones from cholesterol. ACTH is thought to bind to a specific plasma membrane receptor of adrenocortical cells. This in turn increases adenyl cyclase activity, which increases the formation of cAMP (Ney, 1969). The anticonvulsant effect of ACTH is secondary to the increased synthesis and release of corticosteroids from the adrenal cortex.

Corticosteroids

The adrenocorticosteroids have widespread actions on all body tissues, but their action on the CNS, which is pertinent to their anticonvulsant effects, is not clearly understood. The effects of desoxycorticosterone on brain excitability are probably mediated by its influence on sodium transport. Cortisol acts by a different and as yet unknown mechanism. It may act directly on neurons, as do cortisol-binding proteins that have the characteristics of steroid receptors (Ballard et al., 1974).

Desoxycorticosterone experimentally elevates the threshold to electroshock convulsions, and the combination of this steroid and phenytoin results in significant potentiation of anticonvulsant effects (Woodbury, 1952). Aird and Gordon (1951) have reported that steroid therapy potentiates the anticonvulsant effects of other drugs in patients with refractory seizure disorders.

The mechanism of action of steroids in status epilepticus related to cerebral trauma, infections, neoplasms, or vascular accidents is the reduction of cerebral edema associated with the primary cerebral pathology. The clinical benefit is thought to be derived from suppression of the inflammatory response of the brain to injury and to the restoration of capillary integrity.

Although they are not antiepileptic drugs, the corticosteroids exert an antiepileptic effect by restoring homeostasis to the brain, either by an action on sodium ion equilibrium or by reducing the response to brain injury. Other actions are not clearly understood.

Pharmacokinetics

Corticotropin

ACTH is ineffective when administered orally because it is inactivated by proteolytic enzymes in the gastrointestinal tract. It is rapidly absorbed from intramuscular and subcutaneous injection sites, and aqueous suspensions can be given intravenously. ACTH is rapidly metabolized and has a plasma half-life of only 15 minutes. No free ACTH is found in the urine.

Intravenously and intramuscularly in aqueous form, ACTH produces only transient effects on the adrenal cortex. ACTH given in an intramuscular repository form or by continuous intravenous infusion results in maximal stimulation of the adrenal cortex to produce and secrete corticosteroid hormones (Haynes and Larner, 1975).

Corticosteroids

Cortisol, its congeners, and the numerous synthetic analogs are readily absorbed after oral ingestion. Water-soluble esters of cortisol and the synthetic congeners can be given intravenously to achieve high concentrations in body fluids. Prolonged effects can be obtained by intramuscular and subcutaneous injections of repository forms of these steroids.

Cortisol is approximately 90% bound to plasma protein. At low concentrations, it is bound to the globulin fraction of plasma proteins, and in high concentrations, to both globulin and albumin. Free and albumin-bound cortisol are available for hepatic metabolism. Metabolites are conjugated to glucuronic acid and sulfates and are excreted in the urine. The plasma half-life of cortisol and related synthetic corticosteroids is approximately 1.5 hr.

Clinical Use

There is marked variability among studies reporting on the use of corticosteroids or ACTH as anticonvulsant therapy. Considerable controversy over the efficacy and indications for steroids still exists, and evidence is inadequate to conclude that long-term steroid treatment for seizures, except in adrenal insufficiency, is efficacious. Relapse generally occurs when therapy is tapered; seizure exacerbation develops with prolonged treatment. Lacy and Penry (1976) have reported that the mortality rates among children with infantile spasms are no different in steroid-treated children than in those not treated with steroids.

Corticotropin

ACTH is highly purified from the pituitary gland of mammals. It is used as adjunctive therapy in infantile spasms, refractory mixed types of seizures of infancy and childhood, and seizures induced by collagen vascular diseases. It is supplied as an aqueous suspension for parenteral injection and in a repository gel form for subcutaneous or intramuscular injection. It is measured in units, and a usual initial dose is 40 to 80 U/day. In the treatment of infantile spasms, Gamstorp (1970) and Hagberg (1976) recommend that high doses of 120 to 180 U/day be given in the repository form (ACTH-gel). Jeavons and Bower (1974) employ a more moderate dose of 20 to 40 U/day ACTH-gel until a clinical response is seen. The initial dose is continued for 1 month and then tapered over a 3- to 4-month period. Thereafter, a reduced dose of 10 to 20 U every other day can be continued indefinitely.

Corticosteroids

The synthetic analogs of corticosterone and cortisol—prednisolone, prednisone, dexamethasone, and methylprednisolone—are used in the treatment of infantile

TABLE 12.1. *Oral tablet equivalency of synthetic corticosteroids[a]*

Nonproprietary name	U.S. trade name	Tablet (mg)	Daily dose[b] (mg/kg)
Methyl prednisolone	Medrol	4	2
Prednisone	Deltasone	5	2
Prednisolone	Delta-Cortef	5	2
Dexamethasone	Decadron	0.75	0.2

[a]Parenteral doses are roughly equivalent to oral doses.
[b]Initiation of therapy.

spasms, refractory mixed types of seizures of infancy and childhood, refractory seizures secondary to progressive CNS disorders caused by collagen vascular diseases and other encephalitities, and status epilepticus resulting from trauma, neoplasms, cerebrovascular disease, and some parasitic infections (see Chapter 3). Methylprednisolone, prednisone, and prednisolone are available in a wide variety of oral and injectable preparations. Their potency is equal (see Table 12.1).

For the treatment of infantile spasms, Jeavons and Bower (1974) recommend prednisolone or prednisone in a daily dose of 2 mg/kg and dexamethasone in a daily dose of 0.3 mg/kg in divided doses. We recommend intramuscular or intravenous dexamethasone in doses of 0.1 to 0.2 mg/kg or prednisone in doses of 1 to 2 mg/kg for the treatment of status epilepticus secondary to an intracranial lesion caused by trauma, neoplasm, cerebrovascular disease, or parasitic infections, such as cysticercosis or schistosomiasis.

In the treatment of infantile spasms and refractory seizures of infancy and childhood, the calculated daily dose can be continued for 1 month and then tapered to every other day in divided oral doses for several months. If seizure exacerbate, the dose can be increased in an attempt to produce the desired response.

Interactions With Other Drugs

Corticotropin

ACTH stimulates the production of adrenocortical hormones that have a potent effect on all organ systems. Phenytoin and other antiepileptic drugs interact with corticosteroid metabolism and interfere with the effects of these hormones on other organ systems. These interactions are discussed in Chapters 14 and 15.

Corticosteroids

The concurrent administration of steroids and antiepileptic drugs may cause alterations in drug and steroid metabolism (see Chapters 14 and 15).

Toxicity

Corticotropin

The toxic effects of ACTH can be attributed to the increased synthesis of adrenocorticosteroids. Hypersensitivity reactions are rare and range from fever and skin rash to anaphylaxis and death. ACTH can result in sodium retention and a mild degree of hypokalemic alkalosis, which may be more marked than when the synthetic congeners of the corticosteroids are used.

Corticosteroids

Acute toxic reactions following brief periods of steroid therapy rarely occur, although anaphylactoid or other hypersensitivity reactions have been reported. Peptic ulcer perforations and gastrointestinal hemorrhage can occur. Sodium and fluid retention are seen, and congestive heart failure can rapidly develop in susceptible individuals.

Adverse reactions to chronic steroid therapy are usually mild, but one or several may be anticipated. Steroids may produce toxic effects in multiple organ systems:

1. Musculoskeletal system
   a. Weakness and myopathy
   b. Osteoporosis and pathological fractures
2. Gastrointestinal system
   a. Peptic ulcer and esophagitis with possible perforation and hemorrhage
   b. Pancreatitis
3. Skin and subcutaneous tissue
   a. Thinning of the dermis with loss of collagenous tissue
   b. Impaired wound healing
   c. Petechiae and ecchymosis
   d. Suppression of skin test reactions
4. CNS
   a. Exacerbation of convulsions
   b. Behavioral changes and psychological and physiological dependency
   c. Increased intracranial pressure with papilledema and pseudotumor cerebri
5. Endocrine system
   a. Cushing syndrome
   b. Growth retardation in children
   c. Menstrual irregularities
6. Eye
   a. Posterior subcapsular cataracts
   b. Glaucoma
   c. Exophthalmos
7. Metabolic system
   a. Negative nitrogen balance with diffuse tissue wasting
   b. Pseudodiabetic state
8. Fluid and electrolyte disturbances
   a. Sodium and water retention and edema
   b. Congestive heart failure
   c. Hypertension
   d. Potassium loss and hypokalemic alkalosis

These and other adverse reactions resulting from chronic steroid therapy are listed in the package inserts of the various steroid analogs marketed.

PHENACEMIDE

Phenacemide (Phenurone®) was introduced by Gibbs and colleagues (1949) for the treatment of refractory complex partial seizures. Initially, the drug was highly regarded and was characterized by Lennox (1960) as being a triple threat against generalized tonic-clonic, absence, and complex partial seizures. Subsequent evaluations have shown that the toxic effects of this drug may outweigh its usefulness. It is now recommended for severe complex partial seizures that are refractory to other drugs (Forster, 1951; Livingston, 1966; Aird and Woodbury, 1974).

Chemistry

Phenacemide [1-(2-phenylacetyl)-urea] is a straight-chain analog of 5-phenylhydantoin. It has a molecular weight of 178.19. It is slightly soluble in water and soluble in lipids. The pK_a has not been determined.

$$\text{C}_6\text{H}_5\text{—CH}_2\text{—}\overset{\overset{\textstyle O}{\|}}{\text{C}}\text{—NH—}\overset{\overset{\textstyle O}{\|}}{\text{C}}\text{—NH}_2$$

Mechanism of Action

Phenacemide, like phenytoin, prevents the tonic-clonic seizures induced by MES. It also possesses barbiturate-like activity in that it significantly elevates the seizure threshold to electroshock, PTZ, and picrotoxin (Everett, 1949; Swinyard and Toman, 1950). Phenacemide also elevates the seizure threshold for experimental complex partial seizures induced by slow electrical stimulation of the brain (Toman, 1965).

Pharmacokinetics

The drug is readily absorbed from the gastrointestinal tract, reaching peak plasma levels 3 to 5 hr after a single oral dose. Protein binding has not been determined. Phenacemide is metabolized in the liver by hydroxylation of the phenyl group and conjugated to glucuronic acid. The biological half-life is 5 to 12 hr. The metabolite and its glucuronide are excreted in the urine; little or no free drug is found in the urine (Richards et al., 1954).

Clinical Use

Although originally heralded as a breakthrough in antiepileptic therapy, phenacemide is now used only rarely and then in refractory complex partial seizures and other severe, uncontrollable types of seizures. The drug was found to induce severe behavioral aberations and to be highly toxic to most organ systems. It is supplied as 500 mg scored tablets. The dose is calculated as 20 to 40 mg/kg. Therapeutic plasma drug levels have not been established.

Interactions With Other Drugs

Specific interactions between phenacemide and other drugs have not been described (Schmidt and Wilder, 1968).

Toxicity

The major toxic reactions associated with phenacemide overdosage is excitement leading to maniacal behavior. This is followed by sedation, ataxia, and coma in cases of large doses. Other adverse reactions are secondary to depression of the hematopoietic system, hepatic and renal toxicity, and effects on the CNS. Anorexia, weight loss, sedation, insomnia, paresthesias, vertigo, and headaches have been reported. Major personality or behavioral changes, including psychotic reactions of mania, depression and other disorders of thought content, may occur (Craddock, 1955; Livingston, 1966; Aird and Woodbury, 1974). Hepatic and renal function and red and white blood cell counts should be followed when patients are on this drug. Its use is contraindicated in women contemplating pregnancy.

PARALDEHYDE

Paraldehyde (Paracetaldehyde®) was first used in 1882, 30 years before phenobarbital became available. As a hypnotic, it was initially favored for the treatment of abstinence phenomena. Approximately 40 years ago, it was used widely in the treatment of status epilepticus (Treiman and Delgado-Escueta, 1980). In recent years, it has been used primarily for the treatment of alcohol withdrawal phenomena and is extremely effective in preventing and treating withdrawal seizures. It can be administered by any route: oral, rectal, intramuscular, or intravenous. Because of its disagreeable odor and taste, paraldehyde is often rejected by ambulatory patients.

Chemistry

Paraldehyde (2,4,6-trimethyl-1,3,5-trioxane) is a cyclic polyester.

It is supplied as a clear liquid and has a strong aromatic odor. On exposure to air and light, it spontaneously decomposes to acetaldehyde and acetic acid; therefore, it should be stored in an air-tight, dark glass container. It is miscible with water and oil. The drug is supplied in 2 and 5 ml glass ampules.

Mechanism of Action

The mechanism of action of paraldehyde has not been studied extensively. As a rapid-acting hypnotic with anticonvulsant properties, it protects animals against experimentally induced MES seizures. It is clinically effective in treating the convulsions of tetanus, eclampsia, and those resulting from accidental poisoning with convulsant drugs. In therapeutic doses, paraldehyde has little effect on the cardio-respiratory systems, but larger doses may cause respiratory depression and hypotension (Harvey, 1975).

Pharmacokinetics

Paraldehyde is rapidly absorbed from the stomach, rectum, or muscle and can also be given intravenously. Peak plasma and brain levels occur 30 to 60 min after parenteral, oral, or rectal administration. For intravenous use, the drug should be diluted sufficiently to prevent dissolving of plastic tubing or connections. It is largely metabolized by the liver (70 to 80%) to acetaldehyde by depolymerization and is then oxidized by aldehyde dehydrogenase to acetic acid, which is ultimately metabolized to carbon dioxide and water. The remainder of the drug (20 to 30%) is exhaled; its characteristic odor is present on the recipient's breath. Approximately 1 to 2% is found unchanged in the urine.

Clinical Use

Paraldehyde is effective in treating or preventing alcohol withdrawal convulsions and other manifestations of alcoholism. Some prefer it as a drug of choice in these situations because of its safety in therapeutic doses, each of administration by any route, and effectiveness in preventing the additional sequelae of alcohol withdrawal. It has been self-administered by alcoholic patients, who gradually reduce the dose and eventually discontinue the drug over a period of 5 to 10 days following the acute seizure phase.

Paraldehyde is reported to be effective in treating status epilepticus (Browne, 1978*b*; Treiman and Delgado-Escueta, 1980), but we recommend that it be used only when other drugs have failed (see Chapter 3). There are disadvantages to its use by any route other than oral. In status epilepticus, however, the oral route, even by nasogastric tube, is not preferred. Furthermore, paraldehyde increases the acidosis that accompanies status epilepticus.

The first single dose of paraldehyde is usually calculated on the basis of 0.1 to 0.2 ml/kg for the treatment of alcohol or drug withdrawal convulsions or status epilepticus. Additional doses of 0.1 mg/kg can be given as necessary at 2 to 4-hr intervals. In long-term treatment of alcohol or drug withdrawal, doses of 0.05 to 0.1 ml/kg can be continued as necessary every 4 to 6 hr for days. Orally, paraldehyde should be given only to patients who are alert enough to cooperate in taking the medication. Administration to stuporous or comatose patients, even by nasogastric tube, should be avoided, because of the possibility of aspiration and subsequent pulmonary edema.

The intramuscular dose is the same as the oral dose. Injection into a large muscle mass is followed by rapid absorption. Injection into subcutaneous or fat tissue may result in erratic absorption and the formation of sterile abscess. Large nerve trunks should be carefully avoided, as the drug can produce necrosis and neuropathy.

For intravenous injection, ampules of paraldehyde (USP), 2 and 5 cc, can be mixed in normal saline (1 part drug to at least 20 parts normal saline) at the calculated dose (0.1 to 0.2 ml/kg) and injected slowly (0.5 ml/min paraldehyde). Rapid injection can produce pulmonary edema, cardiorespiratory depression, and right-sided heart dilatation.

Interactions With Other Drugs

The dose of paraldehyde should be reduced if the patient is receiving disulfiram (Antabuse®). This drug interferes with the metabolism of paraldehyde and results in increased blood levels of paraldehyde and its first metabolite, acetaldehyde.

Toxicity

If given as a fresh preparation, paraldehyde is relatively safe in the therapeutic dose range. Old or decomposed preparations, which contain acetaldehyde and acetic acid, are probably responsible for most cases of poisoning. These decomposition products can produce acidosis and pulmonary edema. Gastritis, azotemia, oliguria, albuminuria, fatty changes in the liver and kidney with toxic hepatitis and nephrosis, and right-sided heart dilatation have been reported in cases of severe acute and chronic paraldehyde poisoning (Richie and Cohen, 1975).

LIDOCAINE

Lidocaine (Xylocaine®) is used primarily for the production of local anesthesia. It is nonirritating to tissue, and its systemic toxicity is low. It is also an antiarrhythmic agent. The successful treatment of status epilepticus with intravenous lidocaine was reported 25 years ago (Bernhard et al., 1955). Since then, its efficacy and safety in controlling status epilepticus, focal motor status, electroshock convulsions, and the photoconvulsive response have been widely reported (Ottoson, 1955; Bernhard et al., 1956; Taverner and Bain, 1958; Westreich and Kneller, 1972; Lemmen et al., 1978; Morris, 1979). Experimental studies in animals have demonstrated its anticonvulsant activity in MES seizures and alcohol withdrawal convulsions (Essman, 1965; Freund, 1973; Julien, 1973). We have used it successfully in the treatment of refractory status epilepticus for many years.

Chemistry

Structurally, lidocaine [2-(diethylamino)-N-(2,6-dimethylphenyl)-acetamide] consists of a hydrophilic amino group connected by an amide linkage to a relatively lipophilic aromatic residue.

The drug exhibits a pH-dependent solubility in water and lipids (Richie and Cohen, 1975). The pK_a is between 8 and 9; thus it is largely un-ionized in plasma and freely crosses the capillary barrier and penetrates the brain when given intravenously.

Mechanism of Action

The major mechanism of action of lidocaine in preventing cerebral convulsions is the stabilization of neuronal membranes, probably by preventing calcium uptake and blocking movements of sodium and potassium ions in the depolarization-repolarization process. Therapeutic doses and plasma levels of 1 to 4 μg/ml prevent penicillin-induced cortical discharge and block electrically induced experimental seizures (Essman, 1965; Julien, 1973). Plasma levels exceeding 5 μg/ml produce cortical irritability and convulsions. Therapeutic levels of 2 to 5 μg/ml do not significantly alter the EEG and do not significantly interfere with consciousness (Morris, 1979).

Pharmacokinetics

Lidocaine is readily absorbed from intramuscular and subcutaneous injection sites. It is also absorbed from the gastrointestinal tract. Nevertheless, it should be given intravenously in the treatment of status epilepticus. The drug is hydrolyzed and dealkylated in the liver by the microsomal oxidases to monoethylglycine and xylidine, which are partly excreted in the urine. The xylidine metabolite, which is further metabolized to 4-hydroxy-2,6-dimethylanaline, may account for some of its anticonvulsant activity and toxicity. The half-life of lidocaine is 1.5 to 2 hr.

Clinical Use

The major use of lidocaine as an anticonvulsant is in the treatment of status epilepticus. Greenblatt et al. (1976) have recommended an initial dose of 1.4 mg/kg i.v. followed by a continuous infusion of 29 μg/kg/min. A second injection dose of 1 mg/kg can be injected after 30 min. We have used the drug to treat refractory status epilepticus after using intravenous phenytoin (15 mg/kg) and phenobarbital (10 mg/kg). The dose successfully used in this situation was a continuous infusion of 4 mg/kg/hr (see Chapter 3).

The drug is supplied as lidocaine hydrochloride in 0.4 to 4% solutions. This can be mixed with the desired intravenous solution and the rate of infusion calculated to give 4 mg/kg/hr. The drug is supplied with and without epinephrine. The solution of lidocaine containing epinephrine should not be used.

Interactions With Other Drugs

Lidocaine does not potentiate the hypnotic or depressant effects of barbiturates or diazepam. The anticonvulsant effect may be potentiated by therapeutic plasma levels of phenytoin.

Toxicity

An overdose of lidocaine can produce ventricular fibrillation and convulsions. Overdosage can be prevented, however, if large bolus injections of the drug are avoided and the calculated dose and rate of injection are not exceeded. Somnolence and dizziness have been reported (de Jong, 1978).

Pfeifer et al. (1976) have reported a low incidence of serious side effects in a large series of patients who received lidocaine for cardiac arrhythmias. Caution should be exercised in patients with impaired liver function, for the drug is totally metabolized by the microsomal mixed oxidase system (Richie and Cohen, 1975).

KETOGENIC DIET AND MEDIUM-CHAIN TRIGLYCERIDES DIET

Wilder (1921) introduced specific diet therapy beneficial in reducing the frequency of epileptic seizures. He reported that a diet high in fat and low in carbohydrate resulted in ketosis and acidosis similar to that observed in starvation, which for centuries had been known to have anticonvulsant effects. Withrow (1980*b*) has comprehensively and concisely reviewed the ketogenic and medium-chain triglycrides (MCT) diet.

The classic ketogenic diet calls for a daily regimen of protein (1 g/kg), fat to make up the desired caloric requirement, and a minimal amount of carbohydrate, expressed in the following formula:

$$\frac{K}{AK} = \frac{0.9 \text{ (grams fat)} + 0.46 \text{ (grams protein)}}{\text{(grams carbohydrate)} + 0.1 \text{ (grams fat)} + 0.58 \text{ (grams protein)}}$$

where K = ketogenic potential and AK = antiketogenic potential.

A K/AK ratio of > 1.5 produces ketonuria. As the ratio reaches 3 or higher, the increased ketonuria effects seizure control. This formula clearly shows that the diet must be heavily weighted in favor of fat with a minimum of carbohydrate. The ratio of fat to carbohydrate is of more importance than the total amount of fat. The availability of glucose prevents the production of ketones; large quantities of protein are metabolized to glucose.

The original ketogenic diet was modified by the use of MCT (Huttenlocher et al., 1971). Octanoic and decanoic acids are used to make up the majority of the fat in the diet. An advantage of the MCT diet is that more than three times the carbohydrate intake is permitted than in the ketogenic diet, making the former more palatable than the latter.

Chemical and Physiological Changes Induced by the Ketogenic or MCT Diet

After the initiation of a ketogenic diet, ketone bodies increase rapidly in the blood; ketonuria occurs within 1 to 2 days. Ketones rise and reach steady-state blood levels after 15 to 30 days. Plasma beta-hydroxybutyrate (BHB) and aceto-acetate (AA) levels increase from approximately 0.2 to 4 and 0.06 to 1 mM, respectively. The increase in these organic acids results in a lowering of pH with a rise in H^+ concentration and a decrease in bicarbonate concentration. After a period of time, however, the acidosis produced by the ketogenic diet is compensated, and blood pH returns to normal. Bicarbonate levels remain low, and BHB and AA levels remain high. The results have been similar in both experimental and clinical studies (Huttenlocher, 1976).

The effects of the ketogenic diet on body water and electrolytes have been studied, but the data are conflicting and are probably not relevant to clinical efficacy. The MCT diet is reported to have no effect on serum electrolytes (Millichap et al., 1964; Huttenlocher et al., 1971; Appleton and Devivo, 1974).

The ketogenic diet induces a mild hypoglycemia throughout the period of treatment (DeVivo et al., 1973), but the MCT diet rarely reduces plasma glucose levels (Huttenlocher et al., 1971). The ketogenic diet induces significant elevations in all plasma lipids, with steady-state lipidemia occurring after 2 to 3 weeks. A 3:1 ketogenic diet increases plasma cholesterol by approximately 60% and total fatty acids by 80% (Huttenlocher, 1976). In contrast, the MCT diet lowers cholesterol by 5% and increases total plasma fatty acids by only 25%.

The effects of these diets on brain biochemistry are unknown. DeVivo et al. (1978), in studying the effects of chronic ketosis on cerebral metabolism, have concluded that the diet significantly increases brain energy reserves, probably by an inhibition of the enzymes phosphofructokinase pyruvic dehydrogenase and alpha-ketoglutaric dehydrogenase and by augmentation of glycogen synthetase and hexose transport.

Glutamic acid, glutamine, gamma-aminobutyric acid (GABA), alanine, and aspartic acid concentrations are not altered by the ketogenic or MCT diets. Thus modification of excitatory or inhibitory amino acids is not an important factor in the anticonvulsant effect of ketosis.

Mechanisms of Action

The mechanisms of action of the ketogenic and MCT diets are unknown. Reports of their effect on MES seizures in experimental animals have been conflicting (Davenport and Davenport, 1948; Appleton and DeVivo, 1974), but a high fat diet afforded no protection against PTZ-induced seizures (Uhlemann and Neims, 1972).

These diets have no lasting effect on either intracellular or extracellular pH. Davidian et al. (1978) have proposed that ketosis may produce an anticonvulsant effect by placing an additional demand on the proton pumping mechanism that maintains the electrochemical gradient for intracellular H^+. This could result in transient intracellular acidosis, which would occur when additional metabolic demands are made on brain cells (e.g., when electrical seizure activity builds up). Intracellular acidosis is thought to reduce neuronal excitability and prevent seizure discharge.

The only definitive statement that can be made is that the anticonvulsant effect correlates with the level of ketonemia. Higher K/AK ratios correlate with increased antiepileptic activity.

Clinical Use

Seizures of all types are amenable to treatment with these diets, but they have been particularly effective in children with refractory absence, myoclonic, akinetic, and atonic attacks (Millichap et al., 1964; Huttenlocher, 1976; Gordon, 1977; Stephenson et al., 1977). The diet may sometimes be dramatically effective in infantile spasms and in the Lennox-Gastaut syndrome; Livingston et al. (1958) and Livingston (1974), for example, have achieved control in 49% of patients with infantile spasms who were placed on a ketogenic diet.

The 3:1 ketogenic diet consists of 87% of calories from dietary fat, 6% from carbohydrate, and 7% from protein. It may be modified from a K/AK ratio of 1.5:1 to 4:1. The MCT diet consists of 60% of calories from MCTs (octanoic acid, 75%; decanoic acid, 25%), 11% from other dietary fat (9 calories/g), 19% from carbohydrate (4 calories/g), and 10% from protein (4 calories/g).

The major drawback of the diets is compliance. The 3:1 ketogenic diet is unpalatable after long use. The more palatable MCT diet may be continued for longer periods with proper reinforcement. Diet compliance can be determined by checking the urine for ketones, which should be maintained in the 3 to 4 + range when using a dip stick. A dietician should be consulted regularly when these diets are used.

Interactions With Antiepileptic Drugs

The diets may be effectively and safely used with the traditional antiepileptic drugs, but there is little experience with valproic acid.

Toxicity

Other than nausea, vomiting, and lethargy, which occur early in the course of their use, the diets are free of toxicity. Patients are constantly on the verge of acidosis, however, and acid-base homeostasis is stressed. A nontoxic side effect is the odor of ketones on the patient's breath and skin.

13

Drug Monitoring and Seizure Control

With the development of modern analytical techniques, the monitoring of plasma concentrations of antiepileptic drugs has become part of the routine management of the patient with seizures. The clinician is better able to choose a drug dosage that will achieve an optimum therapeutic response with minimal risk of dose-related toxic effects. The monitoring of plasma antiepileptic drug levels has helped prevent the consequences of adverse drug interactions and has reduced the use of multiple drug therapy.

THEORETICAL BASIS

The biological activity of an antiepileptic drug is proportional to the amount of drug that reaches the central nervous system, which in turn is in dynamic equilibrium with plasma drug concentration. Thus the antiepileptic effect of a drug is best estimated by the plasma concentration and not the dosage.

Antiepileptic drug monitoring is helpful in determining patient compliance, preventing dose-related toxic effects, prescribing individual therapy, and achieving a "therapeutic range" of plasma drug levels for each patient. The therapeutic range is a statistical concept, representing the range of plasma drug concentrations associated with optimum clinical control in the majority of patients without producing unacceptable adverse effects. Patients whose seizures are well controlled despite subtherapeutic plasma drug concentrations should not have their dosage increased to raise, or "treat," the plasma level. In some patients, toxic effects may occur at low, or even subtherapeutic, drug concentrations because of individual differences in susceptibility to adverse effects. Chapter 3 (Table 3.2) gives the therapeutic range of concentrations of the major and minor antiepileptic drugs.

Although a correlation exists between dosage and plasma drug levels in individual patients, interindividual correlation may be lacking because of multiple factors (Azarnoff, 1973; Vessell, 1973; Kutt and Penry, 1974). These include:

1. Variable compliance;
2. Timing of the plasma sample in relation to previous dose;
3. Individual differences in absorption, volume of distribution, and elimination;
4. Differences in nature of drug formulation altering bioavailability (e.g., capsule versus suspension);
5. Environmental factors, which may influence drug metabolism;
6. Presence of diseases that may alter absorption, metabolism, or excretion of antiepileptic drugs (e.g., gastrointestinal, cardiac, hepatic, or renal diseases, abnormal protein binding);
7. Drug interactions;
8. Unknown genetic factors;
9. Saturation (zero-order) kinetics of some antiepileptic drugs (e.g., phenytoin); plasma drug concentrations may increase disproportionately to increasing dose.

PLASMA CONCENTRATIONS AND SEIZURE CONTROL

Therapeutic plasma concentrations have been defined for most antiepileptic drugs, so that seizure control can be achieved without excess risk of toxicity. The effective plasma level may vary from patient to patient because seizure severity may differ. This may explain why in some patients seizures are well controlled at subtherapeutic plasma drug levels (Feldman and Pippenger, 1976). The usefulness of antiepileptic drug monitoring in achieving optimum seizure control has been supported by many clinical studies (Lascelles et al., 1970; Buchthal and Lennox-Buchthal, 1972*a,b*; Sherwin and Robb, 1972; Kutt, 1972, 1973, 1974; Kutt and Penry, 1974; Lund, 1974; Cereghino et al. 1975; Livingston et al., 1975; Eadie, 1976). It is important, however, that laboratories offering determination of antiepileptic drugs participate in a quality control program to establish interlaboratory reproducibility (Pippenger et al., 1976).

Phenytoin

The accepted therapeutic range of plasma phenytoin levels is 10 to 20 µg/ml (Chadwick et al., 1977*b*; Bruni, 1979; Penry, 1979). The majority of patients show the most favorable response when phenytoin concentrations are within this range. Therapeutic plasma concentrations generally can be achieved with daily doses of 5 to 7 mg/kg. When plasma concentrations must be raised quickly to therapeutic levels, a loading dose may be given. Initiation of therapy at a constant daily dose will produce therapeutic steady-state concentrations in 5 to 7 days unless saturation kinetics (slow metabolism) have occurred (see Chapter 5).

Phenobarbital

The accepted therapeutic range of plasma phenobarbital levels is 20 to 45 µg/ml (Bruni, 1979). Therapeutic plasma concentrations generally can be achieved with daily doses of 2 to 5 mg/kg and are reached in 2 to 4 weeks.

Mephobarbital

Mephobarbital is rapidly metabolized to phenobarbital. Divided daily doses of 4 to 10 mg/kg mephobarbital result in steady-state phenobarbital levels in 3 to 4 weeks.

Primidone

Primidone is metabolized to two active metabolites: phenobarbital and phenyl-ethylmalonamide. Primidone therapy can best be monitored by measuring plasma levels of phenobarbital, the metabolite responsible for some of the antiepileptic efficacy of primidone. The therapeutic plasma primidone level is 7 to 15 µg/ml (Bruni, 1979) and is most useful in assessing recent ingestion of the drug. Therapeutic plasma concentrations of primidone and phenobarbital are generally achieved with daily doses of 10 to 20 mg/kg. After 2 to 3 weeks of primidone therapy, therapeutic plasma concentrations of phenobarbital are observed.

Carbamazepine

Daily doses of 4 to 20 mg/kg carbamazepine usually result in therapeutic plasma concentrations of 4 to 10 µg/ml. Steady-state concentrations are achieved in 3 to 4 days.

Ethosuximide

Plasma ethosuximide concentrations of 40 to 100 µg/ml are considered optimal for seizure control; however, higher concentrations may be required in some patients. Daily doses of 15 to 35 mg/kg are required to achieve therapeutic plasma levels. Steady-state concentrations are reached after 7 to 10 days.

Methsuximide

Although methsuximide is active physiologically, it is rapidly metabolized by demethylation to *N*-desmethylsuximide, which is primarily responsible for the antiepileptic effect. Constant daily dosing in single or divided doses of 5 to 15 mg/kg methsuximide will produce the steady-state therapeutic range of 10 to 20 µg/ml of *N*-desmethylsuximide in 8 to 10 days. *N*-desmethylsuximide is metabolized by hydroxylation and follows first-order kinetics in the therapeutic range.

Valproic Acid

Therapeutic plasma concentrations of valproic acid range from 50 to 100 µg/ml, although higher levels may be required for optimum seizure control (Booker and

Darcey, 1973; Levy, 1973; Pinder et al., 1977; Bruni et al., 1978*b*). Daily doses of 10 to 60 mg/kg are needed to achieve therapeutic plasma levels. Therapy is initiated at 10 to 15 mg/kg/day and is increased weekly by 5 mg/kg/day. Generally, 4 to 5 weeks are required for the most effective seizure control.

Clonazepam

Therapeutic plasma clonazepam concentrations are not fully established, although we have obtained good seizure control with concentrations of 20 to 80 ng/ml. Therapy in adults should be initiated with daily doses of 0.05 mg/kg; daily doses of 0.1 to 0.2 mg/kg are required to produce effective plasma levels. The time required to reach steady-state concentrations is unknown, but a minimum of 5 days can be predicted from the half-life of 22 to 33 hr.

Trimethadione

Trimethadione is rapidly metabolized to dimethadione, which is responsible for most of the antiepileptic activity. Divided daily doses of 20 to 30 mg/kg trimethadione will produce steady-state therapeutic levels of 500 to 1,000 μg/ml dimethadione within 3 to 4 weeks.

PLASMA CONCENTRATIONS AND TOXICITY

Plasma concentrations of antiepileptic drugs higher than those accepted as therapeutic are usually associated with signs and symptoms of toxicity. The concentration at which adverse effects occur is variable, however, and tolerance to some of the side effects develops over time.

Drug assays done by most laboratories measure the plasma concentration of total (protein bound plus unbound) drug and not the free (unbound) drug only. This limitation must be recognized, since it is only the unbound drug that can act at the site of action of the drug. Toxicity, like efficacy, correlates better with free than with total drug concentration (Booker and Darcey, 1973).

Nystagmus often occurs when plasma phenytoin levels exceed 20 μg/ml, but it may also occur when concentrations are lower. Ataxia of gait may be observed when concentrations are higher than 30 μg/ml, and somnolence may be caused by levels above 40 μg/ml. Behavioral changes may occur at high therapeutic levels.

It is more difficult to determine a toxic plasma level for phenobarbital, because of the large variation among patients. The development of tolerance to the toxic effects is more common than with phenytoin. Plasma phenobarbital concentrations above 60 μg/ml may cause lethargy; nystagmus and gait ataxia may occur at variable concentrations, and a progression of signs and symptoms may not be observed.

At initiation of therapy, primidone, may cause sedation, malaise, and vertigo at subtherapeutic concentrations. Nystagmus may be observed when the therapeutic range of 7 to 15 μg/ml is exceeded. During chronic therapy, behavioral side effects may be related to high primidone levels. Plasma concentrations from the phenobarbital metabolite may also contribute to toxicity.

Side effects of ethosuximide that respond to dosage reduction include sedation, fatigue, headache, dizziness, nausea, vomiting, and singultus. The correlation between signs and symptoms of toxicity and plasma ethosuximide levels is poor. Sedation is the most common side effect of concentrations above 40 to 100 μg/ml.

Initiation of valproic acid therapy may result in mild nausea, vomiting, diarrhea, and fatigue. If the patient is receiving other antiepileptic drugs concurrently, particularly phenobarbital, sedation may also occur. These side effects are generally transient. With plasma concentrations in the high therapeutic range, a resting and postural tremor may develop.

The relationship between toxic side effects and plasma clonazepam levels is not well defined, but drowsiness, ataxia, and behavioral changes may be observed during therapy.

INDICATIONS FOR ANTIEPILEPTIC DRUG MONITORING

Antiepileptic drug monitoring is indicated in the following situations:

1. At initiation of therapy, to determine if a satisfactory plasma drug level has been achieved;

2. When seizures are uncontrolled, to determine compliance, rapid drug metabolism, or whether the seizures are specifically drug resistant;

3. When drug dosage is changed and a new steady-state concentration is achieved;

4. During development of intercurrent illness (e.g., hypoproteinemia; gastrointestinal, hepatic, or renal disease);

5. When drug interaction is suspected (e.g., when a drug is added or withdrawn);

6. When toxic symptoms may be drug related;

7. When unexplained behavioral changes may be caused by severe drug toxicity;

8. During pregnancy, when alterations in drug absorption and metabolism may occur;

9. During prepuberty or puberty, when changes in drug metabolism may require dosage adjustment;

10. During antiepileptic drug clinical trials.

Ideally, plasma drug concentrations should be monitored when the plasma concentration is at steady state and at fixed times in relation to drug administration. This is particularly important in the case of the antiepileptic drugs that have short half-lives (e.g., valproic acid, primidone, carbamazepine).

Further information on antiepileptic drug monitoring may be found in the articles by Levy (1973), Eadie (1976), Brett (1977), Bruni and Wilder (1979c), and Richens and Warrington (1979).

SALIVARY MONITORING OF ANTIEPILEPTIC DRUGS

Although not done routinely, salivary monitoring of antiepileptic drugs has been investigated for the last several years. One of its advantages is the simplicity of collecting saliva samples. In addition, the salivary concentration of most drugs corresponds to the free, biologically active portion of the drug. For salivary monitoring to be useful, a correlation between plasma and salivary concentrations must be present. This is true for most antiepileptic drugs, which are transported by passive diffusion. Constant saliva-to-plasma ratios have been obtained for phenobarbital, phenytoin, ethosuximide, carbamazepine, primidone, and diazepam.

Salivary determinations of protein-bound drugs, such as phenytoin, may be useful when abnormalities of protein binding (e.g., uremia, hypoproteinemia) are suspected. The transport mechanisms into saliva and cerebrospinal fluid are similar, and a correlation exists between drug concentration in the saliva and in the cerebrospinal fluid (Schmidt and Kupferberg, 1975; Troupin and Friel, 1975). Several additional articles on salivary monitoring of antiepileptic drugs may be consulted (Bochner et al., 1974; Cook et al., 1976a; McAuliffe et al., 1977; Horning et al., 1977; Anavekar et al., 1978; Danhof and Breimer, 1978; DiGregorio et al., 1978).

14

Drug Interactions

Significant adverse drug interactions may occur when two or more antiepileptic drugs are administered concurrently. These interactions may result in a decreased or increased effect of one or more of the drugs. Knowledge of potential interactions is necessary for proper dosage adjustment.

Drug interactions are generally classified into two broad groups: pharmacodynamic and pharmacokinetic. Pharmacodynamic interactions occur when the drugs interact at receptor sites. These usually are dose related and may lead to antagonism, enhancement, or synergism of drug effect. Administration of antiepileptic drugs to patients with central nervous system damage may result in a higher incidence of adverse neurological effects. Other factors include age and the presence of disease states.

Pharmacokinetic interactions are caused by alterations in the absorption, protein binding, distribution, metabolism, or excretion of one drug by another. More or less drug is made available at the site of action, which is generally reflected in changes in the plasma concentration of the affected drug.

Drug interactions are an important consideration in epileptic patients because long-term multidrug therapy is often indicated. Furthermore, interactions may occur between antiepileptic drugs and drugs used for other medical conditions. The clinician must be aware of these interactions in order to prevent potential toxicity of some drugs or subtherapeutic effects of others. The patient should be advised about possible drug interactions, and a complete drug history should be obtained.

ABSORPTION

Phenytoin is absorbed slowly from the gastrointestinal tract. It has been suggested that antacids containing calcium, aluminum, or magnesium may reduce absorption

(Kutt, 1975; Richens, 1979). However, a study in two normal volunteers failed to show any changes in the rate and extent of phenytoin absorption (Chapron et al., 1979). Studies in patients on chronic phenytoin therapy, however, do show reduced absorption (Karas and Wilder, 1981). Antihistamines may decrease the absorption of phenytoin. The efficacy of griseofulvin is reduced by phenobarbital because of impaired absorption (Busfield et al., 1963; Rigelman et al., 1970). Phenytoin decreases the absorption of calcium, vitamin C, vitamin D, and folate. The absorption of bishydroxycoumarin is reduced when phenytoin and/or phenobarbital are given concurrently. The absorption of primidone may be impaired by acetazolamide (Syversen et al., 1977).

PROTEIN BINDING

Protein binding interactions are an important consideration when drugs that are highly protein bound are used concurrently. Decreased efficacy or intoxication may ensue, since many antiepileptic drugs have a narrow therapeutic range. Displacement of antiepileptic drugs from protein makes them more readily available for metabolism, resulting in lower plasma concentrations if the drug-metabolizing enzymes have not reached saturation. If hepatic metabolic enzymes are saturated, high plasma drug concentrations may result. Part of the effect of carbamazepine on phenytoin may be attributable to this mechanism (Hansen et al., 1971). The concurrent administration of phenytoin and valproic acid causes transiently lowered total phenytoin levels (Bruni et al., 1979b). Although total plasma phenytoin levels are decreased, the effect is counteracted by increased free phenytoin. Usually no increase in phenytoin dosage is required.

Interactions may occur between phenytoin and other drugs that are highly protein bound: thyroid hormones, tricyclic antidepressants, oral hypoglycemic agents, sulfonamides, salicylates, diazoxide, clofibrate, phenylbutazone, and bishydroxycoumarin (Richens, 1977b, 1979; Bruni and Wilder, 1979b). Valproic acid is also highly protein bound, and an increase in the free portion may result from the coadministration of salicylates or phenylbutazone but not warfarin (Fleitman et al., 1980).

METABOLISM AND EXCRETION

Hepatic parahydroxylation is an important step in the metabolism of antiepileptic drugs. Changes in enzyme activity may lead to altered plasma concentrations. Interactions between the major antiepileptic drugs do occur, and experimental enzyme induction can be produced. In the clinical situation, with combinations of phenobarbital, phenytoin, and primidone, little such effect occurs. The effects of adding phenobarbital to phenytoin are variable (Buchanan and Sholiton, 1972; Cucinell, 1972). We have found that plasma concentrations of individual drugs increase when these drugs are used. As doses of these drugs are increased, enzyme saturation may occur, and metabolism may be slowed; thus any inductive effect tends to be canceled.

Interactions of phenytoin and phenobarbital with methsuximide have been reported (Rambeck, 1979). Methsuximide was found to cause elevated levels of these drugs. Patients receiving phenytoin or phenobarbital also had higher levels of methsuximide and *N*-desmethylmethsuximide, its active metabolite.

Data on interactions between phenytoin and the benzodiazepines are conflicting. Carbamazepine is a powerful inducer of enzymes, and plasma phenytoin levels may be reduced (Cereghino et al., 1973).

In addition to interacting with phenytoin at protein binding sites, valproic acid causes higher plasma concentrations of phenobarbital (Bruni and Wilder, 1979*b*). The data are compatible with the inhibition of phenobarbital metabolism by valproic acid. This interaction should be anticipated in the majority of patients and generally requires a reduction of phenobarbital dosage. Phenytoin, primidone, phenobarbital, and carbamazepine may enhance valproic acid metabolism.

Antiepileptic drugs may interact with other classes of drugs. Compounds that may have reduced therapeutic effects because of hepatic enzyme induction by antiepileptic drugs include steroids, hormone contraceptives, and phenylbutazone. Folic acid therapy may lower phenytoin levels.

Disulfiram and isoniazid inhibit phenytoin metabolism. Phenothiazines, propoxyphene, methylphenidate, phenyramidol, certain antimicrobials, and rarely bishydroxycoumarin increase phenytoin concentrations. Isoniazid inhibits primidone metabolism. Carbamazepine and alcohol may induce hepatic enzymes and thus lower phenytoin concentrations. Urinary alkalinization can markedly increase renal phenobarbital excretion. Phenytoin may cause decreased diuresis with furosamide and inhibit levodopa effect, but the mechanisms are not clear. It may also decrease the quinidine effect by induction of microsomal enzymes.

DRUG POTENTIATION

Drug potentiation, which can occur at the receptor level, can also be expected when drugs from the same class are used. The concurrent administration of primidone and phenobarbital, for example, may result in high plasma phenobarbital levels because a significant portion of primidone is converted to phenobarbital. Drug effects may be markedly potentiated when benzodiazepines are used with barbiturates. Absence status may be precipitated in some patients receiving clonazepam and valproic acid concurrently (Jeavons et al., 1977). Other drug interactions are discussed in the chapters on the individual drugs (Chapters 4–12) and in the chapter on drug toxicity (Chapter 15).

15

Drug Toxicity

Antiepileptic drug toxicity may be the result of either changes in normal physiological functions or a direct toxic action. In the former, antiepileptic drugs may interfere with the normal physiological actions of vitamins, minerals, hormones, amino acids, neurotransmitters, energy metabolism, and cell division. In the latter, a de novo toxic effect is produced. Toxic effects can be classified according to type of reaction, time of appearance of the effect, exaggeration or depression of physiological responses, induced deficiency states, and drug interactions. These effects usually are secondary to the effect of the drug, but adverse reactions may also be caused by toxic metabolites of the parent drug.

The occurrence of antiepileptic drug toxicity is influenced by such factors as genetic and age-related processes, central nervous system (CNS) structural disease, concurrent malnutrition, hypoproteinemia, diseases of the renal, hepatic, or endocrine systems, multiple drug therapy, and prolonged drug use. Although serious toxic reactions to antiepileptic drugs are uncommon considering the number of doses administered, milder forms of toxicity, such as transient drowsiness and gastrointestinal disturbances, are prevalent. The major targets for antiepileptic drug toxicity are the CNS, blood, blood-forming organs, bone, skin, connective tissue, and hepatic, renal, endocrine and immunological systems. The fetus is also subject to teratogenic effects of these drugs.

Toxicity can be most appropriately considered under acute toxic reactions (either dose-related or allergic in nature), idiosyncratic reactions, chronic toxicity, teratogenicity, and toxic drug interactions (Table 15.1). The latter are discussed in Chapter 14. An overview of the basic types of toxic reactions is presented in this chapter, and a more complete account of the pharmacotoxicology of each antiepileptic drug is given in Chapters 4 to 12.

TABLE 15.1. *Toxic reactions of antiepileptic drugs*

Type of reaction	Frequency	Time of occurrence
Acute	+ + + +	Early
Idiosyncratic	+	Early to late
Chronic	+ + +	Late
Teratogenic	+	Prenatal exposure
Drug interactions	+ +	Early to late

ACUTE TOXICITY

Acute toxicity is usually manifested as adverse effects on the CNS, gastrointestinal system, or integumentary system. These effects usually are the result of initial intolerance to a drug or of drug overdosage. Less frequently, they are secondary to an allergic or idiosyncratic reaction.

CNS toxicity may cause mental and behavioral changes, dizziness, nystagmus, ataxia, extrapyramidal systems, seizure exacerbation, somnolence, or coma. Generally, hydantoins initially produce signs of cerebellovestibular dysfunction (nystagmus, ataxia, incoordination, dysarthria, tremor). As toxicity increases, higher cortical function (judgment, concentration, affect, behavior, speech) is altered. With more severe toxicity, pyramidal and extrapyramidal signs may appear (asterexis, dystonia, dyskinesias, myoclonus, ophthalmoplegia). Epileptic seizures may be exacerbated; with profound toxicity, autonomic dysfunction and coma may occur.

Barbiturates generally interfere with reticulocortical activating systems early in the course of treatment and may induce lethargy, somnolence, nystagmus, ataxia, and higher cortical dysfunction. Stupor and coma may occur as toxicity increases. Paradoxically, barbiturates may cause irritability and hyperactivity in children and excitation in the elderly.

The benzodiazepines interfere with reticulocortical arousal systems and may induce early lethargy and somnolence. In patients with decreased cardiopulmonary reserve and in very young patients, cardiorespiratory depression may occur, especially with intravenous administration. Intravenous benzodiazepines may also precipitate tonic status epilepticus.

Carbamazepine interferes with cerebellovestibular, pyramidal, extrapyramidal, and higher cortical function. Signs of toxicity include ataxia, nystagmus, diplopia, and drowsiness. Gastrointestinal disturbances are common, especially if therapy is not initiated gradually.

The succinimides and oxazolidinediones sometimes result in higher cortical dysfunction, with the occurrence of somnolence, lethargy, and emotional instability. Trimethadione may cause hemeralopia, or light blindness.

Ethosuximide does not often produce signs of early CNS toxicity, but methsuximide may cause lethargy, photophobia, somnolence, or hiccups even at low plasma drug levels. Abnormal extrapyramidal movements are rarely seen with ethosuximide.

TABLE 15.2. *Acute toxic reactions of antiepileptic drugs*

System affected	Drug
Neurological	Phenytoin
Higher cortical function	Primidone, phenobarbital, phenytoin
Reticulocortical activating system	Phenobarbital, primidone, diazepam
Pyramidal-extrapyramidal systems	Carbamazepine, phenytoin
Cerebellovestibular system	Phenytoin, carbamazepine
Gastrointestinal	Valproic acid, primidone, carbamazepine
Integumentary	Phenytoin

Valproic acid may result in early CNS toxicity, with the occurrence of lethargy and postural and resting tremor. Sedation, stupor, and coma rarely occur in patients taking valproic acid alone but may occur in those concurrently receiving phenobarbital. Early gastrointestinal disturbances, which are generally mild and transient, may be caused by valproic acid, carbamazepine, and primidone. The occurrence of these effects generally can be minimized by a gradual increase in dose. In large doses, phenytoin may cause nausea and gastric irritation.

All the antiepileptic drugs—in particular phenytoin—may produce allergic skin rashes, but these are uncommon. Table 15.2 summarizes the most common acute toxic reactions and the antiepileptic drugs most often responsible for them. Some reviews of the toxicology of antiepileptic drugs are available (Booker, 1975; Plaa, 1975; Reynolds, 1975*b*; Dam, 1977; Bruni and Wilder, 1979*b*).

IDIOSYNCRATIC REACTIONS

Idiosyncratic drug reactions are genetically determined abnormal responses to drugs. Various mechanisms may be responsible (Levine, 1978), including alterations in (a) an enzyme system normally responsible for drug transformation, (b) functional proteins and enzyme systems not involved in the biotransformation reaction, (c) drug absorption and distribution, and (d) drug receptor proteins.

As shown in Table 15.3, idiosyncratic toxic reactions involving the antiepileptic drugs are all examples of alterations in drug metabolism in genetically susceptible individuals (Booker, 1975). Although rare, these reactions are serious and life threatening. They involve the hemapoietic system, skin, autoimmunological system, liver, kidneys, CNS, and gastrointestinal tract. The pharmacogenetic aspects of drug metabolism have been reviewed (Kutt, 1971; Vessell, 1972).

CHRONIC TOXICITY

Neurological Toxicity

Disturbances of Higher Cortical Functions

Adverse effects of the antiepileptic drugs on cerebral function include behavioral and psychological aberrations, memory disturbances, disturbed sensorimotor perfor-

TABLE 15.3. *Idiosyncratic reactions*

Type and examples	Effect	Inheritance
Alterations of metabolic enzyme system		
Aminolevulinic acid synthetase	Stimulation by phenytoin, resulting in porphyric crisis	Autosomal recessive
Microsomal oxidase	Deficiency, resulting in phenytoin toxicity	Autosomal dominant
Acetyltransferase	Deficiency, resulting in phenytoin toxicity with coadministration of isoniazid	Autosomal recessive
Alterations of functional proteins		
Glucose-3-phosphate dehydrogenase deficiency	Drug-induced hemolytic anemia with primaquine	Sex-linked
Alterations in drug absorption and distribution		
Ceruloplasmin deficiency (Wilson disease)	Excessive distribution of free copper	Autosomal recessive
Abnormalities of drug receptor protein		
Taste receptors	Inability to taste phenylthiourea	Autosomal recessive

mance, seizure exacerbation, and electroencephalographic (EEG) changes. These aspects of toxicity have received relatively little attention because of the difficulty in distinguishing drug-related mental symptoms from symptoms caused by brain injury or seizures themselves. In addition, this aspect is difficult to analyze quantitatively.

It has long been recognized that mental symptoms may occur in epileptic patients. Lennox (1942), for example, proposed the following causes for mental deterioration in epilepsy: (a) heredity, (b) psychological handicaps, (c) brain injury antedating the seizure disorder, (d) epilepsy itself, and (e) drugs. The introduction of new antiepileptic drugs theoretically could contribute to a higher incidence of toxic neurological effects. Antiepileptic drug monitoring, however, can help to avoid toxic plasma concentrations of drugs, although mental aberrations may occur with therapeutic or even subtherapeutic plasma drug concentrations.

It is well known that phenytoin can cause an encephalopathy and seizure exacerbation (Gruber et al., 1940; Levy and Fenichel, 1965; Glaser, 1972). The syndrome of chronic phenytoin encephalopathy is characterized by insidious deterioration of intellect and behavior with or without seizure exacerbation, mild cerebrospinal fluid (CSF) pleocytosis, and moderate increase in CSF protein; the plasma phenytoin concentration may be in the therapeutic or toxic range (Rawson, 1968). This encephalopathy is rare and probably more common in epileptic patients with underlying brain damage (Reynolds and Travers, 1974).

Decreased intellectual performance as a complication of long-term phenytoin use has been reported by numerous investigators (Rosen, 1968; Ideström et al., 1972; Vallarta et al., 1974; Stores, 1975). Epileptic patients with drug toxicity have been shown to have a greater decrease in cognitive and sensorimotor performance than those without (Matthews and Harley, 1975).

The cause of these effects on higher cortical functions is not definitely known, but a direct depressant effect on CNS function and an effect on folate metabolism are probably important. The CSF folate concentration is normally three times higher than the serum folate concentration, and folate plays a major role in CNS function. Long-term folate deficiency associated with antiepileptic drug therapy has been reported to result in mental slowing and apathy, lack of drive, organic brain syndrome, and psychosis, all of which develop in some epileptic patients. Treatment with folic acid improves mental functioning in these patients at the possible expense of increased seizures (Reynolds, 1972, 1975*b*).

Phenytoin therapy, especially in doses yielding toxic plasma concentrations, may result in significant EEG abnormalities (McLellan and Swash, 1974; Ahmad et al., 1975; Perucca, 1976; Iivanainen and Viukari, 1977; Iivanainen et al., 1978). These abnormalities are most frequent in mentally retarded epileptic patients and are more prominent with toxic plasma phenytoin concentrations. These effects include an increase in paroxysmal discharges, slowing of the background activity, impaired reaction to alerting procedures, diffuse slow wave abnormalities, abnormal fast activity, and asymmetries of background activity.

Experimentally, phenobarbital has been associated with brain growth retardation in animals (Schain and Watanabe, 1976; Diaz et al., 1977) and neuronal deficits after prenatal drug exposure (Yanai et al., 1979). The significance of these findings in relation to phenobarbital therapy of children and pregnant epileptic women is unknown. In children, it may be associated with hyperactivity and irritability, and elderly patients may experience paradoxical excitation. Several studies have suggested that behavioral changes, decreased intellectual performance, and disturbed sensorimotor functions may accompany the use of phenobarbital (Hutt et al., 1968; Tchicaloff and Gaillard, 1970; Holdsworth and Whitmore, 1974; MacLeod et al., 1978). It has also been shown that high plasma phenobarbital concentrations can slow short-term memory scanning without impairing long-term memory (MacLeod et al., 1978). Since a significant portion of primidone is metabolized to phenobarbital, the expected side effects are probably similar, although primidone itself and its second most abundant metabolite, phenylethylmalonamide, may be contributory.

It has been suggested that of the major antiepileptic agents effective against generalized tonic-clonic seizures, carbamazepine has the least effect on intellectual and sensorimotor performance. Although a direct psychotropic effect of carbamazepine is unproved, it is important to note its close chemical relationship to the tricyclic antidepressants. In a double-blind study, primidone caused a greater impairment of cognitive function than carbamazepine (Rodin et al., 1976). A psychometric evaluation by Dodrill and Troupin (1977) comparing phenytoin and carbamazepine showed lesser impairment with carbamazepine. In a recent study of 20 epileptic patients with behavioral disorders, carbamazepine reportedly lessened excitement, irritability, hostility, and uncooperativeness (Singh et al., 1977).

The effects of ethosuximide therapy on mental function are not clearly defined, and controversies exist as to whether it impairs intellectual function. No adverse effects occurred in a controlled study of 37 patients (Browne et al., 1975), but earlier studies showed deleterious effects (Guey et al., 1967; Soulayrol and Roger, 1970). It has also been reported that ethosuximide therapy may exacerbate generalized nonconvulsive seizures (Todorov et al., 1978).

Clonazepam has been implicated in such behavioral abnormalities as irritability, aggression, hyperactivity, and difficulty with concentration (Reynolds, 1975b). In the treatment of 22 children with intractable epilepsy, clonazepam therapy was associated with hyperactivity in four children, aggression in two, and depression in two others. A large-scale controlled study on the effects of clonazepam on intellectual function has not been performed.

The long-term effects of valproic acid therapy have not been fully established. One study, however, has shown psychomotor deterioration (Sommerbeck et al., 1977). The effects of antiepileptic drugs on mental function have been reviewed (Trimble and Reynolds, 1976; Trimble, 1979).

Withdrawal Symptoms

The abrupt withdrawal of antiepileptic drugs may result in seizure exacerbation caused by the underlying disorder, or rarely it may precipitate drug withdrawal seizures. In addition, withdrawal symptoms characterized by an organic brain syndrome or extreme anxiety may occur.

Withdrawal seizures may appear upon discontinuation of chronically administered barbiturates, benzodiazepines, and primidone. Barbiturate withdrawal convulsions are more common with short-acting barbiturates (Dam, 1977), but they also can occur after phenobarbital withdrawal. The EEG may show transient paroxysmal high-voltage discharges. The seizures are of the generalized tonic-clonic type. Diazepam is the benzodiazepine most often implicated in withdrawal seizures (Maletzky and Klotter, 1976; Preskorn and Denner, 1977; de Bard, 1979). We have not observed seizures after the withdrawal of carbamazepine or valproic acid.

Cerebellar Dysfunction

In addition to causing reversible cerebellar dysfunction, which is usually dose-related, prolonged treatment with phenytoin may lead to irreversible cerebellar deficits. Cerebellar degeneration has been attributed to large doses of phenytoin or prolonged phenytoin therapy (Utterback, 1958; Hofmann, 1958; Haberland, 1962; Ghatak et al., 1976). Brain-damaged, mentally retarded epileptic patients may be unusually susceptible (Iivanainen et al., 1977). Dam (1972a,b) has noted Purkinje cell degeneration and astrocytic changes in patients on long-term phenytoin therapy, but the changes could be attributed to repeated convulsions and hypoxic episodes (Dam, 1970, 1972a,b). A case has been reported of phenytoin-related cerebellar degeneration in a nonepileptic patient with a CNS tuberculous infection (Rapport and Shaw, 1977). A later study, however, led to the conclusion that permanent damage is related to the cumulative effects of the frequency and chronicity of seizures (Salcman et al., 1978).

In animal studies, Snider and Del Cerro (1967, 1972) have presented electron microscopic evidence of abnormal proliferating spiral membranes arising from Purkinje cells, altered mossy and basket cell terminals, and Bermann astrocyte abnormalities. The authors attributed these changes to phenytoin toxicity. Dam (1972a,b), however, has attributed such changes and those reported by others to fixation artifact, hypoxic changes, or poor quantitative methods of counting Purkinje cells. Thus, although cerebellar cortical degeneration has been found in chronically treated epileptic patients, the relative roles of repeated seizures, hypoxia, and phenytoin therapy are not clear. Considering the number of patients treated with prolonged phenytoin therapy, clinically significant cerebellar deficits are uncommon.

Peripheral Neuropathy

Peripheral neuropathy as a complication of phenytoin therapy has been noted by many investigators (Finkelman and Arieff, 1942; Michaux et al., 1959; Horwitz et al., 1968; Lovelace and Horwitz, 1968; Birket-Smith and Krogh, 1971; Eisen et al., 1974; Chokroverty and Sayeed, 1975). Experimentally, the acute administration of phenytoin has resulted in decreased nerve conduction velocity (LeQuesne et al., 1976). Lovelace and Horwitz (1968) found ankle and knee reflexes absent in 18% of their epileptic patients. Sensory signs, usually involving decreased vibration and, less frequently, disturbances of joint position, touch, and pain, were present in some patients. In more than 50% of those tested, nerve conduction velocities were slow. Eisen et al. (1974) examined patients who had been treated with phenytoin for longer than 10 years. Most showed neurogenic changes and slow nerve conduction. Positive electrodiagnostic studies correlated with high plasma phenytoin levels. In all affected patients, folate and vitamin B_{12} concentrations were normal, which has been the case in most other studies (Eisen et al., 1974, Chokroverty and Sayeed, 1975). These investigators considered positive neurogenic findings to be of two types: (a) transient dysfunction associated with acute toxicity and high phenytoin levels, and (b) a neuropathy accompanying long-term phenytoin therapy.

Clinically significant peripheral neuropathy from phenytoin therapy is relatively rare, although alterations of nerve conduction may be more frequent. If a patient on long-term phenytoin therapy experiences peripheral neuropathy, other causative factors should be excluded before the neuropathy is attributed to phenytoin.

Myasthenia Gravis

A syndrome resembling myasthenia gravis has been attributed to phenytoin therapy (Brumlik and Jacobs, 1974) and trimethadione (Peterson, 1966; Booker et al.,

TABLE 15.4. *Chronic neurotoxicity of antiepileptic drugs*

Adverse reaction	Mechanism	Drug
Higher cortical dysfunction	Possible interference with normal metabolic pathways (? folate deficiency)	Succinimides, primidone, phenobarbital, phenytoin, carbamazepine, benzodiazepines
Withdrawal syndromes	Not fully established	Benzodiazepines, phenobarbital, primidone
Cerebellar dysfunction	Cerebellar degeneration	Phenytoin
Peripheral neuropathy	Interference with nerve conduction	Phenytoin
Myasthenia gravis	Immunological injury	Phenytoin, trimethadione

1970), probably as a result of an immunological reaction. It has been shown that phenytoin may produce defective neuromuscular transmission and a curare-like effect (Norris et al., 1964). In addition to causing a myasthenia gravis-like syndrome, phenytoin may unmask and exacerbate true myasthenia gravis.

Miscellaneous Neurotoxicity

Myopathy has been reported in a patient who developed clinical, biochemical, radiological, and bone biopsy evidence of severe osteomalacia (Findler and Lavy, 1979). The features of this myopathy included the typical myopathic distribution of muscle weakness (trunk and limb-girdle), muscle wasting, absence of normal reflexes, and abnormal levels of creatine phosphokinase. Transient hemiparesis has been reported as a result of overdosage of phenytoin after several weeks of therapy (Findler and Lavy, 1979). Anterior horn cell dysfunction resulting in muscle fasciculations has been observed in one patient (Direkze and Fernando, 1977). These are all isolated case reports, and their relationship to antiepileptic therapy is not definitely established. Table 15.4 summarizes the chronic neurotoxicity of the antiepileptic drugs.

Connective Tissue and Dermatological Effects

A variety of skin rashes, including erythematous, urticarial, acneform, and morbilliform rashes, may be caused by antiepileptic therapy. More rarely, exfoliative dermatitis, erythema multiforme, Stevens-Johnson syndrome, and alopecia may occur. A dermatological reaction to phenytoin is reported in about 5% of children and is slightly less common in adults. A high incidence of skin rashes has been observed in epileptic children (Wilson et al., 1978). This effect seems to be dose related and may disappear with reduction of dosage. Hypersensitivity does not appear to be involved.

Hypertrichosis and chloasma-like pigmentation are recognized side effects of phenytoin, and the exacerbation of acne may occur in children and adults. It is believed that such changes are unrelated to phenytoin dosage, blood levels of the drug, or endocrine dysfunction (Livingston, 1972). Phenytoin stimulation of melanin synthesis might account for the increased pigmentation and darkening of hair color that occurs in many chronically treated patients (Von Krebs, 1964). Hypertrichosis is irreversible but may regress slightly after drug withdrawal. Valproic acid commonly causes mild and transient alopecia, and discontinuation of therapy usually is not required.

Thickening of subcutaneous tissues, coarsening of facial features, enlargement of the lips and nose, and subcutaneous fibrous deposits are often recognized in patients on long-term phenytoin therapy. The term "hydantoin facies" has been used to describe these features, which are more common in institutionalized patients (Falconer and Davidson, 1973).

Gingival Hyperplasia

Gingival hyperplasia has been recognized as a side effect of antiepileptic therapy since the introduction of phenytoin. It occurs in many patients (children more than adults) receiving phenytoin and in a few patients receiving other antiepileptic drugs. The degree of gum hypertrophy has been correlated with daily dosage and serum concentrations of the drugs (Kapur et al., 1973). Poor oral hygiene often plays an important role in its development (Angelopoulos and Goaz, 1972). Phenytoin has been shown to decrease significantly the secretion of salivary immunoglobulin A (IgA), which is the most prominent immunoglobulin in external secretions. It is believed that a deficiency of serum and salivary IgA is the predisposing factor to the gingivitis and gum hypertrophy induced by phenytoin (Aarli, 1976), but this may be disputed (Smith et al., 1979b). Institutionalized epileptic patients, those of low socioeconomic background, and younger patients are more severely affected. Vitamin C malabsorption induced by phenytoin has been implicated as a causative factor in periodontitis (Houck et al., 1972; Stambaugh et al., 1973). Treatment consists of withdrawal of phenytoin, meticulous oral hygiene, and gingivectomy. The benefit of vitamin C therapy is not clear.

Dupuytren Contracture

The association of Dupuytren contracture and antiepileptic therapy was first reported in 1941 (Lund, 1941); the incidence was 50% for males and 32% for females. A later study found a similar incidence (Critchley et al., 1976). The latter study concluded that the incidence increased with the duration of the epilepsy but found no correlation among dosage, number of different antiepileptic drugs used, and the percentage of patients with Dupuytren contracture. If phenobarbital was excluded from consideration, the risk of Dupuytren contracture fell dramatically; only two of 21 patients not receiving phenobarbital were affected.

The pathogenesis of Dupuytren contracture is not clear. Some investigators have noted an increased incidence in both alcoholic and epileptic patients receiving antiepileptic drugs and have suggested altered hepatic function as a possible cause

(Pojer et al., 1972). Both alcohol and antiepileptic drugs stimulate microsomal enzymes, particularly those involved in steroid hydroxylation, bilirubin conjugation, lipid synthesis, and metabolism of certain drugs (Kuntzman, 1969). The incidence of liver enzyme abnormalities, however, was found to be similar in patients with and without Dupuytren disease (Houck et al., 1972), and the investigators proposed a direct effect of antiepileptic drugs on peripheral tissues. Additional studies have shown enhanced wound healing with phenytoin (Shapiro, 1958; Simpson et al., 1965) and proliferation of human and animal fibroblasts in tissue cultures (Houck et al., 1972). Chronic phenytoin administration in animals retards collagen metabolism. Collagenolysis is regulated by cortisol, which depends on a normal pituitary-adrenal axis. Prolonged phenytoin administration inhibits andrenocorticotropic hormone (ACTH) secretion and enhances cortisol or steroid metabolism by microsomal enzyme induction.

Shoulder-Hand Syndrome, Frozen Shoulder

An increased incidence of the shoulder-hand syndrome was found in epileptic patients taking antiepileptic drugs (Van der Korst et al., 1966); 19 of 75 patients with the shoulder-hand syndrome were taking phenobarbital. Frozen shoulder has been found to be a part of Dupuytren disease (Early, 1962).

Pulmonary Fibrosis

Moore (1959) described abnormalities of the pulmonary parenchyma on chest roentgenograms of patients on long-term phenytoin therapy, although this was not confirmed by other workers (Low and Yahr, 1960). However, abnormalities of pulmonary gas exchange may occur without evidence of radiographic abnormalities. An additional case of phenytoin-induced pulmonary toxicity has been reported, and it was suggested that an immune-complex injury occurred (Bayer et al., 1976). Table 15.5 summarizes the adverse dermatological and connective tissue effects of the antiepileptic drugs.

Endocrine Disturbances and Metabolic Effects

At least four endocrine systems are targets for antiepileptic drug effects: bone metabolism, pituitary-adrenal-gonadal axis, thyroid gland, and pancreatic beta cells.

Bone Metabolism

Hypocalcemia, rickets, and osteomalacia are known complications of antiepileptic drug therapy. The hydantoins and, to a lesser extent, the barbiturates, especially phenobarbital, decrease intestinal absorption of calcium by mechanisms not involving cholecalciferol (vitamin D) or its active metabolites (Koch et al., 1972). Calcium metabolism may also alter hepatic vitamin D hydroxylation (Hahn et al., 1972a,b). Antiepileptic drugs induce hepatic microsomal enzymes. This mechanism is thought to be responsible for an increase in the metabolism of vitamin D to

TABLE 15.5. *Dermatological and connective tissue effects of antiepileptic drugs*

Adverse reaction	Mechanism	Drug
Skin rashes	Allergic	All drugs
Urticarial		
Morbilliform		
Acneform		
Erythematous		
Erythema multiforme		
Exfoliative dermatitis		
Stevens-Johnson syndrome		
Gingival hyperplasia	Changes in collagen metabolism and fibroblast proliferation	Primidone, phenytoin, phenobarbital.
Coarse facial features	Changes in collagen metabolism and fibroblast proliferation	Primidone, phenobarbital, phenytoin
Dupuytren disease	Changes in collagen metabolism and fibroblast proliferation	Phenytoin, phenobarbital, primidone
Shoulder-hand syndrome	Changes in collagen metabolism and fibroblast proliferation	Phenobarbital
Pulmonary fibrosis	Immunologic	Phenytoin

inactive compounds, which leads to a decrease in serum 25-hydroxycholecalciferol (the major active metabolite of vitamin D) and subsequently osteomalacia. Phenytoin also inhibits parathyroid hormone-induced release of calcium from bone (Harris et al., 1974). These interactions are pertinent to an understanding of metabolic bone disease induced by antiepileptic drugs (Borgstedt et al., 1972; DeLuca et al., 1972; Christiansen et al., 1973). In many patients receiving phenytoin, serum calcium and serum 25-hydroxycholecalciferol concentrations are decreased, and alkaline phosphatase values are increased (Polypchuk et al., 1978). Reversal of laboratory findings and successful treatment of osteomalacia or rickets can be accomplished with oral hydroxycholecalciferol therapy (Stamp et al., 1972).

Metabolic bone disease is more prominent in institutionalized epileptic patients and in patients on multiple drug therapy. Dietary factors and amount of exposure to sunlight may be contributory factors. In a bone biopsy study, (Bell et al., 1979), an increase in unmineralized bone (osteomalacia) was found in 53% of patients, along with evidence of increased bone resorption (secondary hyperparathyroidism), suggesting that more than one mechanism is operative. In another bone biopsy study (Polypchuk et al., 1978), bone mineral mass was decreased in 44% of 32 patients, but no clinical evidence of metabolic bone disease was found in any.

Hypocalciuria and hypercalcemia have been documented in a study of 86 epileptic patients (Dymling et al., 1979). None of these patients had hypocalcemia, which may be related to their having a sufficient daily intake of calcium and vitamin D or adequate exposure to sunlight, or both. The mechanism responsible for the decreased calcium absorption that occurs in some epileptic patients has not been fully established. In organ cultured embryonic chick duodenum, a direct inhibitory effect of phenytoin on vitamin D-mediated calcium absorption has been demonstrated (Corradino, 1976). Sensitivity of the intestine to exogenous active vitamin D metabolites is normal; thus the inhibition may be related to decreased tissue concentrations of the active metabolites (Mosekilde et al., 1979).

The prevention of metabolic bone disease is difficult, and long-term treatment with vitamin D should be considered in patients with elevated serum alkaline phosphatase and decreases in serum 25-hydroxycholecalciferol or bone mineral mass.

Pituitary-Adrenal-Gonadal Axis

Phenytoin, phenobarbital, and carbamazepine can influence the pituitary-adrenal axis. Large, acutely administered doses of phenytoin initially increase circulating ACTH and cortisol. Chronic administration of phenytoin or phenobarbital leads to a shift in steroid metabolism, with an increase in urinary excretion of 6-hydroxy-cortisol. Phenytoin administration can result in erroneous metyrapone and 2-mg dexamethasone suppression tests (Gharib and Munoz, 1974). Phenytoin and carbamazepine also depress the release of antidiuretic hormone.

Testosterone and estradiol metabolism may be enhanced by antiepileptic drugs because of their hepatic enzyme-inducing properties. Chronic antiepileptic therapy also may be associated with elevated plasma concentrations of sex hormone-binding globulin in males and females (Victor et al., 1977; Barragry et al., 1978). The effect on sexual function of increased testosterone binding to the excess globulin is uncertain. In male rats, phenytoin treatment for 2 months did not affect fertility or testicular histology (Cohn et al., 1978).

Thyroid Function

The decline of serum protein iodine sometimes induced by phenytoin deserves mention, since some features of antiepileptic drug toxicity (lethargy, mental dullness, ataxia, and coarseness of facial features) may be confused with the clinical signs of hypothyroidism. In the absence of hypothyroidism, however, uptake of I^{131} and T_3 by red blood cells is not altered (Cantu and Schwab, 1966), although T_4 levels may be low because of displacement by phenytoin from α_2-globulin and increased clearance (Yeo et al., 1978). Carbamazepine and valproic acid, because of protein binding, may also displace thyroxine from binding sites (DiSalle et al., 1974; Fichsell, 1978). Despite changes in the various measurements of thyroid function, most patients on long-term antiepileptic therapy are clinically euthyroid.

Carbohydrate Tolerance and Insulin Secretion

The majority of patients receiving long-term phenytoin therapy have normal carbohydrate tolerance, but insulin secretion may be impaired in some, especially those with diabetes or prediabetes. The pseudodiabetogenic effect of phenytoin may be manifested by an abnormal glucose tolerance test (Treasure and Toseland, 1971), and acute phenytoin intoxication may be accompanied by extremely high blood glucose levels (Wilder et al., 1973*a*). Experimentally, phenytoin has been shown to cause hyperglycemia (Belton et al., 1965; Peters and Samaen, 1969; Kiser et al., 1970; Levin et al., 1970). The action of antiepileptic drugs on endocrine cells leads to a decrease in hormone secretion. This action may be due to a membrane effect, but no data are available to confirm this mechanism. In one study, carbohydrate intolerance was not observed with either toxic or nontoxic plasma levels of phenytoin (Callaghan et al., 1977). The investigators suggested that impaired insulin release is rarely a consequence of the routine treatment of epilepsy.

Weight gain is a common complication of valproic acid therapy, but its mechanism of production is unknown. A few patients experience an increase in appetite, but this is not the sole explanation. Thyroid function is not clinically disturbed, and carbohydrate metabolism does not appear grossly impaired. This problem has not been fully investigated.

Changes in Lipoprotein Metabolism

Both phenytoin and phenobarbital have been associated with elevated cholesterol levels (Miller and Nestel, 1973; Pelkonen et al., 1975). This may be related to an increase in the synthesis of high density lipoprotein (HDL) cholesterol as a result of hepatic microsomal enzyme induction (Nikkilä et al., 1978). Triglycerides also have been found to be elevated (Gordon et al., 1977). The clinical significance of this change in HDL is uncertain. It has been suggested, however, that HDL is inversely related to the risk of coronary artery disease (Gordon et al., 1977; Miller et al., 1977). Table 15.6 summarizes the adverse endocrine effects of the antiepileptic drugs.

Hematological Effects

The effects of antiepileptic drugs on the hematopoietic system can be classified under neonatal coagulation defects, bone marrow suppression, folate deficiency, and disturbances of platelets.

Neonatal Coagulation Defects

Neonatal coagulation defects have been strongly associated with both phenytoin and phenobarbital (Van Creveld, 1958; Monnet et al., 1968; Solomon et al., 1972). Many affected infants have been born to epileptic mothers receiving a combination of antiepileptic drugs (Kohler, 1966; Evans et al., 1970; Mountain et al., 1970). Phenobarbital has been shown to induce disturbances of the clotting mechanism in both experimental animals and neonates (Van Creveld, 1958; Monnet et al., 1968; Solomon et al., 1974). Infants born to mothers receiving hydantoins or phenobarbital may have clinical signs of intraperitoneal, intrathoracic, or intracranial bleeding within 24 hr of birth. Bleeding is caused by a deficiency of vitamin K-dependent clotting factors. The coagulation abnormalities are similar to those observed with hemorrhagic disease of the newborn in which clinical signs of bleeding

TABLE 15.6. *Endocrine effects of antiepileptic drugs*

Adverse reaction	Mechanism	Drug
Osteomalacia, rickets	Induction of vitamin D metabolism, decreased calcium absorption, inhibition of parathyroid hormone release	Phenytoin, phenobarbital
Hyperglycemia	Inhibition of insulin release	Phenytoin
Water and electrolyte disturbances	Inhibition of antidiuretic hormone release	Phenytoin, carbamazepine
Hirsutism, acne, chloasma	Disturbed sex hormone metabolism	Phenytoin, phenobarbital
Alopecia	Unknown	Valproic acid
Thyroid function tests	Decreased binding of thyroxine, increased peripheral clearance, increased conversion of T_4 to T_3	Phenytoin, valproic acid, carbamazepine
Subnormal metyrapone test	Increased excretion	Phenytoin, phenobarbital, carbamazepine
Failure of low-dose dexamethasone suppression tests	Increased excretion	Phenytoin, phenobarbital, carbamazepine
Weight change	Unknown	Valproic acid
Increase in serum cholesterol	Increased synthesis	Phenytoin, phenobarbital

generally begin 48 to 120 hr after delivery. Phenytoin and phenobarbital cross the placenta, concentrate in the fetal liver, compete with vitamin K, and prevent the production of vitamin K-dependent factors. The neonate's vitamin K balance has a narrow margin of safety because exogenous and intestinal sources of the vitamin are lacking. Very little vitamin K crosses the placenta. It is recommended that a small dose of vitamin K be administered to the mother before delivery or to the infant immediately after birth to prevent this coagulopathy (Kohler, 1966; Davies, 1960; Mountain et al., 1970; Solomon et al., 1972).

Bone Marrow Suppression

Agranulocytosis, pancytopenia, neutropenia, leukopenia, thrombocytopenia, and aplastic anemia occur less frequently with phenytoin, primidone, phenobarbital, and ethosuximide than with other antiepileptic drugs. Numerous reports of hematopoietic depression secondary to carbamazepine have appeared, but they mainly concerned elderly patients who were being treated for trigeminal neuralgia. Similar reports have been much less frequent in younger patients receiving this drug for the control of epileptic seizures (Killian and Fromm, 1968; Pearce and Ron, 1968; Saleh and Mendes de Leon, 1968; Killian, 1969; Prieur et al., 1973; Pisciotta, 1975). Selective erythroid aplasia has been reported with phenytoin (Yunis et al., 1967).

Megaloblastic Anemia and Folate Deficiency

Folate deficiency is a common occurrence in chronically treated epileptic patients; the incidence varies from 27 to 41% (Reynolds, 1972). The clinical significance is uncertain, except in the case of the megaloblastic anemia induced by antiepileptic drugs, which is unassociated with vitamin B_{12} deficiency. This anemia always responds to folic acid therapy. The role that folate plays in nucleoprotein synthesis is such that prolonged deficiency might be expected to result in pathophysiological changes in every organ system. Neuropsychiatric disturbances, neuropathy, congenital defects, and antiepileptic drug toxicity have all been attributed to folate deficiency.

The mechanism by which antiepileptic drugs produce folate deficiency is not clear, although several mechanisms are possible. Folate absorption (Hoffbrand and Necheles, 1968; Hoffbrand and Peters, 1968; Rosenberg et al., 1968), folate coenzyme metabolism (Baker et al., 1962), and tissue use of folate (Yunis et al., 1967) may be altered. The drugs most frequently implicated are phenytoin, phenobarbital, and primidone (Mannheimer et al., 1952; Bademoch, 1954; Chanarin et al., 1960; Druskin et al., 1962; Penny, 1963; Klipstein, 1964; Gibson, 1966; Reynolds et al., 1968; Reynolds, 1972). Most patients treated chronically with antiepileptic drugs have subnormal serum folate levels and normal serum vitamin B_{12} levels, but overt megaloblastic anemia is rare.

Some of the indicators of folate deficiency, other than megaloblastic anemia, include macrocytosis, decreased folate concentrations in the serum, red cells, and spinal fluid, marrow megaloblastosis, decreased serum lactic dehydrogenase, and hypersegmentation of peripheral neutrophils. Theoretically, widespread CNS damage, such as Purkinje cell loss, chronic encephalopathy, and peripheral neuropathy, could result from severe folate deficiency. Such changes, however, have not been reported commonly in patients with antiepileptic drug-induced megaloblastic anemia. Bone marrow megaloblastosis has been reported in a number of patients treated with antiepileptic drugs, but correlation with peripheral macrocytosis was poor (Reynolds, 1972). In the absence of anemia, hypersegmented neutrophils have been found in 10 to 40% of patients with low folate levels, and macrocytosis has been found in 9 to 51% (Hawkins and Meynell, 1958)).

Disturbances of Platelets

Valproic acid may cause mild thrombocytopenia in many patients, but the mechanisms for this are unknown (Sutor and Jesdinsky-Buscher, 1974; Simon and Penry, 1975; Pinder et al., 1977; Bruni and Wilder, 1979a; Neophytides et al., 1979). It is not thought to be related to bone marrow suppression but may be related to increased peripheral destruction of platelets. Rarely, a prolonged bleeding time in the absence of thrombocytopenia is observed. A decreased erythrocyte sedimentation rate (Nutt et al., 1978) and low fibrinogen levels (Dale et al., 1978) have also been observed. We have not found any of these abnormalities to be clinically significant. Inhibition of the secondary phase of platelet aggregation may occur

TABLE 15.7. *Hematological effects of antiepileptic drugs*

Adverse reactions	Mechanism	Drug
Neonatal coagulopathy	Deficiency of vitamin K – dependent factors	Phenytoin, phenobarbital, primidone
Agranulocytosis, neutropenia, pancytopenia, leukopenia, thrombocytopenia, aplastic anemia	Bone marrow suppression	Carbamazepine
Erythroid aplasia	Suppression of erythroid series	Phenytoin
Megaloblastosis, folate deficiency, megaloblastic anemia	Altered folate absorption, folate coenzyme metabolism, tissue use of folate	Phenytoin, phenobarbital, primidone
Thrombocytopenia, inhibition of secondary phase platelet aggregation	Unknown	Valproic acid
Hypofibrinogenemia	Unknown	Valproic acid
Lowered erythrocyte sedimentation rate	? Hypofibrinogenemia	Valproic acid

(Stores, 1975), but this is generally of no clinical importance. The significance of these changes in the patient undergoing surgery is not known. In the patient undergoing major surgery, coagulation function should be screened; if abnormalities are found, valproic acid should be temporarily discontinued if possible.

Table 15.7 summarizes the hematological side effects of antiepileptic therapy.

Immunological Effects

Immunological disorders caused by antiepileptic drugs may result in acute allergic reactions or chronic toxicity. Lymphadenopathy resembling a malignant lymphoma may occur after chronic therapy (Bjornberg and Holst, 1967). Whether the occurrence of a true malignant transformation occurs in epileptic patients is uncertain. It has been suggested, however, that an etiological relationship might exist between phenytoin therapy and malignant lymphoma (Charlton and Lunsford, 1971). Occasionally, the syndrome has occurred with the administration of primidone and phensuximide. This syndrome may be related to decreased immunological surveillance, since it has been found that a number of phenytoin-treated patients have depressed cellular and humoral immunity (Sorrell et al., 1971). The reduced production of IgA in some patients has been confirmed (Slavin et al., 1974). It has been suggested that IgA deficiency is more likely to develop in phenytoin-treated patients possessing the HLA-A$_2$ histocompatibility antigen (Shakir et al., 1978). As mentioned above, salivary IgA may be decreased in patients with gingival hyperplasia (Aarli, 1976), but decreased salivary IgA has not been found, despite a decrease in plasma IgA (Smith et al., 1979b).

Hydantoin drugs have been reported to induce a lupus-like syndrome (Smith et al., 1979b), and antinuclear antibodies have also been implicated (Alarcon-Segovia et al., 1972). The presence of antinuclear antibodies has been confirmed, and lymphocytotoxins of the IgM class have also been been found (Ooi et al., 1977).

These findings may have importance in the genesis of an altered immune state of epileptic patients receiving phenytoin. A carbamazepine-induced lupus-like syndrome also has been observed. Deposits of plasma proteins have been found in biopsies from patients receiving carbamazepine or phenytoin. Dermatological side effects were not noted (Permin and Sestoft, 1977). These most often consisted of IgA deposits, but IgM deposits were also found. The changes were similar to those seen in patients with systemic or drug-induced lupus erythematosus with or without lesions.

Hepatic Dysfunction

The significance of hepatic enzyme induction by antiepileptic drugs is unknown, and no definite proof exists that this may result in a higher incidence of hepatic tumors in humans. In animals, however, phenobarbital can induce hepatic enzymes. The enzyme induction of the fetal liver does not result in an increased incidence of tumors in neonates of epileptic mothers.

Hepatitis from phenytoin or phenobarbital is uncommon and is usually on an immunological basis (Welton, 1950; Harinasuta and Zimmerman, 1968; Martin and Rickers, 1972; Dhar et al., 1974; Evans et al., 1976; Parker and Shearer, 1979). This is generally associated with a skin rash, fever, lymphadenopathy, and eosinophilia. Potentially fatal hepatic necrosis can occur at any time during the course of therapy. Carbamazepine can also cause hepatic dysfunction, which is generally reversible but may rarely be fatal (Zucker et al., 1977).

The hepatotoxicity of valproic acid has been reported, but most patients were also taking other antiepileptic drugs (Willmore et al., 1978). Rare fatal cases have been reported (Suchy et al., 1979). The mechanism of toxicity is uncertain, but chemicals related in structure to valproic acid are hepatotoxic.

Renal Toxicity

Trimethadione is the only antiepileptic drug that has a significant incidence of renal toxicity (Wells, 1957). Albuminuria and the nephrotic syndrome may occur. Rarely, renal failure may result from a hypersensitivity reaction to phenytoin (Michael and Mitch, 1976).

TERATOGENICITY

The incidence of congenital malformations in children born of epileptic mothers is about three times that in offspring of nonepileptic mothers. The role played by antiepileptic drugs is not clear. Congenital anomalies have occurred in 6% of newborn offspring from drug-treated epileptic mothers, 4.2% of newborns from untreated epileptic mothers, and 2% of offspring from nonepileptic mothers (Speidel and Meadow, 1972; Janz, 1975). Most epileptic patients receive multiple drug therapy, and interpretation of potential individual drug teratogenesis is difficult. A higher incidence of anomalies has been found in infants born to mothers receiving combined treatment with phenytoin and phenobarbital than with phenytoin or phenobarbital alone (Fedrick, 1973). Many investigators have demonstrated that the epileptic woman on antiepileptic therapy is at a higher risk of delivering an affected child (Speidel and Meadow, 1972; South, 1972; Monson et al., 1973; Miller and Nevin, 1973; Annegers et al., 1974). It has also been shown that women with epilepsy have a higher incidence of complications during pregnancy and labor (Bjerkedal and Bahna, 1973).

Malformations associated with antiepileptic drugs are, in descending order of frequency, cleft lip and palate, abnormalities of the heart, skeleton, and CNS, hypospadias, and intestinal atresia. A fetal hydantoin syndrome has also been described (Hanson et al., 1976), but it is not universally accepted as a distinct entity.

No single drug appears to be more teratogenic than the others; however, no malformation has been definitely attributed to carbamazepine (Niebyl et al., 1979) or valproic acid. The latter is teratogenic in experimental animals (Whittle, 1976), but its role in human teratogenesis is unknown because experience with its use is still limited.

The mechanism of antiepileptic drug-induced malformation is unknown, but it may be related to chromosomal abnormalities (Herha and Obe, 1977), folate deficiency (Herbert, 1968; Arakawa, 1970; Meadow, 1970), or a combined effect of folate deficiency and tissue concentration of phenytoin (DeVore and Woodbury, 1977).

Many questions relating to pregnancy and teratogenicity of the antiepileptic drugs remain unanswered. The practical question is whether treatment should be continued during pregnancy. The risk of problems resulting from antiepileptic drug therapy during pregnancy would appear to be minor, provided the patient receives medical care by a physician who anticipates potential problems and takes appropriate action. Careful clinical evaluation and antiepileptic drug monitoring should be part of the routine follow-up. Antiepileptic drugs should be maintained at the lowest plasma concentrations that will offer satisfactory seizure control. A recent report summarizes the current thinking on congenital malformations in epileptic patients (Meadow, 1979); the conclusions are:

1. An increased incidence, but not the cause, is firmly established.

2. No increase in congenital malformations is observed in children born before the onset or after remission of the epilepsy or in children of an epileptic mother not taking antiepileptic medication (contradicted in some studies).

3. The father's epilepsy is not a major factor in the contribution to congenital malformations.

4. It is unlikely that the frequency or severity of seizures during pregnancy has an important effect on the incidence of major congenital malformations.

5. The incidence of epilepsy in children of parents with epilepsy is increased.

6. There is no suggestion that antiepileptic drugs or seizures during pregnancy contribute to the increased incidence of epilepsy in the offspring.

16

Quantitative Laboratory Analysis of Antiepileptic Drugs

Within the past 10 years, the quantitation of antiepileptic drugs in plasma and other biological fluids has advanced from a problem solvable by only a few and only with much time and effort, to a generally accepted and necessary, routine clinical procedure, performed accurately in many laboratories throughout the world by a number of sensitive and selective methodologies. Few specific problems in chemical analysis have commanded such widespread attention and concentrated, cooperative effort on the part of analytical chemists, pharmacologists, physicians, and other physical and biological scientists. The rewards of this effort are now reflected in national and international quality control programs, such rapid methods of analysis that the results can be made available to a physician during the patient's visit, and techniques so simple to perform that an inexperienced technician can be trained in a few hours. This advanced state of the art, however, does not in itself guarantee precise and accurate clinical data. Reliable laboratories still devote much time to the selection, evaluation, and improvement of methods, and consistently accurate results can always be traced to a conscientiously applied quality control program.

METHODS

Three basic methodologies are currently used for the analysis of antiepileptic drugs: spectrophotometry, immunoassay, and chromatography. Of these, only the chromatographic methods are versatile, specific, and sensitive enough to be applied to all the currently used drugs and their metabolites over the full concentration range of interest for each. However, because only a research laboratory or a laboratory specializing in antiepileptic drug analysis would be concerned with this capability, there is a definite place for the more limited techniques. Two major reference works on the use and analysis of antiepileptic drugs are available (Woodbury et al., 1972; Pippenger et al., 1978). The first covers much of the early work in pharmacology and analysis. The second updates the earlier work and deals mainly with quantitation and good laboratory practice, and should be considered a necessity for anyone involved in anticonvulsant drug analysis.

Spectrophotometry

Spectrophotometry, the earliest method of antiepileptic drug analysis, is based on the absorption of light of a specified wave length by a chemical substance in solution. Under certain conditions, this absorbance is proportional to the concentration of the species of interest. Some chemical species are capable of absorbing light of a certain wavelength (energy) and then reemitting light of lower energy (longer wavelength). This property of fluorescence can also be used for quantitation and can impart greater sensitivity to an analysis; rather than measuring a relatively small difference in high light intensities, the emitted light intensity is measured with respect to a zero light level or nonemitting blank. In absorbance spectrophotometry, the light source, sample cell, and photodetector are in line; in fluorescence spectrophotometry, the photodetector is at a right angle to the line of the light source and sample cell.

Only phenobarbital, phenytoin, and carbamazepine can be analyzed by spectrophotometric techniques. Because of sample size restrictions and interferences from commonly used drugs, only the phenytoin and carbamazepine methods have sufficient specificity and sensitivity to be generally useful. Good reviews of early work on phenytoin and phenobarbital (Wallace and Hamilton, 1974) and carbamazepine (Fellenberg and Pollard, 1976a,b) are available. The methods of Goldbaum (1952) for phenobarbital, Wallace et al. (1965) for phenytoin, and Beyer and Klinge (1969) for carbamazepine are the forerunners of modern practical techniques.

The state of the art for quantitative analysis of phenytoin and carbamazepine is reflected in the articles by Fellenberg et al. (1975) and Fellenberg and Pollard (1976a), respectively. These methods have been combined (Fellenberg and Pollard, 1976b) to allow assay of both drugs in a single, small (0.1 to 0.2 ml) sample. Because the phenobarbital assay is not so specific or sensitive, it is not generally useful for therapeutic monitoring (Wallace and Hamilton, 1974). Fluorometric methods for phenytoin (Dill and Glazko, 1972; Dill et al., 1976) and carbamazepine (Meilink, 1974) have been reported. The phenytoin assay involves a simple extension of Wallace's procedure and is based on the fluorescence of benzophenone in concentrated sulfuric acid.

The primary advantages of spectrophotometric methods are as follows: (a) after extraction and reaction procedures are performed, relatively little time is required to take the actual measurements; and (b) the instruments are generally available, inexpensive, and need not be dedicated solely to anticonvulsant analysis. Disadvantages include (a) the lack of selectivity in the case of phenobarbital, and (b) the inability to monitor all anticonvulsants. It is generally accepted procedure to analyze samples in duplicate since spectrophotometry does not incorporate some type of internal standardization, as do the chromatographic techniques. Also, the analyst must be continually conscious of technique, since the methods require precise transfer of volumes. This can be a significant source of error, especially when volatile organic solvents are involved.

Immunoassay

The immunochemical techniques that have been applied to anticonvulsant analysis are radioimmunoassay (RIA) and homogeneous enzyme immunoassay. These and other immunoassay techniques are based on a competitive binding reaction between an analyte and some labeled analyte-macromolecule complex for an antibody that has been produced specifically for the system. In the typical immunoassay, the drug or hapten is made immunogenic (capable of stimulating antibody production) by covalently bonding it to some large molecule, usually a protein. The complex (antigen) is injected into an animal in an attempt to produce antibodies that will bind specifically to the antigen and also to the original hapten. If this occurs, the animal serum then becomes an analytical reagent. The second reagent is an antigen solution, adjusted to the approximate concentration of the hapten in the system to be analyzed. The activity of the antibody reagent (animal serum) is adjusted to bind 20 to 70% of the antigen in the absence of hapten. In the presence of hapten, a competition between the antigen and hapten for antibody binding sites results in an increase of unbound antigen in proportion to the concentration of hapten. The final consideration is that there must be some method of measuring the unbound antigen.

In RIA, the antigen is made radioactive so that it is only necessary to measure the radioactivity. Since both bound and unbound antigen are radioactive, however, they must first be separated. This is usually accomplished by a simple protein precipitation. In the enzyme multiplied immunoassay technique (EMIT®),[1] no separation step is necessary because only the unbound antigen acts to produce a measurable response. The antigen is a drug-enzyme complex formed with glucose-6-phosphate dehydrogenase and is only active when it is not bound to antibody. In the unbound state, the antigen catalyzes the oxidation of glucose-6-phosphate to 6-phosphoglucono-δ-lactone with the accompanying reduction of NAD^+ to NADH. The rate of increase of NADH is measured spectrophotometrically at 340 nm. Since each molecule of enzyme catalyzes many oxidation reactions (EMIT), the method contains a built-in chemical amplification system that greatly increases the sensitivity.

---

[1]Syva Company, Palo Alto, California 94394.

Cook et al. (1976*b*) and Cook (1978) have reviewed the procedures for the production of antigens that will produce specific antibodies, along with other important considerations in the development and use of immunoassays. Excellent reviews of immunoassay techniques are available (Brattin and Sunshine, 1973; Hawker, 1973; Bidanset, 1974; Sharpe et al., 1976; Wisdom, 1976; Pippenger, 1976), the latest being those by Felber (1978) on RIA and Curtis and Patel (1978) on EMIT. Fernandez and Loeb (1975) and Rodbard et al. (1969) discuss the logit transform used to linearize the sigmoid curve that is characteristic of immunoassays.

Although RIA procedures have been reported for phenytoin (Tigelaar et al., 1973; Cook et al., 1976*a,b*; Paxton et al., 1977), phenobarbital (Cook et al., 1976*a,b*), and clonazepam (Dixon et al., 1975), only phenytoin and phenobarbital reagent kits are commercially available. A comprehensive guide to radioassay has been published (American Association of Clinical Chemists, 1978) and includes data on sample size, sensitivity, incubation time, sources of RIA kits, literature references, and a problem solving guide. Since a considerable amount of skill, knowledge of chemical synthesis and immunological techniques, and chemical and biological resources are necessary for the successful development of immunoassay procedures, it is reasonable to assume that only the commercially available tests will be of interest. Also, only laboratories having the counting equipment, licensure, and expertise available for the performance of these assays will be interested, since their versatility and general applicability to a comprehensive antiepileptic drug monitoring program are severely limited.

The advantages of RIA lie in the sensitivity and simplicity of the technique, which consists only of addition of reagents to a small specimen (0.1 ml), incubation (45 to 60 min), separation of free and bound antigen (protein precipitation), and counting. The free drug may be determined in small samples of plasma, saliva, tissue, or plasma ultrafiltrate. The disadvantages of RIA arise from its applicability to only two drugs, the need for expensive radioactivity monitoring equipment (gamma ray spectrometer for ^{125}I or liquid scintillation counter for ^3H), licensure (for ^{125}I use), and technical personnel specially trained in radioisotope methodology. More versatile, faster, simpler, and less expensive techniques are available for anticonvulsant analysis.

A primary example of the last statement is the EMIT. In the last 5 years, it has become the most used assay in the United States for antiepileptic drug analysis (Dijkhuis et al., 1979). Based on a morphine assay first described by Rubenstein et al. (1972), the method involves a simple mixing of reagents and monitoring of the absorbance change of the mixture over a short time (45 sec). The measurement phase is performed in a specially modified spectrophotometer, the output of which is recorded by a timer-calculator designed to read the absorbance at specific times after sample introduction and to calculate the difference ($A_{45sec} - A_{15sec}$).

The advantages of the EMIT include commercial availability of complete instrument systems and reagents for analysis of the six major antiepileptic drugs (phenobarbital, primidone, phenytoin, carbamazepine, ethosuximide, and valproic acid) and adaptability to automated clinical analyzer systems (Hardin et al., 1976;

Howell et al., 1978; Malkus et al., 1978; Urquhart et al., 1979). In addition, minimal training and technical expertise are needed to run the assay, which requires only 50 μl plasma or serum for four single drug determinations, and a preparation and analysis time of about 90 sec for each determination after calibration. The small sample size makes this an ideal technique for pediatric samples and for monitoring free drug levels in plasma ultrafiltrates (Booker and Darcy, 1973) and saliva (McAuliffe et al., 1977).

The versatility of the technique is limited, however, as reflected by the relatively narrow concentration ranges covered by normal calibration curves and by its applicability to only six drugs. These factors, along with the ever-present danger of malfunction in a "black box" type system that does not lend itself to on-site troubleshooting, makes a chromatographic back-up system a requirement to handle the extremes of concentrations, or more likely, the drugs and metabolites that are not covered. The primary disadvantage of EMIT is the high cost of reagents. The cost is always doubled for each drug, since duplicate assays are necessary, and may be tripled if the initial determination finds the level outside the normal calibration range, requiring sample dilution and reanalysis. A less tangible but nevertheless real factor is the effect of the repetitive simplicity of the technique on the attitude and interest of the technician. Employee morale and analytical quality both may be negatively affected.

Adaptation of the method to an automated analyzer (Abbott ABA-100, Dupont ACA, Perkin Elmer KA-150, CentrifiChem, Gemsaec, Gilford System 3400, 3402, and 3500) can totally negate the latter objection and also reduce reagent cost per test by about 60%. An international quality control study (Dijkhuis et al., 1979) has indicated that reduction of reagent volume to less than 20 μl (normal volume, 50 μl) results in unacceptable coefficients of variation in most cases. Generally, in comparison with chromatographic methods (Booker and Darcy, 1975; Schmidt, 1976; Spiehler et al., 1976; Schmidt et al., 1977), the EMIT system gave equal or greater coefficients of variation. However, few differences would have resulted in a change in clinical interpretation. Nandedkar et al. (1978) and others have noted a "bottom of the bottle" effect and recommend mixing the last milliliter or so of reagent with the next new bottle to eliminate the problem. Recently, two independent groups (Flachs and Rasmussen, 1980; McDonald and Kabra, 1980) reported apparently increased phenytoin levels in patients with renal disease when samples were analyzed by EMIT. They concluded that cross-reaction of the EMIT reagents with the increased conjugated 5-(*p*-hydroxyphenyl)-5-phenylhydantoin (HPPH) in plasma of the uremic patients was responsible. This theory has not been confirmed.

Chromatography

Chromatographic techniques are based on differential migration and transport of analytes through a bed of sorbent material (stationary phase) in a second carrier phase (mobile phase), which may or may not contribute to the separation. For the present discussion, these include thin-layer, gas-liquid, and high-performance liquid chromatography (TLC, GLC, and HPLC, respectively). Resolution is affected by selection of the stationary phase and, if applicable, the mobile phase to achieve different solute (analyte) velocities for each component. Solute velocities are determined by the relative affinities of sample components for the two phases. A solute that prefers the mobile phase will move faster through the chromatographic bed than one that prefers the stationary phase. The usual problem, however, is the separation of solutes that vary only slightly in their preference for the phases and, therefore, move with similar velocities. Up-to-date references on theory and practice include those by Touchstone and Dobbins (1978) on TLC, Grob (1977) on GLC, and Snyder and Kirkland (1979) on HPLC. The most complete work on chromatographic theory in general is still the monograph by Giddings (1965).

Chromatographic techniques differ from spectrophotometric and immunoassay methods by allowing the use of internal standards. These are compounds that are added to calibration samples and unknowns at constant concentration and are chemically and chromatographically similar to the species of interest. Dudley (1978) has reviewed the use of internal standards in quantitation of anticonvulsants. In short, an internal standard is chosen that can be chromatographically separated from the analyte but otherwise will undergo the same chemical reactions and behave like the analyte during the prechromatographic procedures, i.e., solvent extraction, evaporation. The ratio of the detector response, peak height or area (Janik, 1975), of the analyte to that of the internal standard is the parameter used for calibration and quantitation. A correctly chosen internal standard, therefore, will "track" the analyte through all structural changes or handling losses that occur.

Thin-Layer Chromatography

In TLC, the stationary phase is coated on a flat sheet of glass, metal, or plastic and is commonly a small-particle silica gel. The samples to be analyzed usually are treated by solvent extraction, and the concentrated extracts are spotted on the plate by microsyringe in a line parallel to the bottom of the plate. The plate then is placed in a chamber in contact with the mobile phase, which rises up the plate by capillary action, carrying with it the components of the sample according to their relative affinities for the mobile and stationary phases. After development, the sample components in the form of spots or bands are visualized by exposing the plate to either ultraviolet light and watching for absorption or fluorescence or to some chemical reagent that produces a colored product. Quantitation can be either off-line, in which case the spots are scraped from the plate, eluted from the stationary phase, and assayed by some other technique, or on-line, in which case the spots are detected *in situ* by a densitometer that monitors transmitted, reflected, or fluorescent light. Frei (1972) and Kirchner (1973) have evaluated the various densitometric methods and reviewed the sources of error in each.

TLC was first used by Huisman (1966) as an adjunct to a spectrophotometric technique (Dill et al., 1956) to expand the range of drugs that could be assayed. Pippenger et al. (1969) reported a three-eluent screening system that allowed qualitative and semiquantitative analysis of phenobarbital, primidone, phenytoin, mephenytoin, normephenytoin, and phenylethylmalonamide. However, gas chromatographic methods, also introduced around this time, rapidly became the focus of most research. Nevertheless, because of improvements in densitometric instruments and thin-layer media, some newer TLC methods deserve attention. Hundt and Clark (1975) have assayed carbamazepine and its epoxide and diol metabolites by directly spotting 1 μl plasma and, after development, converting the analytes to fluorescent derivatives by exposure to HCl gas and ultraviolet light.The authors claim limits of detection of 0.1 and 0.05 μg/ml for the parent drug and epoxide, respectively. Other workers have developed methods for simultaneous determination of phenobarbital, primidone, mephenytoin, phenytoin, carbamazepine, and carbamazepine epoxide (Wad et al., 1977; Wad and Rosenmund, 1978) and the benzodiazepine anticonvulsants clonazepam and diazepam and their metabolites (Wad et al., 1976; Wad and Hanifl, 1977).

The advantage of TLC is its capability of providing rapid, qualitative analysis of many samples at very low cost. When the method is made quantitative, the cost of the instrumentation required generally exceeds that of gas or liquid chromatography, and the level of expertise must increase to the point where the simplicity of the technique is lost. In addition, because the scanning step alone can approach the elution time of the other chromatographic methods, the time gained in the simultaneous development of many samples is also lost. Therefore, as with RIA, unless the equipment and personnel are already available, TLC is not competitive with gas or liquid chromatography.

Gas-Liquid Chromatography

From 1970 to 1976, most of the articles on antiepileptic drug analysis reported new or modified GLC assays. GLC allows integrated purification and qualitative and quantitative analysis of sample components in the microgram to picogram range. Coupling this with the capability of performing simultaneous, broad spectrum analysis of any biological fluid or tissue, and a variety of sensitive, selective detection systems makes gas chromatography one of the most powerful techniques available for drug and metabolite analysis.

Basically, a gas chromatograph consists of three parts: (a) an injection port, usually a simple septum injector, (b) a column oven, and (c) a detector; all have separate temperature controls and various associated electronics. The oven control should be accurately programmable to heat the column at a constant rate during a chromatographic run, if necessary. To prevent sample decomposition, the column, where the actual separation takes place, should be glass; it should be well packed with a high quality packing material that has been proved effective for the intended application. The packing material consists of a thin layer of a thermally stable liquid of low volatility (stationary phase), coated upon a porous solid support (diatomaceous earth), that has been carefully treated to insure inertness and sized to insure regularity in the packed bed. Numerous books cover all phases of gas chromatographic theory and instrumentation, but the chapter by Gibbs and Gibbs (1978) is one of the most complete and concise treatments of practical GLC.

Four detection systems have been used in antiepileptic drug analysis. The most common is the flame ionization detector (FID), which consists of a hydrogen-oxygen flame burning atop an insulated jet at the column outlet, and a collector electrode. A high voltage is applied between the jet and the collector. Organic compounds that elute from the column ionized in the flame, decrease the resistance in the electrode gap, and cause an increase in current, which is measured. The FID is nonselective and is generally applicable in the high nanogram and microgram range.

The alkali FID (AFID), also called the thermionic emission or nitrogen-phosphorous detector, is a modified FID that can be made selective to nitrogen or phosphorous compounds by varying the polarity of the electrodes and adjusting the fuel-to-oxidizer ratio of the flame gases. The modification consists of the addition of an electrically heated, alkali metal-impregnated glass or ceramic bead located above the flame jet. Flame gases are adjusted to give a low flame temperature, generally resulting in transfer of the flame zone from the jet to the bead. Thus ionization does not occur until the compounds enter the bead area containing a plasma of thermally produced alkali metal ions which selectively ionizes nitrogen-containing compounds, as in the case of antiepileptic drugs. Because of this selectivity, interferences from normal plasma constituents, such as fatty acids, are eliminated. Olah et al. (1979) have reviewed the early literature and mechanisms of operation of the AFID. This detector was first applied to antiepileptic drug analysis by Goudie and Burnett (1973). The increased sensitivity of this detector allowed analysts to develop methods requiring as little as 50 μl plasma.

The electron capture detector (ECD) has been used for many years for analysis of halogen-containing compounds. In antiepileptic drug analysis, assay of benzodiazepines is the major application. Modern ECDs operate in a constant current mode, giving a linear dynamic range of four or five orders of magnitude. Basically, the carrier gas (nitrogen or argon + 5% methane) is ionized by beta emission from a radioactive ^{63}Ni source, producing a standing or steady-state current between two electrodes. This current is maintained by regular, constant amplitude voltage pulses applied to the electrodes. If a compound having a high electron affinity passes through the detector, free electrons produced by carrier gas ionization are removed and current is reduced. The voltage pulse circuitry operates in a feedback loop that causes an increase in pulse rate to maintain the constant standing current. The pulse frequency is proportional to the concentration of the electron absorber in the detector. Sensitivity limits for the ECD extend into the low picogram range, allowing analysis of nanogram drug levels in 50 to 100 μl plasma.

The fourth detection system, which is discussed only briefly, is the mass spectrometer (MS). Although sensitive and specific, it will not soon become a routine part of clinical analysis because of the cost and the expertise needed to maintain the instrument and interpret results. The MS can be interfaced directly to a gas chromatograph or, with much more difficulty and expense, to a liquid chromatograph. It is used to identify and quantitate chemical substances by creating ions and ion fragments of molecules and separating these products according to mass-to-charge ratio (m/z). Various means of fragmentation are available, and various signals may be monitored, depending on the type of information desired. Selected ion monitoring allows the analyst to choose a particular ion or ions and disregard all others.

Horning et al. (1974) have described combined GC-MS analyses for antiepileptic drugs. In the most recent application of the MS, the gas chromatograph has been eliminated. Schier et al. (1980) have analyzed valproic acid, ethosuximide, phenobarbital, mephobarbital, primidone, phenytoin, and carbamazepine simultaneously in the equivalent of 20 μl plasma by extracting the drugs into chloroform and, after concentration of the extract, vaporizing an aliquot directly into the ionization chamber of a MS operated in the chemical ionization mode. Magnitudes of the molecular ion peaks for each drug are used for quantitation, based on stable isotope analogs of several drugs, which function as internal standards.

Some of the earliest procedures that were developed for pharmacokinetic studies introduced internal standards that are still in use today. Buchanan et al. (1969) established 2,2,3-trimethylsuccinimide for ethosuximide analysis, and Chang and Glazko (1970) reported the use of 5-(p-methylphenyl)-5-phenylhydantoin (MPPH), which became the primary standard for multiple drug analysis during the early years of method development. Pippenger and Gillen (1969) introduced the idea of simultaneous multiple drug analysis and mentioned the possible use of temperature programing to optimize retention.

The two reports that had the most influence on the early development of antiepileptic drug assays were published almost simultaneously by Kupferberg (1970) and MacGee (1970). They introduced the on-column methylation reagents trimethylphenylammonium hydroxide (TMPAH), reported by Brochmann-Hanssen and Oke (1969), and tetramethylammonium hydroxide (TMAH), reported by Robb and Westbrook (1963) and Stevenson (1966). The Kupferberg technique, later modified to include carbamazepine (Kupferberg, 1972), used an efficient extraction and allowed simultaneous analysis of phenobarbital, primidone, and phenytoin. The extraction procedure was long, requiring about 3 hr. The final residue could be dissolved in a dilute methylating reagent (0.1 mole/liter), however, minimizing the degradation of phenobarbital, a problem mentioned by Stevenson (1966) and later studied by numerous investigators (Osiewicz et al., 1974; Wu, 1974; Wang et al., 1976; Callery and Leslie, 1977). MacGee's novel use of concentrated (2.0 moles/liter) methylating reagent as an extractant paved the way for the rapid extraction procedures that followed.

Solow and Green (1972) used MacGee's extraction without modification but adapted the chromatographic step by temperature programing to analyze the barbiturate, succinimide, and hydantoin drugs. The solvent (toluene) used to remove the drugs from plasma extracts only 71% of the phenytoin, 46% of the phenobarbital, and 8% of the primidone (Perchalski and Wilder, 1978b). Perchalski et al. (1973) introduced an initial ether extraction to maintain the efficiency of the Kupferberg method and used concentrated TMPAH (1.5 moles/liter) to maintain the speed of the MacGee method. Unfortunately, phenobarbital could not be quantified directly using MPPH as internal standard because, in addition to formation of the expected *N,N*-dimethylphenobarbital, there was also extensive degradation to *N*-methyl- and *N-N*-dimethy-α-phenylybutyramide. This problem was effectively although unconventionally solved by adding the responses for the three products after correcting for peak width differences and using the sum as the total phenobarbital response.

The problem of phenobarbital degradation was finally solved by Gibbs and Gibbs (1974), who introduced 5-ethyl-5-(*p*-methylphenyl)-barbituric acid (MPB) as a specific standard. Solow et al. (1974), Dudley et al. (1977), and Perchalski and Wilder (1978*b*) have shown that, although the relative amounts of the three derivatives are variable and unpredictable for each of these barbiturates, the ratios of the N,N-dimethyl derivatives and the butyramide derivatives are reproducible and linear over the concentration range of interest. Dudley et al. (1977) also introduced the methylprimidone analog, which should be used if the extraction efficiency for primidone is low. This occurs if toluene or mixtures of toluene and a more polar solvent (ether, ethyl acetate) are used to extract the drugs from plasma or if a dilute methylating reagent is used for the final extraction.

The on-column methylation techniques are generally applicable to analysis of the succinimide, barbiturate, and hydantoin anticonvulsants. Carbamazepine has been included (Roger et al., 1973), but most investigators agree that degradation reactions that occur are not reproducible unless an automatic injection system is used (Darcey et al., 1978). Some workers have tried the higher tetraalkylammonium homologs to achieve increased retention and resolution, separation of *N*-methyl anticonvulsants from their demethylated metabolites (mephobarbital, mephenytoin, phensuximide, methsuximide), cleaner chromatograms, and fewer side reactions (Friel and Troupin, 1974; Pecci and Giovanniello, 1975; Kumps and Mardens, 1975). These methods have not become popular, however, probably because of the unavailability of commercial reagents. An extensive review of pyrolytic alkylation has been published (Kossa et al., 1979) and covers most of the anticonvulsant applications in addition to mechanisms and problems associated with the technique.

An off-column akylation technique that solved some of the problems of on-column alkylation was introduced by Greeley (1974). The new method required formation of an ion pair with the acidic drug and a strong organic base (TMAH) in a moderately polar solvent (methanol: *N,N*-dimethylacetamide) and then reaction with any of the alkyl iodides to give the desired product. The quaternary ammonium iodide precipitated out during the reaction; thus a fairly clean, unreactive solution of the alkylated drugs was injected. The advantages of decreased injection temperature, prolonged column life, and elimination of side reactions were immediately apparent. Vandemark and Adams (1976) combined the techniques of MacGee and Greeley with the sensitive, selective AFID to analyze a number of drugs in 50-μl plasma samples.

The only other gas chromatographic system that has been developed for broad spectrum simultaneous antiepileptic drug analysis involves no derivatization but requires a column packing material specially developed, prepared, and tested for the purpose. Several reports on the use of this phase[2] have appeared (Godolphin and Thoma, 1978; Hewitt et al., 1978; Thoma et al., 1978). Even though the column is capable of resolving a large number of drugs in a standard mixture, analysis of plasma samples is hindered by several natural plasma constituents (cholesterol, fatty acids) unless more extensive extraction procedures are used. The difficulties of underivatized analysis have been noted by Darcey et al. (1978) and include necessarily higher column temperatures that lead to shortened column life, evidenced by peak tailing and nonreproducibility of analyses and degradation of labile compounds.

Several antiepileptic drugs are most easily analyzed singly without derivatization. Including them in a longer chromatographic run to achieve "simultaneous" analysis introduces more problems than it solves. These drugs are valproic acid, trimethadione and its major metabolite dimethadione, and ethosuximide. Valproic acid is measured by a modification (Kupferberg, 1978) of the Dill procedure for ethosuximide (Glazko and Dill, 1972), which expectedly allows simultaneous determination of the latter with the proper column (SP-1000). Following deproteinization with perchloric acid (10%), the acid and an appropriate internal standard (cyclohexane carboxylic acid, cyclopentylacetic acid) are extracted into chloroform, which is evaporated carefully to 30 to 50 µl after addition of 80 µl amyl acetate. If desired, appropriate internal standards can be added for the barbiturates and hydantoins at the beginning of the analysis, and the amyl acetate residue can be taken up in toluene, which can then be extracted with TMAH or TMPAH for subsequent analysis by on-column methylation (Perchalski and Wilder, 1974*b*). Several modifications of the procedure of Dijkhuis and Vervloet (1974), which involves extraction of valproic acid into a small volume of a halogenated solvent and direct injection, have been published (Wood et al., 1977; Berry and Clarke, 1978; Levy et al., 1978), along with a simple acidification of plasma (20 µl) with 10 µl of 1 M HCl containing the internal standard, followed by direct injection (Jakobs et al., 1978). All chromatography is done on acidified polyester (EGA, DEGS) or polyglycol phases (SP-1000).

Although derivatization offers no real advantage, valproic acid also has been analyzed by on-column methylation (Varma and Hoshino, 1979), off-column butylation by the Greeley technique (Holshoff and Roseboom, 1979), and as the *p*-bromophenacyl ester (Gupta et al., 1979). This last report gives a complete list of references on valproic acid analysis. An extensive and careful study of many of the problems associated with the analysis of valproic acid has been done by Hershey et al. (1979). New internal standards were synthesized and evaluated, and non-hygroscopic barium salts were prepared for use as primary standards.

The initial optimized analysis of trimethadione and dimethadione was reported by Booker and Darcy (1971). Under the normal extraction conditions employed in

---

[2] SP-2510-DA, Supelco, Inc., Bellefonte, Pennsylvania 16823.

cluding charcoal adsorption (Adams and Vandemark, 1976), solvent extraction (Adams et al., 1978), simple deproteinization (Kabra et al., (1977), and a combination of deproteinization and solvent extraction (Perchalski et al., 1979). Increased column temperature has been used to maximize resolution and sensitivity and to minimize pressure and retention (Perchalski and Wilder, 1979).

Although an understanding of the physical and chemical processes that occur in a liquid chromatography column and an appreciation of the theory of liquid chromatography would require considerable study, the use of modern liquid chromatography instrumentation is extremely simple. The basic equipment can be less expensive than that required for any of the other techniques. Most drugs and metabolites are analyzed without derivatization on a single system with simple variation of mobile phase elution strength to maximize throughput.[5] For example, samples containing only phenobarbital and phenytoin can be chromatographed in less than 5 min with 45% acetonitrile on Spherisorb ODS (internal standard: MPPH).

QUALITY CONTROL

The particular methods that a laboratory selects are determined by the needs of those who use the service and the resources available to those who offer the service. No method can be expected to yield consistently accurate results, however, unless it is based on daily intralaboratory and periodic interlaboratory quality control. It is also possible for a laboratory to generate satisfactory quality control data on a daily basis and still not be producing accurate patient data. A monthly comparison of results with other laboratories will alert laboratory personnel to this possibility so that the problem (e.g., impure drug standards, inaccurate weighing) can be isolated and solved.

The drive in this country to increase laboratory awareness of the need for continuous quality control began with the blind survey of Pippenger et al., (1976) in 1974. Shortly thereafter, the Epilepsy Foundation of America provided funds for the establishment of the Antiepileptic Drug Quality Control Program, which has been continued by the American Association of Clinical Chemists. This service provides three monthly quality control samples, in addition to a continuing education program for laboratory personnel. A follow-up report indicated considerable improvement in the quality of reported results (Pippenger et al., 1977). Recently, Juel (1979) has summarized the data obtained in the College of American Pathologists Therapeutic Drug Monitoring Interlaboratory Survey Program, established in 1978. Dijkhuis et al. (1979) have reported the results of an international survey in which samples were sent to participants in the four major quality control programs in the United States and Europe. Data for phenobarbital, primidone, phenytoin, ethosuximide, carbamazepine, valproic acid, clonazepam, and carbamazepine epoxide were summarized according to the method of determination. With the exception of valproic acid, which was determined only by GLC, the only technique that was

---

[5] Number of samples that can be analyzed in a specific period of time.

recommended for all determinations was HPLC. Neither GLC nor EMIT gave acceptable results at all concentrations for all drugs. With proper training and control in the laboratory, however, these methods produce clinically reliable data.

Although quality control should begin when a blood sample is drawn and end when the result is recorded in the patient's medical record, the problems of most concern to the laboratory are methodology and calibration. Pippenger and Kutt (1978) have reviewed the errors associated with all phases of the analytical process, from sampling to reporting. Assuming that a method has been selected based on need and resources, the calibration phase is left. Accurate calibration requires accurate standard solutions of the species of interest in the biological matrix of interest—plasma, saliva, cerebrospinal fluid, urine. Lyophilized plasma controls are available,[6] as are methanolic drug stock solutions (Supelco, Inc.). Pure drug substances, metabolites, and internal standards are available from a number of vendors.[7] Dudley et al. (1977) have outlined procedures for preparing plasma standards and internal standards from alcoholic stock solutions. If stock solutions are made from pure drug substances, care must be used in weighing (to 0.01 mg) and dilution, and complete dissolution must be achieved.

A final consideration that can influence the quality of results is technician training and attitude. It is not easy to find dedicated people who will perform routine assays well over a long period of time. Although it is not always practical, interaction between the laboratory and the patient's physician will generally improve patient care and generate interest that will lead to better long-term performance.

---

[6] Syva Corp., Palo Alto, California 94394.
[7] Applied Science Laboratories, State College, Pennsylvania 16801; Aldrich Chemical Company; Supelco, Inc.

Bibliography

Aarli, J. A. (1976): Phenytoin-induced depression of salivary IgA and gingival hyperplasia. *Epilepsia,* 17:283–291.

Adams, R. F. (1977): The determination of anticonvulsants in biological samples by use of high pressure liquid chromatography. *Adv. Chromatogr.,* 15:131–168.

Adams, R. F., Schmidt, G. J., and Vandemark, F. L. (1978): A micro liquid column chromatography procedure for twelve anticonvulsants and some of their metabolites. *J. Chromatogr.,* 145:275–284.

Adams, R. F., and Vandemark, F. L. (1976): Simultaneous high pressure liquid chromatographic determinations of some anticonvulsants in serum. *Clin. Chem.,* 22:25–31.

Agurell, S., Berlin, A., Ferngren, H., and Hellström, B. (1975): Plasma levels of diazepam after parenteral and rectal administration in children. *Epilepsia,* 16:277–283.

Ahmad, S., Laidlaw, J., Houghton, G. W., and Richens, A. (1975): Involuntary movements caused by phenytoin intoxication in epileptic patients. *J. Neurol. Neurosurg. Psychiatry,* 38:225–231.

Aicardi, J., and Brarton, J. (1971): A pneumoencephalographic demonstration of brain atrophy following status epilepticus. *Dev. Med. Child Neurol.,* 13:660–667.

Aicardi, J., and Chevrie, J. J. (1970): Convulsive status epilepticus in infants and children. A study of 239 cases. *Epilepsia,* 11:187–197.

Aird, R. B., and Gordon, G. S. (1951): Anticonvulsant properties of desoxycorticosterone. *JAMA,* 145:715–719.

Aird, R. B., and Woodbury, D. M. (1974): *The Management of Epilepsy.* Charles C Thomas, Springfield, Illinois.

Alarcon-Segovia, D., Fishbein, E., Reyes, P. A., Dies, H., and Shevadosky, S. (1972): Antinuclear antibodies in patients on anticonvulsant therapy. *Clin. Exp. Immunol.,* 12:39–47.

American Association of Clinical Chemists (1978): Radioassay Subcommittee of the Standards Committee. The chemist's guide to radioassay products. *Clin. Chem.,* 24:1221–1280.

Anavekar, S. N., Saunders, R. H., Wardell, W. M., Shoulson, I., Emmings, F. G., Cook, C. E., and Grinderi, A. J. (1978): Parotid and whole saliva in the prediction of serum total and free phenytoin concentrations. *Clin. Pharmacol. Ther.,* 24:629–637.

Anders, M. W. (1971): Enhancement and inhibition of drug metabolism. *Annu. Rev. Pharmacol.,* 11:37–56.

Angelopoulos, A. P., and Goaz, P. W. (1972): Incidence of diphenylhydantoin gingival hyperplasia. *Oral Surg.*, 34:898–906.

Anlezark, G., Horton, R. W., Meldrum B. S., and Sawaya, M. C. B. (1976): Anticonvulsant action of ethanolamine-o-sulphate and di-n-propylacetate and the metabolism of gamma aminobutyric acid (GABA) in mice with audiogenic seizures. *Biochem. Pharmacol.*, 25:413–417.

Annegers, J. F., Elveback, L. R., Hauser, W. A., and Kurland, L. T. (1974): Do anticonvulsants have a teratogenic effect? *Arch. Neurol.*, 31:364–373.

Annegers, J. F., Hauser, W. A., Elveback, L. R., and Kurland, L. T., (1979): The risk of epilepsy following febrile convulsions. *Neurology*, 29:297–303.

Appleton, D. B., and DeVivo, D. C. (1974): An animal model for the ketogenic diet. *Epilepsia*, 15:211–227.

Arakawa, T. (1970): Congenital defects in folate utilization. *Am. J. Med.*, 45:265–270.

Arnold, K., and Gerber, N. (1970): The rate of decline of diphenylhydantoin in human plasma. *Clin. Pharmacol. Ther.*, 11:121–134.

Arnold, K., Gerber, N., and Levy, G. (1978): Absorption and dissolution of sodium diphenylhydantoin capsules. *Can. J. Pharm. Sci.*, 5:89–92.

Aston, R., and Domino, E. F. (1961): Differential effects of phenobarbital, pentobarbital, and diphenylhydantoin on motor cortical and reticular thresholds in the rhesus monkey. *Psychopharmacologia*, 2:304–317.

Atwell, S. H., Green, V. A., and Haney, W. G. (1975): Development and evaluation of method for simultaneous determination of phenobarbital and diphenylhydantoin in plasma by high-pressure liquid chromatography. *J. Pharm. Sci.*, 64:806–809.

Ayala, G. F., and Johnston, D. (1980): Phenytoin: Electrophysiological studies in simple neuronal systems. In: *Antiepileptic Drugs: Mechanisms of Action, Advances in Neurology, Vol. 27.*, edited by G. H. Glaser, J. K. Penry, and D. M. Woodbury, pp. 339–351. Raven Press, New York.

Ayala, G. F., Lin, S., and Johnston, D. (1977): The mechanism of action of diphenylhydantoin on invertebrate neurons: I. Effects on basic membrane properties. *Brain Res.*, 121:245–258.

Azarnoff, D. L. (1973): Application of blood level data to clinical trials. *Clin. Pharmacol. Ther.*, 16:183–188.

Badenoch, J. (1954): The use of labelled B_{12} and gastric biopsy in the investigation of anemia. *Proc. R. Soc. Med.*, 47:426–427.

Baird, E. S., and Hailey, D. M. (1972): Plasma levels of diazepam and its major metabolite following intramuscular administration. *Br. J. Anaesth.*, 45:546–548.

Baker, H., Frank, O., Hutner, S. H., Aaronson, S., Ziffer, H., and Sobotna, H. (1962): Lesions in folic acid metabolism induced by primidone. *Experientia*, 18:224–226.

Ballard, P. L., Baxter, J. D., Higgins, S. J., Rousseau, G. C., and Tomkins, G. M. (1974): General presence of glucocorticoid receptors in mammalian tissues. *Endocrinology*, 94:998–1002.

Bancaud, J., Bordas-Ferrer, M., and Geier, S. (1972): Use of diazepam in topographic definition of an epileptogenic zone. Effects on seizures provoked by electrical stimulation of the cortex. *Electroencephalogr. Clin. Neurophysiol.*, 33:535.

Barker, J. L. (1975): CNS depressants: Effects on post-synaptic pharmacology. *Brain Res.*, 92:35–56.

Barnes, S. E., Bland, D., Cole, A. P., and Evans, A. R. (1976): The use of sodium valproate in a case of status epilepticus. *Dev. Med. Child Neurol.*, 18:236–238.

Barragry, J. M., Makin, H. L. J., Trafford, D. J. H., and Scott, D. F. (1978): Effect of anticonvulsants on plasma testosterone and sex hormone binding globulin levels. *J. Neurol. Neurosurg. Psychiatry*, 41:913–914.

Baumel, I. P., Gallagher, B. B., and Mattson, R. H. (1972): Phenylethylmalonamide (PEMA). An important metabolite of primidone. *Arch. Neurol.*, 27:34–41.

Baumel, I. P., Gallagher, B. B., DiMicco, J., and Goico, H. (1973): Metabolism and anticonvulsant properties of primidone in the rat. *J. Pharmacol. Exp. Ther.*, 186:305–314.

Bayer, A. S., Targan, S. R., Pitchon, H. E., and Guze, L. B. (1976): Dilantin toxicity: Miliary pulmonary infiltrates and hypoxemia. *Ann. Intern. Med.*, 85:475–476.

Beerman, B., and Edhag, O. (1978): Depressive effects of carbamazepine on idioventricular rhythm in man. *Br. Med. J.*, 2:171–172.

Bell, R. D., Pakcy, C., Zerwekh, J., Barilla, D. E., and Vasco, M. (1979): Effect of phenytoin on bone and vitamin D metabolism. *Ann. Neurol.*, 5:374–378.

Belton, N. R., Etheridge, J. E., and Millichap, J. G. (1965): Effects of convulsions and anticonvulsants on blood sugar in rabbits. *Epilepsia*, 6:243–249.

Bente, H. B. (1978): Nitrogen-selective detectors: Application to quantitation of antiepileptic drugs. In: *Antiepileptic Drugs: Quantitative Analysis and Interpretation*, edited by C. E. Pippenger, J. K. Penry, and H. Kutt, pp. 139–145. Raven Press, New York.

Bernhard, G. C., Bohm, E., and Höjeberg, S. (1955): A new treatment of status epilepticus, intravenous injections of a local anesthetic (lidocaine). *Arch. Neurol. Psychiatry*, 74:208–214.

Bernhard, G. C., Bohm, E., Höjeberg, S., and Melin, K. A. (1956): The effect of intravenous Xylocaine on the cortical seizure activity evoked by intermittent photic stimulation in epileptics. *Acta Psychiatr. Neurol. Scand.*, 31:185–193.

Berry, D. J., and Clarke, L. A. (1978): Determination of valproic acid (dipropylacetic acid) in plasma by gas liquid chromatography. *J. Chromatogr.*, 156:301–307.

Beyer, K. H., and Klinge, D. (1969): Zum spektrophotometrischen Nachweis von carbamazepin. *Arzneim. Forsch.*, 19:1759–1760.

Bidanset, J. H. (1974): Drug analysis by immunoassays. *J. Chromatogr. Sci.*, 12:293–296.

Bird, C. A. K., Griffin, B. P., Miklaszewska, J. M., and Galbraith, A. W. (1966): Tegretol (carbamazepine): A controlled trial of a new anticonvulsant. *Br. J. Psychiatr.*, 112:737–742.

Birket-Smith, E., and Krogh, E. (1971): Motor nerve conduction velocity during diphenylhydantoin intoxication. *Acta Neurol. Scand.*, 47:265–271.

Birket-Smith, E., Lund, M., Mikkelsen, B., Vestermark, S., Zander-Olsen, P., and Holm, P. (1973): A controlled trial of R05-4023 (clonazepam) in the treatment of psychomotor epilepsy. *Acta Neurol. Scand. [Suppl. 53]*, 49:18–25.

Bius, D. L., Teague, B. L., and Dudley, K. H. (1979*a*): Simultaneous gas chromatographic determination of trimethadione and dimethadione in human plasma. *Ther. Drug Monit.*, 1:495–506.

Bius, D. L., Teague, B. L., and Dudley, K. H. (1979*b*): Gas chromatographic determination of carbamazepine in plasma. *Ther. Drug Monit.*, 1:525–544.

Bjerkedal, T., and Bahna, L. (1973): The course and outcome of pregnancy in women with epilepsy. *Acta Obstet. Gynecol. Scand.*, 52:245–248.

Bjornberg, A., and Holst, R. (1967): Generalized lymphadenopathy as a drug reaction to hydantoin. *Acta Neurol. Scand.*, 43:399–402.

Blom, S. (1962): Trigeminal neuralgia: Its treatment with a new anticonvulsant drug (G-32883). *Lancet*, 1:839–840.

Bochner, F., Hooper, W. D., and Sutherland, J. M. (1974): Diphenylhydantoin concentrations in saliva. *Arch. Neurol.*, 31:57–59.

Bochner, F., Hooper, W. D., Sutherland, J. M., Eadie, M. J., and Tyrer, J. H. (1973): The renal handling of diphenylhydantoin and 5-(p-hydroxyphenyl)-5-phenylhydantoin. *Clin. Pharmacol. Ther.*, 14:791–796.

Bogue, J. Y., and Carrington, H. C. (1953): The evaluation of "mysoline"; a new anticonvulsant drug. *Br. J. Pharmacol.*, 8:230–236.

Booker, H. E. (1972*a*): Trimethadione and other oxazolidinediones: Chemistry and methods for determination. In: *Antiepileptic Drugs*, edited by D. M. Woodbury, J. K. Penry, and R. P. Schmidt, pp. 385–388. Raven Press, New York.

Booker, H. E. (1972*b*): Trimethadione and other oxazolidinediones: Relation of plasma levels to clinical control. In: *Antiepileptic Drugs*, edited by D. M. Woodbury, J. K. Penry, and R. P. Schmidt, pp. 403–407. Raven Press, New York.

Booker, H. E. (1975): Idiosyncratic reactions to the antiepileptic drugs. *Epilepsia*, 16:171–181.

Booker, H. E., Chun, R. W. M., and Sanguino, M. (1970): Myasthenia gravis syndrome associated with trimethadione. *JAMA*, 212:2262–2263.

Booker, H. E., and Darcey, B. (1971): Simultaneous determination of trimethadione and its metabolite, dimethadione by gas liquid chromatography. *Clin. Chem.*, 17:607–609.

Booker, H. E., and Darcey, B. (1973): Serum concentrations of free diphenylhydantoin and their relationship to clinical intoxication. *Epilepsia*, 14:177–184.

Booker, H. E., and Darcey, B. A. (1975): Enzymatic immunoassay vs. gas-liquid chromatography for determination of phenobarbital and diphenylhydantoin in serum. *Clin. Chem.*, 21:1766–1768.

Borgstedt, A. D., Bryson, M. F., Young, L. W., and Forbes, G. B. (1972): Long-term administration of antiepileptic drugs and the development of rickets. *J. Pediatr.*, 81:9–15.

Bower, B. (1978): The treatment of epilepsy in children. *Br. J. Hosp. Med.*, 19:8–19.

Braestrup, C., and Squires, R. F. (1978): Brain specific benzodiazepine receptors. *Br. J. Psychiatry*, 133:249–260.

Brattin, W. J., and Sunshine, I. (1973): Immunoassays for drugs in biological samples. *Am. J. Med. Technol.*, 39:223–230.

Brennan, R. W., Dehejia, H., Kutt, H., Verebly, K., and McDowell, F. (1970): Diphenylhydantoin intoxication attendant to slow inactivation of isoniazid. *Neurology*, 20:687–693.

Brett, E. (1977): Implications of measuring anticonvulsant blood levels in epilepsy. *Dev. Med. Child Neurol.*, 19(2):245–251.

Brillman, J., Gallagher, B. B., and Mattson, R. H. (1974): Acute primidone intoxication. *Arch. Neurol.*, 30:255–258.

Brochmann-Hanssen, E., and Oke, T. O. (1969): Gas chromatography of barbiturates, phenolic alkaloids and xanthine bases: Flash heater methylation by means of trimethylanilinium hydroxide. *J. Pharm. Sci.*, 58:370–371.

Browne, T. R. (1978a): Clonazepam. *N. Engl. J. Med.*, 299:812–816.

Browne, T. R. (1978b): Drug therapy reviews: Drug therapy of status epilepticus. *Am. J. Hosp. Pharm.*, 35:915–922.

Browne, T. R., Dreifuss, F. E., Dyken, P. R., Goode, D. J., Penry, J. K., Porter, R. J., White, B. G., and White, P. T. (1975): Ethosuximide in the treatment of absence (petit mal) seizures. *Neurology*, 25:515–524.

Browne, T. R., and Penry, J. K. (1973): Benzodiazepines in the treatment of epilepsy: A review. *Epilepsia*, 14:277–310.

Brumlik, J., and Jacobs, R. S. (1974): Myasthenia gravis associated with diphenylhydantoin therapy for epilepsy. *Can. J. Neurol. Sci.*, 1:127–129.

Bruni, J. (1979): Recent advances in drug therapy for epilepsy. *Can. Med. Assoc. J.*, 120:817–824.

Bruni, J., Gallo, J. M., Lee, C. S., Perchalski, R. J., and Wilder, B. J. (1980c): Interactions of valproic acid with phenytoin. *Neurology*, 30:1233–1236.

Bruni, J., Gallo, J. M., and Wilder, B. J. (1979a): Effect of phenytoin on protein binding of valproic acid. *Can. J. Neurol. Sci.*, 6:453–454.

Bruni, J., and Wilder, B. J. (1979a): Valproic acid: Review of a new antiepileptic drug. *Arch. Neurol.*, 36:393–398.

Bruni, J., and Wilder, B. J. (1979b): The toxicology of antiepileptic drugs. In: *Handbook of Clinical Neurology, Vol. 37, Part II: Intoxications of the Nervous System*, edited by P. J. Vinken and G. W. Bruyn, pp. 199–222. North Holland, Amsterdam.

Bruni, J., and Wilder, B. J. (1979c): Antiepileptic drug monitoring. *J. Fla. Med. Assoc.*, 66:697–699.

Bruni, J., Wilder, B. J., Bauman, A. W., and Willmore, L. J. (1980a): Clinical efficacy and long term effects of valproic acid therapy on spike-and-wave discharges. *Neurology*, 30:42–46.

Bruni, J., Wilder, B. J., Perchalski, R. J., Hammond, E. J., Villarreal, H. J. (1980b): Valproic acid and plasma levels of phenobarbital. *Neurology*, 30:94–97.

Bruni, J. Wilder, B. J., Willmore, L. J., and Barbour, B. (1979b): Valproic acid and plasma levels of phenytoin. *Neurology*, 29:904–905.

Bruni, J., Wilder, B. J., Willmore, L. J., Perchalski, R. J. and Villarreal, H. J. (1978a): Steady-state kinetics of valproic acid in epileptic patients. *Clin. Pharmacol. Ther.*, 24:324–332.

Bruni, J., Wang, L. H., Marbury, T. C., Lee, C. S., and Wilder, B. J. (1979c): Protein binding of valproic acid in uremic patients. *Neurology*, 30:557–559.

Bruni, J., Wilder, B. J., Willmore, L. J., Villarreal, H. J., Thomas, M., and Crawford, M. (1978b): Clinical efficacy of valproic acid in relation to plasma levels. *Can. J. Neurol. Sci.*, 5:385–387.

Bruni, J., Willmore, L. J., and Wilder, B. J. (1979d): Treatment of postanoxic intention myoclonus with valproic acid. *Can. J. Neurol. Sci.*, 6:39–42.

Buchanan, R. A., Fernandez, L., and Kinkel, A. W. (1969): Absorption and elimination of ethosuximide in children. *J. Clin. Pharmacol.*, 9:393–398.

Buchanan, R. A., Kinkel, A. W., and Smith, T. C. (1973): The absorption and excretion of ethosuximide. *Int. J. Clin. Pharmacol. Ther. Toxicol.*, 7:213–218.

Buchanan, R. A., Kinkel, A. W., Turner, J. L., and Heffelinger, J. C. (1976): Ethosuximide dosage regimens. *Clin. Pharmacol. Ther.*, 19:143–147.

Buchanan, R. A., and Sholiton, L. J., (1972): Diphenylhydantoin: Interactions with other drugs. In: *Antiepileptic Drugs*, edited by D. M. Woodbury, J. K. Penry, and R. P. Schmidt, pp. 181–191. Raven Press, New York.

Buchthal, F., and Lennox-Buchthal, M. A. (1972a): Phenobarbital: Relation of serum concentration to control of seizures. In: *Antiepileptic Drugs*, edited by D. M. Woodbury, J. K. Penry, and R. P. Schmidt, pp. 335–343. Raven Press, New York.

Buchthal, F., and Lennox-Buchthal, M. A. (1972b): Diphenylhydantoin: Relation of anticonvulsant effect to concentration in serum. In: *Antiepileptic Drugs*, edited by D. M. Woodbury, J. K. Penry, and R. P. Schmidt, pp. 193–209. Raven Press, New York.

Busfield, D., Child, K. J., Atkinson, R. M., and Tomich, E. G. (1963): An effect of phenobarbital on blood levels of griseofulvin in man. *Lancet*, 2:1042–1043.

Butler, T. C. (1953): Quantitative studies of the physiological disposition of 3-methyl-5-ethyl-5-phenyl hydantoin (Mesantoin) and 5-phenyl hydantoin (Nirvanol). *J. Pharmacol. Exp. Ther.*, 109:340–345.

Butler, T. C. (1956): The metabolic hydroxylation of phenobarbital. *J. Pharmacol. Exp. Ther.*, 116:326–336.

Butler, T. C. (1978): Some quantitative aspects of the pharmacology of phenobarbital. In: *Antiepileptic Drugs: Quantitative Analysis and Interpretation*, edited by C. E. Pippenger, J. K. Penry, and H. Kutt, pp. 261–271. Raven Press, New York.

Butler, T. C., Kuroiwa, Y., Waddell, W. J., and Poole, D. T. (1966): Effects of 5-,5-dimethyl-2,4-oxazolidinedione (DMO) on acid-base and electrolyte equilibria. *J. Pharmacol. Exp. Ther.*, 152:62–66.

Callaghan, N., Feely, M., O'Callaghan, M., Duggan, B., McGarry, J., Cramer, B., Wheelen, J., and Seldrup, J. (1977): The effects of toxic and non-toxic serum phenytoin levels on carbohydrate tolerance and insulin levels. *Acta Neurol. Scand.*, 56:563–571.

Callaghan, N., O'Callaghan, M., Duggan, B., and Feely, M. (1978): Carbamazepine as a single drug in the treatment of epilepsy. A prospective study of serum levels and seizure control. *J. Neurol. Neurosurg. Psychiatry*, 41:907–912.

Callery, P. S., and Leslie, J. (1977): Thermal decomposition of 1,3 dimethyl derivative of phenobarbital in trimethylanilinium hydroxide. *J. Pharm. Sci.*, 66:578–580.

Camfield, C. (1980): Clinical trials of phenobarbital. Presented at NIH Consensus Development Conference on Febrile Seizures. Bethesda, Maryland, May 19–21.

Camfield, P. R., Barnell, P., Camfield, C. S., and Tibbles, J. A. R. (1979): Pancreatitis due to valproic acid. *Lancet*, 1:1198–1199.

Camfield, P. R., Camfield, C. S., Shapiro, S. H., and Cummings, C. (1980): The first febrile seizure—antipyretic instruction plus either phenobarbital or placebo to prevent recurrence. *J. Pediatr.*, 97:16–21.

Cammer, W., Fredman, T., Rose, A. L., and Norton, W. T. (1976): Brain carbonic anhydrase: Activity in isolated myelin and the effect of hexachlorophene. *J. Neurochem.*, 27:165–171.

Cantu, R. C., and Schwab, R. S. (1966): Ceruloplasmin rise and protein bound iodine fall in human serum during diphenylhydantoin (Dilantin) administration. *Trans. Am. Neurol. Assoc.*, 91:201–203.

Carraz, G., Fau, R., Chateau, R., and Bonnin, J. (1964): Communication à propos des premiers essais cliniques sur l'activité anti-épileptique de l'acide n-dipropylacétique (sel de Na+). *Ann. Med. Psychol.*, 122:577–585.

Carroll, W. M., and Walsh, P. J. (1978): Functional independence in post-anoxic myoclonus: Contribution of L-5HTP sodium valproate and clonazepam. *Br. Med. J.*, 2:1612.

Cavazzuti, G. B. (1975): Prevention of febrile convulsions with dipropylacetate (Depakene). *Epilepsia*, 16:647–648.

Cereghino, J. J., Brock, J. T., Van Meter, J. C., Penry, J. K., and Smith, L. D. (1975): The efficacy of carbamazepine combinations in epilepsy. *Clin. Pharmacol. Ther.*, 18:733–741.

Cereghino, J. J., Brock, J. T., Van Meter, J. C., Penry, J. K., Smith, L. D., and White, B. G. (1974): Carbamazepine for epilepsy. *Neurology*, 24:401–410.

Cereghino, J. J., Van Meter, J. C., Brock, J. T., Penry, J. K., Smith, L. D., and White, B. J. (1973): Preliminary observations of serum carbamazepine concentration in epileptic patients. *Neurology*, 23:357–366.

Chadwick, D., Hallett, M., Harris, R., Jenner, P., Reynolds, E. H., and Marsden, C. D. (1977a): Clinical, biochemical, and physiological features distinguishing myoclonus responsive to 5-hydroxytryptophan, tryptophan with a monoamine oxidase inhibitor, and clonazepam. *Brain*, 100:455–487.

Chadwick, D., Vydelingum, L., Galbraith, A., and Reynolds, E. H. (1977b): The value of serum phenytoin levels in new referrals with epilepsy. One drug in the treatment of epilepsy. In: *Antiepileptic Drug Monitoring*, edited by C. Gardner-Thorpe, D. Janz, H. Meinardi, and C. E. Pippenger, pp. 187–196. MCS Consultants, Tunbridge Wells.

Chamberlain, H. R., Waddell, W. J., and Butler, T. C. (1965): A study of the product of demethylation of trimethadione in the control of petit mal epilepsy. *Neurology*, 15:449–454.

Chanarin, I., Laidlaw, J., Loughridge, L. W., and Mollin, D. L. (1960): Megaloblastic anaemia due to phenobarbitone. The convulsant action of therapeutic doses of folic acid. *Br. Med. J.*, 1:1099–1102.

Chang, T., Burkett, A. R., and Glazko, A. J. (1972a): Ethosuximide: Biotransformation. In: *Antiepileptic Drugs*, edited by D. M. Woodbury, J. K. Penry, and R. P. Schmidt, pp. 425–429. Raven Press, New York.

Chang, T., Dill, W. A., and Glazko, A. J. (1972b): Ethosuximide: Absorption, distribution, and excretion. In: *Antiepileptic Drugs*, edited by D. M. Woodbury, J. K. Penry, and R. P. Schmidt, pp. 417–423. Raven Press, New York.

Chang, T., and Glazko, A. J. (1970): Quantitative assay of 5,5-diphenylhydantoin (Dilantin) and 5-(p-hydroxyphenyl)-5-phenylhydantoin by gas liquid chromatography. *J. Lab. Clin. Med.*, 75:145–155.

Chang, T., and Glazko, A. J. (1972): Diphenylhydantoin: Biotransformation. In: *Antiepileptic Drugs*, edited by D. M. Woodbury, J. K. Penry, and R. P. Schmidt, pp. 149–162. Raven Press, New York.

Chapron, D. J., Kramer, P. A., Mariano, S. L., and Hohnadel, D. C. (1979): Effect of calcium and antacids on phenytoin bioavailability. *Arch. Neurol.*, 36:436–438.

Charlton, M. H., and Lunsford, D. (1971): The role of diphenylhydantoin in the causation of malignant lymphoma. *Minerva Med.*, 62:43.

Chen, G., Portman, R., Ensor, C. R., and Bratton, A. C. (1951): The anticonvulsant activity of α-phenylsuccinimides. *J. Pharmacol. Exp. Ther.*, 103:54–61.

Chen, G., Weston, J. K., and Bratton, A. J. (1963): Anticonvulsant activity and toxicity of phensuximide, methsuximide, and ethosuximide. *Epilepsia*, 4:66–76.

Chokroverty, S., and Sayeed, Z. A. (1975): Motor nerve conduction study in patients on diphenylhydantoin therapy. *J. Neurol. Neurosurg. Psychiatry*, 38:1235–1239.

Chou, D. T., and Wang, C. S. (1977): Unit activity of amygdala and hippocampal neurons: Effects of morphine and benzodiazepines. *Brain Res.*, 126:427–440.

Christiansen, C., Rodbro, P., and Lund, M. (1973): Incidence of anticonvulsant osteomalacia and effect of vitamin D: Controlled therapeutic trial. *Br. Med. J.*, 4:695–701.

Cohn, D. F., Axelrod, T., Hommonnai, Z. T., Paz, G., Streifler, M., and Kraicer, P. Z. (1978): Effect of diphenylhydantoin on the reproductive function of the male rat. *J. Neurol. Neurosurg. Psychiatry*, 41:858–860.

Conney, A. H. (1967): Pharmacological implications of microsomal enzyme induction. *Pharmacol. Rev.*, 19:317–366.

Cook, C. E. (1978): Radioimmunoassay. In: *Antiepileptic Drugs: Quantitative Analysis and Interpretation*, edited by C. E. Pippenger, J. K. Penry, and H. Kutt, pp. 163–173. Raven Press, New York.

Cook, C. E., Amerson, E., Poole, W. K., Lesser, P., and O'Tuama, L. (1976a): Phenytoin and phenobarbital concentrations in saliva and plasma measured by radioimmunoassay. *Clin. Pharmacol. Ther.*, 18:742–747.

Cook, C. E., Christensen, H. D., Amerson, E. W., Kepler, J. A., Tallent, C. R., and Taylor, G. F. (1976b): Radioimmunoassay of anticonvulsant drugs: Phenytoin, phenobarbital and primidone. In: *Quantitative Analytic Studies in Epilepsy*, edited by P. Kellaway and I. Petersen, pp. 37–58. Raven Press, New York.

Cordoba, E. F., and Strobos, R. R. J. (1956): N-methyl-a,a-methylphenylsuccinimide in psychomotor epilepsy. *Dis. Nerv. Syst.*, 17:383–385.

Corradino, R. A. (1976): Diphenylhydantoin: Direct inhibition of the vitamin D_3-mediated calcium absorptive mechanism in organ cultured duodenum. *Biochem. Pharmacol.*, 25:863–864.

Craddock, W. L. (1955): Use of phenacemide in epilepsy, with analysis of fatal reactions and case report. *JAMA*, 159:1437–1441.

Cranford, R. E., Patrick, B., Anderson, C. B., and Kostick, B. (1978): Intravenous phenytoin: Clinical and pharmacokinetic aspects. *Neurology*, 28:874–880.

Critchley, E. M. R., Vakil, S. D., Hayward, H. W., and Owen, V. M. H. (1976): Dupuytren's disease in epilepsy: Result of prolonged administration of anticonvulsants. *J. Neurol. Neurosurg. Psychiatry*, 39:498–503.

Crowther, D. L. (1964): Infantile spasm: Response of "salaam seizures" to hydrocortisone. *Calif. Med.*, 100:97–102.

Cucinell, S. A. (1972): Phenobarbital: Interactions with other drugs. In: *Antiepileptic Drugs*, edited by D. M. Woodbury, J. K. Penry, and R. P. Schmidt, pp. 319–327. Raven Press, New York.

Curless, R. G., Walson, P. D., and Carter, D. (1975): Phenytoin kinetics in children. *Neurology*, 26:715–720.

Curtis, E. G., and Patel, J. A. (1978): Enzyme multiplied immunoassay technique: A review. *CRC Crit. Rev. Clin. Lab. Sci.*, 9:303–320.

Dale, B. M., Purdie, G. H., and Rischbieth, R. H. (1978): Fibrinogen depletion with sodium valproate. *Lancet*, 1:1316.

Dam, M. (1970): Number of Purkinje cells in patients with grand mal epilepsy treated with diphenylhydantoin. *Epilepsia*, 11:313–320.

Dam, M. (1972*a*): Diphenylhydantoin: Neurological aspects of toxicity. In: *Antiepileptic Drugs*, edited by D. M. Woodbury, J. K. Penry, and R. P. Schmidt, pp. 227–235. Raven Press, New York.

Dam, M. (1972*b*): The density and ultrastructure of the Purkinje cells following diphenylhydantoin treatment in animals and man. *Acta Neurol. Scand.*, 48:13–63.

Dam, M. (1977): Chronic toxicity of antiepileptic drugs. In: *Advances in Epileptology*, edited by H. Meinardi and A. J. Rowan, pp. 330–341. Swets and Zeitlinger, Amsterdam.

Dam, M., and Olesen, O. V. (1966): Intramuscular administration of phenytoin. *Neurology*, 16:288–292.

Danhof, M., and Breimer, D. D. (1978): Therapeutic drug monitoring in saliva. *Clin. Pharmacokinet.*, 3:39–57.

Darcey, B. A., Solow, E. B., and Pippenger, C. E. (1978): Gas-liquid chromatographic quantitation of phenytoin, phenobarbital, primidone, and carbamazepine. In: *Antiepileptic Drugs: Quantitative Analysis and Interpretation*, edited by C. E. Pippenger, J. K. Penry, and H. Kutt, pp. 67–74. Raven Press, New York.

Davenport, V. D., and Davenport, H. W. (1948): The relation between starvation, metabolic acidosis and convulsive seizures in rats. *J. Nutr.*, 36:139–151.

Davidian, N. M., Butler, T. C., and Poole, D. T. (1978): The effect of ketosis induced by medium chain triglycerides on intracellular pH of mouse brain. *Epilepsia*, 19:369–378.

Davies, P. P. (1960): Coagulation defects due to anticonvulsant drug treatment in pregnancy. *Lancet*, 1:413.

de Bard, M. L. (1979): Diazepam withdrawal syndrome: A case with psychosis, seizure and coma. *Am. J. Psychiatry*, 136(1):104–105.

DeBeer, P., and Dijkhuis, I. C. (1976): Analysis of carbamazepine in serum: Comparative study on several methods. *Pharmaceutisch Weekblad*, 111:93–102.

DeJong, R. H. (1978): Toxic effects of local anesthetics. *JAMA*, 239:1166–1168.

Delgado-Escueta, A. V., and Horan, M. P. (1980): Phenytoin: Biochemical membrane studies. In: *Antiepileptic Drugs: Mechanisms of Action, Advances in Neurology, Vol. 27*, edited by G. H. Glaser, J. K. Penry, and D. M. Woodbury, pp. 377–398. Raven Press, New York.

DeLorenzo, R. J. (1980): Phenytoin: Calcium- and calmodulin-dependent protein phosphorylation and neurotransmitter release. In: *Antiepileptic Drugs: Mechanisms of Action, Advances in Neurology. Vol. 27*, edited by G. H. Glaser, J. K. Penry, and D. M. Woodbury, pp. 399–414. Raven Press, New York.

DeLuca, K., Masotti, R. E., and Partington, M. W. (1972): Altered calcium metabolism due to anticonvulsant drugs. *Dev. Med. Child Neurol.*, 14:318–321.

de Silva, J. A. F. (1978): Electron capture-GLC in the quantitation of 1,4-benzodiazepines. In: *Antiepileptic Drugs: Quantitative Analysis and Interpretation*, edited by C. E. Pippenger, J. K. Penry, and H. Kutt, pp. 111–138. Raven Press, New York.

de Silva, J. A. F., Bekersky, I., Puglisi, C. V., Brooks, M. A., and Weinfeld, R. E. (1976): Determination of 1,4-benzodiazepines and diazepin-2-ones in blood by electron capture gas-liquid chromatography. *Anal. Chem.*, 48:10–19.

DeVivo, D. C., Leckie, M. P., Ferrendelli, J. S., and McDougal, D. B., Jr. (1978): Chronic ketosis and cerebral metabolism. *Ann. Neurol.*, 3:331–337.

DeVivo, D. C., Pagliara, A. S., and Prensky, A. L. (1973): Ketotic hypoglycemia and the ketogenic diet. *Neurology*, 23:640–644.

DeVore, G. R., and Woodbury, D. M. (1977): Phenytoin: An evaluation of several teratogenic mechanisms. *Epilepsia*, 18:387–396.

DeWeer, P. (1980): Phenytoin: Blockage of resting sodium channels. In: *Antiepileptic Drugs: Mechanisms of Action, Advances in Neurology, Vol. 27*, edited by G. H. Glaser, J. K. Penry, and D. M. Woodbury, pp. 353–361. Raven Press, New York.

Dhar, G. J., Ahamed, P. N., Pierach, C. A., and Howard, R. B. (1974): Diphenylhydantoin-induced hepatic necrosis. *Postgrad. Med.*, 56:128–134.

Dianese, G. (1979): Prophylactic diazepam in febrile convulsions (letter). *Arch. Dis. Child.*, 54:244–245.

Diaz, J., and Schain, R. J. (1978): Phenobarbital: Effects of long-term administration on behavior and brain of artificially reared rats. *Science*, 199:90–91.

Diaz, J., Schain, R., and Bailey, B. G. (1977): Phenobarbital induced brain growth retardation in artificially reared rat pups. *Biol. Neonate*, 32:77–82.

Diaz, P. M. (1974): Interaction of pentylenetetrazol and trimethadione on the metabolism of serotonin in brain and its relation to the anticonvulsant action of trimethadione. *Neuropharmacology*, 13:615–621.

DiGregorio, G. J., Piraino, A. J., and Ruch, E. (1978): Diazepam concentrations in parotid saliva, mixed saliva, and plasma. *Clin. Pharmacol. Ther.*, 24:720–725.

Dijkhuis, I., DeJong, H. J., Richens, A., Pippenger, C. E., Leskinen, E. E. A., and Nyberg, A. P. W. (1979): Joint international quality control programme on the determination of antiepileptic drugs. *Pharmaceutisch Weekblad*, 1:151–184.

Dijkhuis, I. C., and Vervloet, E. (1974): Rapid determination of the antiepileptic drug di-n-propylacetic acid in plasma. *Pharm. Weekblad Sci.*, 109:42–45.

Dill, W. A., and Glazko, A. J. (1972): Fluorometric assay of diphenylhydantoin in plasma or whole blood. *Clin. Chem.*, 18:675–676.

Dill, W. A., Kazenko, A., Wolf, L. M., and Glazko, A. J. (1956): Studies on 5,5-diphenylhydantoin (Dilantin) in animals and man. *J. Pharmacol. Exp. Ther.*, 118:270–279.

Dill, W. A., Leung, A., Kinkel, A. W., and Glazko, A. J. (1976): Simplified fluorometric assay for diphenylhydantoin in plasma. *Clin. Chem.*, 22:908–911.

Direkze, M., and Fernando, P. S. L. (1977): Transient anterior horn cell dysfunction in diphenylhydantoin therapy. *Eur. Neurol.*, 15:131–134.

DiSalle, E., Pacifici, G. M., and Morselli, P. L. (1974): Studies on plasma protein binding of carbamazepine. *Pharmacol. Res. Commun.*, 6:193–202.

Dixon, W. R., Young, R. L., Ning, R., and Liebman, A. (1975): Radioimmunoassay of the anticonvulsant agent clonazepam. *Pharmacologist*, 17:251.

Dodrill, C. B., and Troupin, A. S. (1977): Psychotropic effects of carbamazepine in epilepsy: A double-blind comparison with phenytoin. *Neurology*, 27:1023–1028.

Domek, N. S., Barlow, C. F., and Roth, L. J. (1960): An ontogenetic study of phenobarbital-C^{14} in cat brain. *J. Pharmacol. Exp. Ther.*, 130:285–293.

Dreifuss, F. E., Penry, J. K., Rose, S. W., Kupferberg, H. J., Dyken, P., and Sato, S. (1975): Serum clonazepam concentrations in children with absence seizures. *Neurology*, 25:255–258.

Druskin, M. S., Wallen, M. H., and Bonagura, L. (1962): Anticonvulsant associated megaloblastic anemia. *N. Engl. J. Med.*, 267:483–485.

Dudley, K. H. (1978): Internal standards in gas-liquid chromatographic determination of antiepileptic drugs. In: *Antiepileptic Drugs: Quantitative Analysis and Interpretation*, edited by C. E. Pippenger, J. K. Penry, and H. Kutt, pp. 19–34. Raven Press, New York.

Dudley, K. H., Bius, D. L., Kraus, B. L., and Boyles, L. W. (1977): Gas chromatographic on-column methylation technique for the simultaneous determination of antiepileptic drugs in blood. *Epilepsia*, 18:259–276.

Duffy, F. H., and Lombroso, C. T. (1978): Treatment of status epilepticus. In: *Clinical Neuropharmacology, Vol. 3*, edited by H. L. Klawans, pp. 41–56. Raven Press, New York.

Dumermuth, G., and Kovacs, E. (1973): The effect of clonazepam (RO 5-4023) in the syndrome of infantile spasms with hypsarrhythmia and in petit mal variant or Lennox syndrome. *Acta Neurol. Scand.* 49, Suppl. 53:26–28.

Dymling, J. F., Lidgren, L., and Walloe, A. (1979): Biochemical variables related to calcium metabolism in epileptics. *Acta Med. Scand.*, 205:401–404.

Eadie, M. J. (1976): Plasma level monitoring of anticonvulsants. *Clin. Pharmacokinet.*, 1:52–66.

Eadie, M. J., and Tyrer, J. H. (1980): *Anticonvulsant Therapy. Pharmacological Basis and Practice.* Churchill Livingstone, Edinburgh.

Early, P. F. (1962): Population studies in Dupuytren's contracture. *J. Bone Joint Surg.*, 44B:602–613.

Eichelbaum, M., Bertilsson, L., Rane, E., and Sjoquist, F. (1976): Autoinduction of carbamazepine metabolism in man. In: *Antiepileptic Drugs and Enzyme Induction*, edited by A. Richens and F. P. Woodford, pp. 147–158. Associated Scientific Publishers, Amsterdam.

Eisen, A. A., Woods, J. F., and Sherwin, A. L. (1974): Peripheral nerve function in long-term therapy with diphenylhydantoin. *Neurology*, 24:411–417.

Emson, P. C. (1976): Effects of chronic treatment with amino-oxyacetic acid or sodium n-dipropylacetate on brain GABA levels and development and regression of cobalt epileptic focus in rats. *J. Neurochem.*, 27:1489–1494.

Engel, J., Ludwig, B. I., and Fetell, M. (1978): Prolonged partial complex status epilepticus: EEG and behavioral observations. *Neurology*, 28:863–869.

Englander, R. N., Johnson, R. N., and Hanna, G. R. (1977): Ethosuximide and bicuculline: Inhibition in petit mal epilepsy. *Neurol. Neurocir. Psiquiatr.*, 18:265–275.

Epilepsy Foundation of America (1975): *Basic Statistics on the Epilepsies.* F. A. Davis, Philadelphia.

Epstein, M. H., and O'Connor, J. S. (1966): Destructive effects of prolonged status epilepticus. *J. Neurol. Neurosurg. Psychiatry*, 29:251–254.

Espir, M. L. E., Benton, P., Will, E., Hayes, M. J., and Walker, G. (1976): Sodium valproate (Epilim): Some clinical and pharmacological aspects. In: *Clinical and Pharmacological Aspects of Sodium Valproate (Epilim) in the Treatment of Epilepsy*, edited by N. J. Legg, pp. 145–151. MCS Consultants, Tunbridge Wells.

Esplin, D. W., and Curto, E. M. (1957): Effects of trimethadione on synaptic transmission in the spinal cord: Antagonism of trimethadione and pentylenetetrazol. *J. Pharmacol. Exp. Ther.*, 121:457–467.

Essman, W. B. (1965): Xylocaine induced protection against electrically induced convulsions in mice. *Arch. Int. Pharmacodyn. Ther.*, 157:166–173.

Evans, A. R., Forrester, R. M., and Discombe, C. (1970): Neonatal hemorrhage following maternal anticonvulsant therapy. *Lancet*, 1:517–518.

Evans, J. R. (1973): Simultaneous measurement of diphenylhydantoin and phenobarbital in serum by high pressure liquid chromatography. *Anal. Chem.*, 45:2428–2429.

Evans, W. E., Self, T. H., and Weisburst, M. R. (1976): Phenobarbital induced hepatic dysfunction. *Drug Intell. Clin. Pharmacol.*, 10:439–443.

Everett, G. M. (1949): Pharmacological studies of phenacetylurea (Phenurone), an anticonvulsant drug. *Fed. Proc.*, 8:289.

Eymard, P., Simiand, J., Teoule, R., Polverelli, M., Werbenec, J. P., and Broll, M. (1971): Etude de la répartition et de la résorption du dipropylacetate de sodium marqué au 14C chez le rat. *J. Pharmacol.*, 2:359–368.

Faero, O., Kastrup, K. W., Nielsen, E. L., Melchior, J. C., and Thorn, I. (1972): Successful prophylaxis of febrile convulsions with phenobarbital. *Epilepsia*, 13:279–285.

Fahn, S. (1978): Post-anoxic action myoclonus: Improvement with valproic acid. *N. Engl. J. Med.*, 299:313–314.

Falconer, M. A. (1972): Febrile convulsions in early childhood. *Br. Med. J.*, 2:292.

Falconer, M. A., and Davidson, S. (1973): Coarse features in epilepsy as a consequence of anticonvulsant therapy. *Lancet*, 2:1112–1114.

Fedrick, J. (1973): Epilepsy and pregnancy: A report from the Oxford Record Linkage Study. *Br. Med. J.*, 2:442–448.

Felber, J. P. (1978): Radioimmunoassay in the clinic chemistry laboratory. *Adv. Clin. Chem.*, 20:130–179.

Feldman, R. G., and Pippenger, C. E. (1976): The relation of anticonvulsant drug levels to complete seizure control. *J. Clin. Pharmacol.*, 16:51–59.

Feldman, S. (1974): Drug distribution. *Med. Clin. North Am.*, 58:917–926.

Fellenberg, A. J., Magarey, A., and Pollard, A. C. (1975): An improved benzophenone procedure for the micro-determination of 5,5-diphenylhydantoin in blood. *Clin. Chim. Acta*, 59:155–160.

Fellenberg, A. J., and Pollard, A. C. (1976a): A rapid and sensitive spectrophotometric procedure for the micro-determination of carbamazepine in blood. *Clin. Chim. Acta*, 69:423–428.

Fellenberg, A. J., and Pollard, A. C. (1976b): A rapid spectrophotometric procedure for the simultaneous micro-determination of carbamazepine and 5,5-diphenylhydantoin in blood. *Clin. Chim. Acta*, 69:429–431.

Fernandez, A. A., and Loeb, H. G. (1975): Practical applications of radioimmunoassay theory. A simple procedure yielding linear calibration curves. *Clin. Chem.*, 21:1113–1120.

Ferrandes, B., and Eymard, P. (1973): Methode rapide d'analyse quantitative du dipropyl-acetate de sodium dans le serum au le plasma. *Ann. Pharm. Fr.*, 31:279–282.

Ferrandes, B., and Eymard, P. (1977): Metabolism of valproate sodium in rabbit, rat, dog, and man. *Epilepsia*, 18:169–182.

Ferrari, R. A., and Arnold, A. (1961): The effect of central nervous system agents on rat-brain-γ-aminobutyric acid level. *Biochim. Biophys. Acta*, 52:361–367.

Ferrendelli, J. A. (1980): Phenytoin: Cyclic nucleotide regulation in the brain. In: *Antiepileptic Drugs: Mechanisms of Action, Advances in Neurology, Vol. 27*, edited by G. H. Glaser, J. K. Penry, and D. M. Woodbury, pp. 429–433. Raven Press, New York.

Ferrendelli, J. A., and Kinscherf, D. A. (1977): Phenytoin: Effects on calcium flux and cyclic nucleotides. *Epilepsia*, 18:331–348.

Ferrendelli, J. A., and Kupferberg, H. J. (1980): Antiepileptic drugs: Succinimides. In: *Antiepileptic Drugs: Mechanisms of Action, Advances in Neurology, Vol. 27*, edited by G. H. Glaser, J. K. Penry, and D. M. Woodbury, pp. 587–595. Raven Press, New York.

Festoff, B. W., and Appel, S. H. (1968): Effect of diphenylhydantoin on synaptosome sodium-potassium-ATPase. *J. Clin. Invest.*, 47:2752–2758.

Fichsel, H. (1978): Effect of anticonvulsant drugs on thyroid hormones. *Epilepsia*, 19:111–112.

Findler, G., and Lavy, S. (1979): Transient hemiparesis: A rare manifestation of diphenyl-hydantoin toxicity. *J. Neurosurg.*, 50:685–687.

Fingl, E. (1972): General principles: Absorption, distribution and elimination: Practical pharmacokinetics. In: *Antiepileptic Drugs*, edited by D. M. Woodbury, J. K. Penry, and R. P. Schmidt, pp. 7–21. Raven Press, New York.

Fingl, E. (1978): Principles of drug absorption, distribution, and metabolism. In: *Antiepileptic Drugs: Quantitative Analysis and Interpretation*, edited by C. E. Pippenger, J. K. Penry, and H. Kutt, pp. 221–236. Raven Press, New York.

Finkelman, M. P., and Arieff, A. J. (1942): Untoward effects of phenytoin sodium in epilepsy. *JAMA*, 118:1209–1212.

Fishman, M. A. (1979): Febrile seizures: The treatment controversy. *J. Pediatr.*, 94:177–184.

Flachs, H., and Rasmussen, J. M. (1980): Renal disease may increase apparent phenytoin in serum as measured by enzyme multiplied immunoassay. *Clin. Chem.*, 26:361.

Flegel, K. M., and Cole, C. H. (1977): Inappropriate anticiuresis during carbamazepine treatment. *Ann. Int. Med.*, 87:722–723.

Fleitman, J. S., Bruni, J., Perrin, J. H., and Wilder, B. J. (1980): Albumin binding interaction of sodium valproate. *J. Clin. Pharmacol.*, 20:514–517.

Forster, F. M. (1951): Therapy in psychomotor epilepsy. *JAMA*, 145:211–215.

Fowler, L. J., Beckford, J., and John, R. A. (1975): An analysis of the kinetics of the inhibition of rabbit brain γ-aminobutyrate amino transferase by sodium n-dipropylacetate and some other simple carboxylic acids. *Biochem. Pharmacol.*, 24:1267–1270.

Fowler, M. (1957): Brain damage after febrile convulsions. *Arch. Dis. Child.*, 32:67–76.

Freeman, J. M. (1978): Febrile seizures: An end to confusion. *Pediatrics*, 61:806–808.

Frei, R. W. (1972): A critical study of some parameters in quantitative in situ investigations of thin layer chromatography by light absorption methods. *J. Chromatogr.*, 64:285–295.

French, E. G., Rey-Bellet, J., and Lennox, W. G. (1958): Methsuximide in psychomotor and petit-mal seizures. *N. Engl. J. Med.*, 285:892–894.

Freund, G. (1973): The prevention of ethanol withdrawal seizures in mice by lidocaine. *Neurology*, 23:91–93.

Frey, H. H., and Loescher, W. (1976): Di-n-propylacetate profile of anticonvulsant activity in mice. *Arzneim. Forsch.*, 26:299–301.

Frey, H. H., and Loescher, W. (1978): Distribution of valproate across the interface between blood and cerebrospinal fluid. *Neuropharmacology*, 17:637–642.

Friel, P., and Green, J. R. (1973): Quantitative assay for carbamazepine serum levels by gas-liquid chromatography. *Clin. Chim. Acta*, 43:69–72.

Friel, P., and Troupin, A. S. (1975): Flash heater ethylation of some antiepileptic drugs. *Clin. Chem.*, 21:751–754.

Frigerio, A., Baker, K. M., and Belvedere, G. (1973): Gas chromatographic degradation of several drugs and their metabolites. *Anal. Chem.*, 45:1846–1851.

Frigerio, A., and Morselli, P. L. (1975): Carbamazepine: Biotransformation. In: *Complex Partial Seizures and Their Treatment, Advances in Neurology, Vol. 11*, edited by J. K. Penry and D. D. Daly, pp. 295–308. Raven Press, New York.

Friis, M. L., and Christiansen, J. (1978): Carbamazepine, carbamazepine-10, 11-epoxide and phenytoin concentrations in brain tissue of epileptic children. *Acta Neurol. Scand.*, 58:104–108.

Friis, M. L., Christiansen, J., and Hvidberg, E. F. (1977): Brain concentrations of carbamazepine and carbamazepine-10,11-epoxide concentrations in human brain. *Br. J. Clin. Pharmacol.*, 4:535–540.

Fromm, G. H., and Killian, J. M. (1967): Effect of some anticonvulsant drugs on spinal trigeminal nucleus. *Neurology*, 17:275–280.

Fromm, G. H., and Kohli, C. M. (1972): The role of inhibitory pathways in petit mal epilepsy. *Neurology*, 22:1012–1020.

Gallagher, B. B. (1972): Trimethadione and other oxazolidinediones: Toxicity. In: *Antiepileptic Drugs*, edited by D. M. Woodbury, J. K. Penry, and R. P. Schmidt, pp. 409–412. Raven Press, New York.

Gallagher, B. B., Baumel, I. P., and Mattson, R. H. (1972): Metabolic disposition of primidone and its metabolites in epileptic subjects after single and repeated administration. *Neurology*, 22:1186–1192.

Gallagher, B. B., Smith, D. B., and Mattson, R. H. (1970): The relationship of the anticonvulsant properties of primidone to phenobarbital. *Epilepsia*, 11:293–301.

Gallagher, D. W., Thomas, J. W., and Tallman, J. F. (1978): Effect of GABAergic drugs on benzodiazepine binding site sensitivity in rat cerebral cortex. *Biochem. Pharmacol.*, 27:2745–2749.

Gamble, J. A. S., Mackay, J. S., and Dundee, J. W. (1973): Blood diazepam levels: Preliminary results. *Br. J. Anaesth.*, 45:926–927.

Gamstorp, I. (1970): *Pediatric Neurology*. Meredith Corporation, New York.

Gastaut, H. (1970): Clinical and electroencephalographical classification of epileptic seizures. *Epilepsia*, 11:102–113.

Gastaut, H. (1973): *Dictionary of Epilepsy, Part I: Definitions*. World Health Organization, Geneva.

Gastaut, H., Nacquet, R., Poire, R., and Tassinari, C. A. (1965): Treatment of status epilepticus with diazepam (Valium). *Epilepsia*, 6:167–182.

Gauchel, G., Gauchel, F. D., and Birkhofer, L. (1973): A micro-method for the determination of carbamazepine in blood by high speed liquid chromatography. *Z. Klin. Chem. Klin. Biochem.*, 11:459–460.

Gellis, S. S. (1978): *The Yearbook of Pediatrics*. Yearbook Medical Publishers, Chicago.

Gharib, H., and Munoz, J. M. (1974): Endocrine manifestations of diphenylhydantoin therapy. *Metabolism*, 23:515–524.

Ghatak, N. R., Santoso, R. A., and McKinney, W. M. (1976): Cerebellar degeneration following long-term phenytoin therapy. *Neurology*, 26:818–820.

Gibaldi, M., and Levy, G. (1976): Pharmacokinetics in clinical practice. *JAMA*, 235:1864–1867, 1987–1992.

Gibbs, F. A., Everett, G. M., and Richards, R. K. (1949): Phenurone in epilepsy. *Dis. Nerv. Syst.*, 10:47–49.

Gibbs, E. L., and Gibbs, T. J. (1974): Gas liquid chromatographic determination of anti-epilepsy drugs and their active metabolites in blood. Gibbs Laboratory Reports, February 20, 1974.

Gibbs, E. L., and Gibbs, T. J. (1978): Instrumentation for gas-liquid chromatographic analysis of antiepileptic drugs: Quality control. In: *Antiepileptic Drugs: Quantitative Analysis and Interpretation*, edited by C. E. Pippenger, J. K. Penry, and H. Kutt, pp. 55–66. Raven Press, New York.

Gibson, I. I. J. M. (1966): Anemia associated with phenobarbital. *Postgrad. Med. J.*, 42:53–54.

Giddings, J. C. (1965): *Dynamics of Chromatography*. Marcel Dekker, New York.

Gilbert, J. C., and Wyllie, M. G. (1974): The effect of the anticonvulsant ethosuximide on adenosine triphosphatase activities of synaptosomes prepared from rat cerebral cortex. *Br. J. Pharmacol.*, 52:139P–140P.

Gillette, J. R., and Pang, K. S. (1977): Theoretic aspects of pharmacokinetic drug interactions. *Clin. Pharmacol. Ther.*, 22:623–639.

Glaser, G. H. (1972): Diphenylhydantoin: Toxicity. In: *Antiepileptic Drugs*, edited by D. M. Woodbury, J. K. Penry, and R. P. Schmidt, pp. 219–226. Raven Press, New York.

Glazko, A. J. (1972): Diphenylhydantoin: Chemistry and methods for determination. In: *Antiepileptic Drugs*, edited by D. M. Woodbury, J. K. Penry, and R. P. Schmidt, pp. 103–112. Raven Press, New York.

Glazko, A. J. (1973): Diphenylhydantoin metabolism. A prospective review. *Drug Metab. Dispos.*, 1:711–714.

Glazko, A. J., Chang, T., Baukema, J., Bill, W. A., Goulet, J. R., and Buchanan, R. A. (1969): Metabolic disposition of diphenylhydantoin in normal human subjects following intravenous administration. *Clin. Pharmacol. Ther.*, 10:495–504.

Glazko, A. J., and Dill, W. A. (1972): Ethosuximide: Chemistry and methods for determination. In: *Antiepileptic Drugs*, edited by D. M. Woodbury, J. K. Penry, and R. P. Schmidt, pp. 413–415. Raven Press, New York.

Gloor, P., and Testa, G. (1974): Generalized penicillin epilepsy in the cat: Effects of intracarotid and intravertebral pentylenetetrazol and amobarbital injections. *Electroencephalogr. Clin. Neurophysiol.*, 36:499–515.

Godin, Y., Heiner, L., Mark, J., and Mandel, P. (1969): Effects of di-n-propylacetate, an anticonvulsant compound, on GABA metabolism. *J. Neurochem.*, 16:869–873.

Godolphin, W., and Thoma, J. (1978): Quantitation of anticonvulsant drugs in serum by gas chromatography on the stationary phase SP-2510. *Clin. Chem.*, 24:483–485.

Goldbaum, L. R. (1952): Determination of barbiturates. *Anal. Chem.*, 24:1604–1607.

Goldberg, M. A. (1980a): Phenobarbital: Binding. In: *Antiepileptic Drugs: Mechanisms of Action, Advances in Neurology, Vol. 27*, edited by G. H. Glaser, J. K. Penry, and D. M. Woodbury, pp. 501–504. Raven Press, New York.

Goldberg, M. A. (1980*b*): Phenytoin: Binding. In: *Antiepileptic Drugs: Mechanisms of Action, Advances in Neurology, Vol. 27*, edited by G. H. Glaser, J. K. Penry, and D. M. Woodbury, pp. 323–337. Raven Press, New York.

Goldberg, M. A., and Crandall, P. H. (1978): Human brain binding of phenytoin. *Neurology*, 28:881–885.

Goldberg, M. A., and Todoroff, T. (1976): Diphenylhydantoin binding to brain lipids and phospholipids. *Biochem. Pharmacol.*, 25:2079–2083.

Goldberg, M. A., and Todoroff, T. (1978): Human brain binding of phenytoin. *Neurology*, 28:881–885.

Goldstein, D. B. (1979): Sodium bromide and sodium valproate: Effective suppressants of ethanol withdrawal reactions in mice. *J. Exp. Pharmacol. Ther.*, 208:223–227.

Gompertz, D., Tippett, P., Bartlett, K., and Baillie, T. (1977): Identification of urinary metabolites of sodium dipropylacetate in man: Potential sources of interferences in organic acid screening procedures. *Clin. Chim. Acta*, 74:153–160.

Gordon, N. (1977): Medium-chain triglycerides in a ketogenic diet. *Dev. Med. Child Neurol.*, 19:535–538.

Gordon, T., Castelli, W. P., Hjortland, M. C., Kanner, W. B., and Dawber, T. R. (1977): High-density lipoprotein as a protective factor against coronary heart disease. The Farmington Study. *Am. J. Med.*, 62:707–714.

Goudie, J. H., and Burnett, D. (1973): A gas chromatographic method for the simultaneous determination of phenobarbital, primidone, and phenytoin using a nitrogen detector. *Clin. Chim. Acta*, 43:423–429.

Goulet, J. R., Kinkel, A. W., and Smith, T. C. (1976): Metabolism of ethosuximide. *Clin. Pharmacol. Ther.*, 20:213–218.

Gowers, W. R. (1885): Epilepsy and other chronic convulsive disorders. *American Academy of Neurology Reprint Series, Vol. 1*, Dover Publications, New York.

Gram, L., Flachs, H., Würtz-Jorgensen, A., Parnas, J., and Anderson, B. (1979): Sodium valproate, serum levels and clinical effect in epilepsy. A controlled study. *Epilepsia*, 20:303–312.

Greeley, R. H. (1974): New approach to derivatization and gas-chromatographic analysis of barbiturates. *Clin. Chem.*, 20:192–194.

Greenblatt, D. J., Allen, M. D., MacLaughlin, D. S., Harmatz, J. S. and Shader, R. I. (1978): Diazepam absorption: Effect of antacids and food. *Clin. Pharmacol. Ther.*, 24:600–609.

Greenblatt, D. J., Bolognini, V., Koch-Weser, J., and Harmatz, J. S. (1976): Pharmacokinetic approach to the clinical use of lidocaine intravenously. *JAMA*, 236:273.

Greenblatt, D. J., and Koch-Weser, J. (1975): Clinical pharmacokinetics. *N. Engl. J. Med.*, 293:702–705, 964–970.

Grob, R. L., editor (1977): *Modern Practice of Gas Chromatography*. Wiley, New York.

Gruber, C. M., Haury, V. G., and Drake, M. E. (1940): The toxic actions of sodium diphenylhydantoinate (Dilantin) when injected intraperitoneally and intravenously in experimental animals. *J. Pharmacol. Exp. Ther.*, 68:433–436.

Guberman, A., Gloor, P., and Sherwin, A. L. (1975): Response of generalized penicillin epilepsy in the cat to ethosuximide and diphenylhydantoin. *Neurology*, 25:758–764.

Guerrero-Figueroa, R., Rye, M. M., and Heath, R. G. (1969a): Effects of two benzodiazepine derivatives on cortical and subcortical epileptogenic tissues in the cat and monkey. I. Limbic system structures. *Curr. Ther. Res.*, 11:27–39.

Guerrero-Figueroa, R., Rye, M. M., and Heath, R. G. (1969b): Effects of two benzodiazepine derivatives on cortical and subcortical epileptogenic tissues in the cat and monkey. II. Cortical and centrencephalic structures. *Curr. Ther. Res.*, 11:40–50.

Guey, J., Charles, C., Coquery, C., Roger, J., and Soulayrol, R. (1967): Study of psychological effects of ethosuximide (Zarontin) on 25 children suffering from petit mal epilepsy. *Epilepsia*, 8:129–141.

Gugler, R., and Mueller, G. (1978): Plasma protein binding of valproic acid in healthy subjects and in patients with renal disease. *Br. J. Clin. Pharmacol.*, 5:441–446.

Gugler, R., Schell, A., Eichelbaum, N., Fröscher, W., and Sculz, H. V. (1977): Disposition of valproic acid in man. *Eur. J. Clin. Pharmacol.*, 12:125–132.

Gugler, R., Shoeman, D. W., Huffman, D. H., Cohlmia, J. B., and Lazarnoff, D. (1975): Pharmacokinetics of drugs in patients with nephrotic syndrome. *J. Clin. Invest.*, 55:1182–1189.

Gupta, R. N., Eng, F., and Gupta, M. L. (1979): Gas chromatographic analysis of valproic acid as phenacyl esters. *Clin. Chem.*, 25:1303–1305.

Haberland, C. (1962): Cerebellar degeneration with clinical manifestations in chronic epileptic patients. *Psychiatr. Clin.*, 143:29–44.

Haefely, W. E. (1978): Central actions of benzodiazepines: General introduction. *Br. J. Psychiatry*, 133:231–238.

Hagberg, B. (1976): The nosology of epilepsy in infancy and childhood. In: *Epileptic Seizures-Behavior-Pain*, edited by W. Birkmayer, pp. 51–64. Hans Huber, Vienna.

Hahn, T. J., Birge, S. J., Scharp, C. R., and Avioli, L. V. (1972a): Phenobarbital-induced alterations in vitamin D metabolism. *J. Clin. Invest.*, 51:741–748.

Hahn, T. J., Henden, B. A., Scharp, C. R., and Haddad, J. G., Jr., (1972b): Effect of chronic anticonvulsant therapy on serum 25-hydroxycalciferol levels in adults. *N. Engl. J. Med.*, 287:900–904.

Halpern, L. M., and Julien, R. M. (1972): Augmentation of cerebellar Purkinje cell discharge rate after diphenylhydantoin. *Epilepsia*, 13:377–385.

Hamilton, D. V. (1978): Carbamazepine and heart block. *Lancet*, 1:1365.

Hamilton, H. E., and Wallace, J. E. (1978): Ultraviolet spectrophotometric quantitation of phenytoin and phenobarbital. In: *Antiepileptic Drugs: Quantitative Analysis and Interpretation*, edited by C. E. Pippenger, J. K. Penry, and H. Kutt, pp. 175–183. Raven Press, New York.

Handley, R., and Stewart, A. S. R. (1952): Mysoline: A new drug in the treatment of epilepsy. *Lancet*, 1:742–744.

Hansen, J. M., Siersbaek-Nielsen, K., and Skovsted, L. (1971): Carbamazepine-induced acceleration of diphenylhydantoin and warfarin metabolism in man. *Clin. Pharmacol. Ther.*, 12:539–543.

Hanson, J. W., Myrianthopoulos, N. C., Harvey, M. A. S., and Smith, D. W. (1976): Risks to the offspring of women treated with hydantoin anticonvulsants, with emphasis on the fetal hydantoin syndrome. *J. Pediatr.*, 89:662–668.

Hardin, E., Passey, R. B., Gillium, R. L., Fuller, J. B., and Lawrence, D. (1976): Clinical laboratory evaluation of the Perkin-Elmer KA-150 enzyme analyzer. *Clin. Chem.*, 22:434–438.

Harding, G. F. A., Herrick, C. E., and Jeavons, P. M. (1978): A controlled study of the effect of sodium valproate on photosensitive epilepsy and its prognosis. *Epilepsia*, 19:555–566.

Harinasuta, U., and Zimmerman, H. J. (1968): Diphenylhydantoin sodium hepatitis. *JAMA*, 203:1015–1018.

Harris, M., Jenkins, M. V., and Wills, M. R. (1974): Phenytoin inhibition of parathyroid hormone-induced bone resorption in vitro. *Br. J. Pharmacol.*, 50:405–408.

Harvey, D. J., Glazener, L., Stratton, C., Nowlin, J., Hill, R. M., and Horning, M. G. (1972): Detection of a 5-(3,4-dihydroxy-1,5-cyclohexadine-1-yl)-metabolite of phenobarbital and mephobarbital in rat, guinea pig and human. *Res. Commun. Chem. Pathol. Pharmacol.*, 3:557–565.

Harvey, P. K. P. (1976): Some aspects of the neurochemistry of Epilim. In: *Clinical and Pharmacological Aspects of Sodium Valproate (Epilim) in the Treatment of Epilepsy*, edited by N. J. Legg, pp. 130–135. MCS Consultants, Tunbridge Wells.

Harvey, P. K. P., Bradford, H. F., and Davison, A. N. (1975): The inhibitory effect of sodium n-dipropylacetate on the degradative enzymes of the GABA shunt. *FEBS Lett.*, 52:251–254.

Harvey, S. C. (1975): Hypnotics and sedatives. In: *The Pharmacological Basis of Therapeutics*, edited by L. S. Goodman and A. Gilman, pp. 102–136. MacMillan, New York.

Hassan, M. N., and Parsonage, M. J. (1977): Experience in the long-term use of carbamazepine (Tegretol) in the treatment of epilepsy. In: *Epilepsy, The Eighth International Symposium*, edited by J. K. Penry, pp. 35–44. Raven Press, New York.

Hauptmann, A. (1912): Luminal bei Epilepsie. *Munch. Med. Wochenschr.*, 59:1907–1909.

Hawk, G. L., and Franconi, L. C. (1978): High pressure liquid chromatography in quantitation of antiepileptic drugs. In: *Antiepileptic Drugs: Quantitative Analysis and Interpretation*, edited by C. E. Pippenger, J. K. Penry, and H. Kutt, pp. 153–162. Raven Press, New York.

Hawker, C. D. (1973): Radioimmunoassay and related methods, review. *Anal. Chem.*, 45:878A–890A.

Hawkins, C. F., and Meynell, M. J. (1958): Macrocytosis and macrocytic anemia caused by anticonvulsant drugs. *Q. J. Med.*, 27:45–63.

Haynes, R. C., and Larner, J. (1975): Adrenocorticotropic hormone; adrenocortical steroids and their synthetic analogs; inhibitors of adrenocortical steroid biosynthesis. In: *The Pharmacological Basis of Therapeutics*, edited by L. S. Goodman and A. Gilman, pp. 1472–1506. MacMillan, New York.

Hazlett, D. R., Ward, G. W., Jr., and Madison, D. S. (1974): Pulmonary function loss in diphenylhydantoin therapy. *Chest*, 66:660–664.

Heckmatt, J. Z., Houston, A. B., Clow, D. J., Stephenson, J. B. P., Dodd, K. L., Lealman, G. T., and Logan, R. W. (1976): Failure of phenobarbital to prevent febrile convulsions. *Br. J. Med.*, 1:559–561.

Heinemann, L. I., and Lux, H. D. (1973): Effects of diphenylhydantoin on extracellular (K+) in cat cortex. *Electroencephalogr. Clin. Neurophysiol.*, 34:735.

Helin, I., Nilsson, K. O., Bjerre, I., and Vegfors, P. (1977): Serum sodium and osmolality during carbamazepine treatment in children. *Br. Med. J.*, 2:558.

Herbert, V. (1968): Inborn errors in folate metabolism—a cause of mental retardation. *Ann. Int. Med.*, 68:956–958.

Herha, J., and Obe, G. (1977): Chromosomal damage in patients with epilepsy: Possible mutagenic properties of long-term antiepileptic drug treatment. In: *Epilepsy, The Eighth International Symposium*, edited by J. K. Penry, pp. 87–94. Raven Press, New York.

Hershey, A. E., Patton, J. R., and Dudley, K. K. (1979): Gas chromatographic method for the determination of valproic acid in human plasma. *Ther. Drug Monit.*, 1:217–241.

Herzberg, L. (1978): Carbamazepine and bradycardia. *Lancet*, 1:1097–1098.

Hewitt, T. E., Sievers, D. L., and Kessler, G. (1978): Improved gas chromatographic analysis for anticonvulsants. *Clin. Chem.*, 1854–1856.

Hill, R., Horning, M., and Horning, E. (1973): Identification of transplacentally acquired anticonvulsant agents in the neonate. In: *Methods of Analysis of Anti-epileptic Drugs*, edited by J. W. A. Meijer, H. Meinardi, C. Gardner-Thorpe, and E. Van der Kleijn, pp. 146–147. American Elsevier, New York.

Hillbom, M. E. (1975): The prevention of ethanol withdrawal seizures in rats by dipropyl-acetate. *Neuropharmacology*, 14:755–761.

Hillestad, L., Hansen, T., and Melson, H. (1974): Diazepam metabolism in normal man. II. Serum concentration and clinical effect after oral administration and cumulation. *Clin. Pharmacol. Ther.*, 16:485–489.

Hoffbrand, A. V., and Necheles, T. H. (1968): Mechanism of folate deficiency in patients receiving phenytoin. *Lancet*, 2:528–530.

Hoffbrand, A. V., and Peters, T. J. (1968): Subcellular localization of folate conjugase in guinea-pig intestinal mucosa. *J. Physiol.*, 202:40P.

Hofmann, W. W. (1958): Cerebellar lesions after parenteral Dilantin administration. *Neurology*, 8:210–214.

Holdsworth, L., and Whitmore, K. (1974): A study of children with epilepsy attending ordinary schools. *Dev. Med. Child Neurol.*, 16:747–758.

Holm, E., Kelleter, R., Heinemann, H., and Hamann, K. F. (1970): Elektrophysiologiche analyse der wirkungen von carbamazepine auf das (Gehirn) der katze. *Pharmakopsychiatr. Neuropsychopharmakol.*, 3:187–200.

Hooper, W. D., Bochner, F., Eadie, M. J., and Tyrer, J. H. (1974): Plasma protein binding of diphenylhydantoin. Effects of sex hormones, renal and hepatic disease. *Clin. Pharmacol. Ther.*, 15:276–282.

Hooper, W. D., Dubetz, D. K., Bochner, F., Cotter, L. M., Smith, G. A., Eadie, M. J., and Tyrer, J. H. (1975): Plasma protein binding of carbamazepine. *Clin. Pharmacol. Ther.*, 17:433–440.

Horning, M. G., Brown, L., Nowlin, J., Lertratanangkoon, K., Kellaway, P., and Zion, T. E. (1977): Use of saliva in therapeutic drug monitoring. *Clin. Chem.*, 23:157–164.

Horning, M. G., Lertratanangkoon, K., Nowlin, J., Stillwell, W. G., Stillwell, R. N., Zion, T. E., Kellaway, P., and Hill, R. M. (1974): Anticonvulsant drug monitoring by GC-MS-COM techniques. *J. Chromatogr. Sci.*, 12:630–635.

Horning, M. G., Stratton, C., Nowlin, J., Harvey, D. J., and Hill, R. M. (1973): Metabolism of 2-ethyl-2-methyl succinimide in the rat and human. *Drug Metab. Dispos.*, 1:569–576.

Horton, R. W., Anlezark, G. M., Sawaya, M. C. B., and Meldrum, B. S. (1977): Monoamine and GABA metabolism and the anticonvulsant action of di-n-propylacetate and ethanol-amine-o-sulphate. *Eur. J. Pharmacol.*, 41:387–397.

Horwitz, S. J., Klipstein, F. A., and Lovelace, R. E. (1968): Relation of abnormal folate metabolism to neuropathy developing during anticonvulsant drug therapy. *Lancet*, 1:563–565.

Houck, J. C., Cheng, R. F., and Waters, M. D. (1972): Diphenylhydantoin: Effects on connective tissue and wound repairs. In: *Antiepileptic Drugs*, edited by D. M. Woodbury, J. K. Penry, and R. P. Schmidt, pp. 267–274. Raven Press, New York.

Houghton, G. W., and Richens, A. (1975): The effect of benzodiazepines and pheneturide on phenytoin metabolism in man. *Br. J. Pharmacol.*, 1:334–335.

Houghton, G. W., Richens, A., Toseland, P. A., Davidson, S., and Falconer, M. A. (1975): Brain concentrations of phenytoin, phenobarbital, and primidone in epileptic patients. *Eur. J. Clin. Pharmacol.*, 9:73–78.

Howell, B. F., Schaffer, R., and Sasse, E. A. (1978): Enzyme immunoassay adapted for use with a digital kinetic analyzer. *Clin. Chem.*, 24:1284.

Huang, C. Y., McLeod, J. G., Sampson, D., and Hensley, W. J. (1974): Clonazepam in the treatment of epilepsy. *Med. J. Aust.*, 2:5–8.

Huisman, J. W. (1966): The estimation of some important anticonvulsant drugs in serum. *Clin. Chim. Acta*, 13:323–328.

Hulshoff, A., and Roseboom, H. (1979): Determination of valproic acid (di-n-propylacetic acid) in plasma by gas-liquid chromatography with pre-column butylation. *Clin. Chim. Acta*, 93:9–13.

Hundt, H. K. L., and Clark, E. C. (1975): Thin-layer chromatography for determination of carbamazepine and two of its metabolites in serum. *J. Chromatogr.*, 107:49–54.

Hunter, R. A. (1959): Status epilepticus: History, incidence, and problems. *Epilepsia*, 1:62–188.

Hutt, S. J., Jackson, P. M., Belsham, A., and Higgins, G. (1968): Perceptual-motor behavior in relation to blood phenobarbital level: A preliminary report. *Dev. Med. Child Neurol.*, 10:626–632.

Huttenlocher, P. R. (1976): Ketonemia and seizures: Metabolic and anticonvulsant effects of two ketogenic diets in childhood epilepsy. *Pediatr. Res.*, 10:536–540.

Huttenlocher, P. R., Wilbourn, A. J., and Signore, J. M. (1971): Medium-chain triglycerides as a therapy for intractable childhood epilepsy. *Neurology*, 21:1097–1103.

Hvidberg, E. F., and Dam, M. (1976): Clinical pharmacokinetics of anticonvulsants. *Clin. Pharmacokinet.*, 1:161–188.

Hvidberg, E. F., and Sjö, O. (1975): Clinical pharmacokinetic experiences with clonazepam. In: *Clinical Pharmacology of Antiepileptic Drugs*, edited by H. Schneider, pp. 242–246. Springer-Verlag, Berlin.

Ideström, C. M., Schalling, D., Carlquist, U., and Sjöqvist, F. (1972): Acute effects of diphenylhydantoin in relation to plasma levels: Psychological studies. *Psychol. Med.*, 2:111–120.

Iivanainen, M., and Viukari, M. (1977): Serum phenytoin, seizures and electroencephalography. *Lancet*, 1:860–861.

Iivanainen, M., Viukari, M., and Helle, E. P. (1977): Cerebellar atrophy in phenytoin-treated mentally retarded epileptics. *Epilepsia*, 18:375–386.

Iivanainen, M., Viukari, M., Seppäläinen, A. M., and Helle, E. P. (1978): Electroencephalography and phenytoin toxicity in mentally retarded epileptic patients. *J. Neurol. Neurosurg. Psychiatry*, 41:272–277.

Iverson, L. L. (1979): The chemistry of the brain. *Sci. Am.*, September, 134–149.

Jaeken, J., Corbeel, L., Casaer, P., Carchon, H., Eggermont, E., and Eeckels, R. (1977): Dipropylacetate (Valproate) and glycine metabolism. *Lancet*, 2:617.

Jakobs, C., Bojasch, M., and Hanefeld, F. (1978): New direct method for determination of valproic acid in serum by gas liquid chromatography. *J. Chromatogr.*, 146:494.

Jakobs, C., and Loscher, W. (1978): Identification of metabolites of valproic acid in serum of humans, dog, rat, and mouse. *Epilepsia*, 19:591–602.

Jalling, B. (1968): Plasma and cerebrospinal fluid concentrations of phenobarbital in infants given single doses. *Dev. Med. Child Neurol.*, 10:626–632.

Jalling, B. (1974): Plasma and cerebrospinal fluid concentrations of phenobarbital in infants given single doses. *Dev. Med. Child Neurol.*, 16:781–793.

Jan, J. E., Riegl, J. A., Crichton, J. M., and Dunn, H. G. (1971): Nitrazepam in the treatment of epilepsy in childhood. *Can. Med. Assoc. J.*, 104:571–575.

Janik, A. (1975): What is the best measure of the detector signal: The peak area or the peak height? *J. Chromatogr. Sci.*, 13:93–96.

Janz, D. (1961): Conditions and causes of status epilepticus. *Epilepsia*, 2:170–177.

Janz, D. (1964): Status epilepticus and frontal lobe lesions. *J. Neurol. Sci.*, 1:446–457.

Janz, D. (1975): Teratogenic risk of antiepileptic drugs. *Epilepsia*, 16:159–169.

Janz, D., and Kautz, G. (1964): The aetiology and treatment of status epilepticus. *Ger. Med. Mon.*, 9:451–456.

Jeavons, P. M. (1977): Nosological problems of myoclonic epilepsies in childhood and adolescence. *Dev. Med. Child Neurol.*, 19:3–8.

Jeavons, P. M., and Bower, B. D. (1974): Infantile spasms. In: *Handbook of Clinical Neurology*, edited by P. J. Vinken and G. W. Bruyn, pp. 219–234. American Elsevier, New York.

Jeavons, P. M., Bower, B. D., and Dimitrakondi, M. (1973): Long-term prognosis of 150 cases of "West Syndrome." *Epilepsia*, 14:153–164.

Jeavons, P. M., Clark, J. E., and Maheshwari, M. D. (1977): Treatment of generalized epilepsies of childhood and adolescence with sodium valproate (Epilim). *Dev. Med. Child Neurol.*, 19:9–25.

Jenner, P., Chadwick, D., Reynolds, E. H., and Marsden, C. D. (1975): Clonazepam-induced changes in 5-hydroxytryptamine metabolism in animals and man. *J. Pharmacol. [Suppl.]*, 27:38.

Jordan, B. J., Shillingford, J. S., and Steed, K. P. (1976): Preliminary observations on the protein-binding and enzyme-inducing properties of sodium valproate (Epilim). In: *Clinical and Pharmacological Aspects of Sodium Valproate (Epilim) in the Treatment of Epilepsy*, pp. 112–118. MCS Consultants, Tunbridge Wells.

Juel, R. (1979): The 1978 College of American Pathologists therapeutic drug monitoring interlaboratory survey program. *Am. J. Clin. Pathol.*, 72:306–319.

Julien, R. M. (1972): Cerebellar involvement in the antiepileptic action of diazepam. *Neuropharmacology*, 11:683–691.

Julien, R. M. (1973): Lidocaine in experimental epilepsy: Correlation of anticonvulsant effect with blood concentrations. *Electroencephalogr. Clin. Neurophysiol.*, 34:639–645.

Julien, R. M., and Fowler, G. W. (1977): A comparative study of the efficacy of newer antiepileptic drugs on experimentally-induced febrile convulsions. *Neuropharmacology*, 16:719–724.

Julien, R. M., and Hollister, R. P. (1975): Carbamazepine: Mechanism of action. In: *Complex Partial Seizures and Their Treatment, Advances in Neurology, Vol. 11*, edited by J. K. Penry and D. D. Daly, pp. 263–277. Raven Press, New York.

Jusko, W. J. (1972): Pharmacokinetic principles in pediatric pharmacology. *Pediatr. Clin. North. Am.*, 19:81–100.

Jusko, W. J., and Gretch, M. (1976): Plasma and tissue protein binding of drugs in pharmacokinetics. *Drug Metab. Rev.*, 5:43–140.

Juul-Jensen, P. (1968): Frequency of recurrence after discontinuation of anticonvulsant therapy in patients with epileptic seizures. *Epilepsia*, 9:11–16.

Juul-Jensen, P., and Denny-Brown, D. (1966): Epilepsia partialis continua. *Arch. Neurol.*, 15:563–578.

Kabra, P. M., Stafford, B. E., and Marton, L. J. (1977): Simultaneous measurement of phenobarbital, phenytoin, primidone, ethosuximide, and carbamazepine in serum by high pressure liquid chromatography. *Clin. Chem.*, 23:1284–1288.

Kallberg, N., Agurell, S., Ericsson, O., Bucht, E., Jalling, B., and Boreus, L. O. (1975): Quantitation of phenobarbital and its main metabolites in human urine. *Eur. J. Clin. Pharmacol.*, 9:161–168.

Kaplan, S. A., Alexander, K., Jack, M. L., Puglisi, C. V., deSilva, J. A. F., Lee, T. L., and Weinfeld, R. E. (1974): Pharmacokinetic profiles of clonazepam in dog and humans and of flunitrazepam in dog. *J. Pharmacol. Sci.*, 63:527–532.

Kapur, R. N., Girgis, S., Little, T. M., and Mossotti, R. E. (1973): Diphenylhydantoin-induced gingival hyperplasia: Its relationship to dose and serum level. *Dev. Med. Child Neurol.*, 15:483–487.

Karas, B. J., and Wilder, B. J. (1981): Dilantin and antacid drug interaction. *(Unpublished data.)*

Karlov, V. A., Gerber, E. L., and Voronkin, G. V. (1974): The pathomorphology of status epilepticus. *Zh. Nevropatol. Psikhiatr.*, 74:1659–1666.

Kas, S., and Orszagh, J. (1976): Clinical study of status epilepticus: Review of 111 statuses. *Acta Univ. Carol.*, 22:133–178.

Kauffman, R. E., Habersant, R., and Lansky, L. (1977): Kinetics of primidone metabolism and excretion in children. *Clin. Pharmacol. Ther.*, 22:200–205.

Keller, A. D., and Fulton, J. F. (1931): The action of anesthetic drugs on the motor cortex of monkeys. *Am. J. Physiol.*, 47:537.

Killian, J. M. (1969): Tegretol in trigeminal neuralgia with special reference to hematopoietic side effects. *Headache*, 9:58–63.

Killian, J. M., and Fromm, G. H. (1968): Carbamazepine in the treatment of neuralgia. Use and side effects. *Arch Neurol.*, 19:129–136.

Killian, J. M., and Fromm, G. H. (1970): A double-blind comparison of nitrazepam versus diazepam in myoclonic seizure disorders. *Dev. Med. Child Neurol.*, 13:32–39.

Kiørboe, E., Paludan, J., Trolle, E., and Overvad, E. (1964): Zarontin (Ethosuximide) in the treatment of petit mal and related disorders. *Epilepsia*, 5:83–89.

Kirchner, J. G. (1973): Thin-layer chromatographic quantitative analysis. *J. Chromatogr.*, 82:101–115.

Kiser, J. S., Vargas-Cordon, M., Brendel, K., and Bressler, R. (1970): The in vitro inhibition of insulin secretion by diphenylhydantoin. *J. Clin. Invest.*, 49:1942–1948.

Klipstein, F. A. (1964): Subnormal serum folate and macrocytosis associated with anticonvulsant drug therapy. *Blood*, 23:68–86.

Klotz, U., and Antonin, K. H. (1977): Pharmacokinetics and bioavailability of sodium valproate. *Clin. Pharmacol. Ther.*, 21:736–743.

Klotz, U., Antonin, K. H., Brugel, H., and Bieck, P. R. (1977): Disposition of diazepam and its major metabolite desmethyldiazepam in patients with liver disease. *Clin. Pharmacol. Ther.*, 21:430–436.

Knudsen, F. U. (1977): Plasma diazepam after rectal administration in solution and by suppository. *Acta Paediatr. Scand.*, 66:563–567.

Knudsen, F. U., and Vestermark, S. (1978): Prophylactic diazepam or phenobarbital in febrile convulsions: A prospective, controlled study. *Arch. Dis. Child.*, 53:660–663.

Kober, A., Sjoholm, I., Borga, O., and Oder-Cederlof, I. (1979): Protein binding of diazepam and digitoxin in uremic and normal serum. *Biochem. Pharmacol.*, 28:1037–1042.

Koch, H. U., Kraft, D., VonHerrath, D., and Schaefer, K. (1972): Influences of diphenylhydantoin and phenobarbital on intestinal calcium transport in the rat. *Epilepsia*, 13:829–834.

Kohler, H. G. (1966): Hemorrhage in the newborn of epileptic mothers. *Lancet*, 1:267.

Kossa, W. C., MacGee, J., Ramachandran, S., and Webber, A. J. (1979): Pyrolytic methylation/gas chromatography: A short review. *J. Chromatogr. Sci.*, 17:177–187.

Kosteljanetz, M., Christiansen, J., Dam, A. M., Hansen, B. S., Lyon, B. B., Pedersen, H., and Dam, M. (1979): Carbamazepine vs phenytoin. A controlled clinical trial in focal motor and generalized epilepsy. *Arch. Neurol.*, 36:22–24.

Krupp, P. (1969): The effects of Tegretol on some elementary neuronal mechanisms. *Headache*, 9:46–53.

Kuhara, T., and Matsumoto, I. (1974): Metabolism of branched medium chain length fatty acids. I. ω-Oxidation of sodium dipropylacetate in rats. *Biomed. Mass Spectrom.*, 1:291–294.

Kumps, A., and Mardens, Y. (1975): A rapid gas liquid chromatographic determination of serum phenobarbital and diphenylhydantoin. *Clin. Chim. Acta*, 62:371–376.

Kuntzman, R. (1969): Drugs and enzyme induction. *Ann. Rev. Pharmacol.*, 9:21–36.

Kupferberg, H. J. (1970): Quantitative estimation of diphenylhydantoin, primidone, and phenobarbital in plasma by gas-liquid chromatography. *Clin. Chim. Acta*, 29:283–288.

Kupferberg, H. J. (1972): GLC determination of carbamazepine in plasma. *J. Pharm. Sci.*, 61:284–286.

Kupferberg, H. J. (1978): Gas liquid chromatographic quantitation of valproic acid. In: *Antiepileptic Drugs: Quantitative Analysis and Interpretation*, edited by C. E. Pippenger, J. K. Penry, and H. Kutt, pp. 147–151. Raven Press, New York.

Kupferberg, H. J., Yonekawa, W. D., Lacy, J. R., Porter, R. J., and Penry, J. K. (1977): Comparison of methsuximide and phensuximide metabolism in epileptic patients. In: *Antiepileptic Drug Monitoring*, edited by C. Gardner-Thorp, D. Janz, I. T. Meinardi, and C. E. Pippenger, pp. 173–180. Pitman Medical, Kent, England.

Kusske, J A., Ojeman, G. A., and Ward, A. A., Jr. (1972): Effects of lesions in ventricular anterior thalamus on experimental focal epilepsy. *Exp. Neurol.*, 34:279–290.

Kutt, H. (1971): Biochemical and genetic factors regulating Dilantin metabolism in man. *Ann. NY Acad. Sci.*, 179:704–722.

Kutt, H. (1972): Diphenylhydantoin: Relation of plasma levels to clinical control. In: *Antiepileptic Drugs*, edited by D. M. Woodbury, J. K. Penry, and R. P. Schmidt, pp. 211–218. Raven Press, New York.

Kutt, H. (1973): Pharmacodynamics and pharmacokinetic measurements of antiepileptic drugs. *Clin. Pharmacol. Ther.*, 16:243–250.

Kutt, H. (1974): The use of blood levels of antiepileptic drugs in clinical practice. *Pediatrics*, 53:557–560.

Kutt, H. (1975): Interactions of antiepileptic drugs. *Epilepsia*, 16:393–402.

Kutt, H. (1978): Clinical pharmacology of carbamazepine. In: *Antiepileptic Drugs: Quantitative Analysis and Interpretation*, edited by C. E. Pippenger, J. K. Penry, and H. Kutt, pp. 297–305. Raven Press, New York.

Kutt, H., and Penry, J. K. (1974): Usefulness of blood levels of antiepileptic drugs. *Arch. Neurol.*, 31:283–288.

Kutt, H., Winters, W., Scherman, R., and McDowell, F. (1964): Diphenylhydantoin and phenobarbital toxicity. The role of liver disease. *Arch. Neurol.*, 11:649–656.

Labram, C. (1975): Dangerous combinations: Phenytoin and disulfiram. *Concours. Med.*, 97:6490–6493.

Lacy, J. R., and Penry, J. K. (1976): *Infantile Spasms*. Raven Press, New York.

Lai, A. A., Levy, R. H., and Cutler, R. E. (1978): Time-course of interaction between carbamazepine and clonazepam in normal man. *Clin. Pharmacol. Ther.*, 24:316–323.

Lance, J. W., and Anthony, M. (1977): Sodium valproate and clonazepam in the treatment of intractable epilepsy. *Arch. Neurol.*, 34:14–17.

Lascelles, P. T., Kocen, R. S., and Reynolds, E. H. (1970): The distribution of plasma phenytoin levels in epileptic patients. *J. Neurol. Neurosurg. Psychiatry*, 33:501–505.

Laxer, K. D., Robertson, L. T., Julien, R. M., and Dow, R. S. (1980): Phenytoin: Relationship between cerebellar function and epileptic discharges. In: *Antiepileptic Drugs: Mechanisms of Action, Advances in Neurology, Vol. 27*, edited by G. H. Glaser, J. K. Penry, and D. M. Woodbury, pp. 415–427. Raven Press, New York.

Lemmen, L. J., Klassen, M., and Duiser, B. (1978): Intravenous lidocaine in the treatment of convulsions. *JAMA*, 239:2025.

Lennox, W. G. (1942): Brain injury, drugs and environmental causes of mental decay in epilepsy. *Am. J. Psychiatry*, 99:174–180.

Lennox, W. G. (1947): Tridione® in the treatment of epilepsy. *JAMA*, 134:138–143.

Lennox, W. G. (1960): *Epilepsy and Related Disorders*. Little, Brown and Company, Boston.

Lennox-Buchthal, M. A. (1976): A summing up: Clinical session. In: *Brain Dysfunction in Infantile Febrile Convulsions*, edited by M. A. B. Brazier and F. Coceani, pp. 327–351. Raven Press, New York.

Leppik, I. E., and Sherwin, A. (1977): Anticonvulsant activity of phenobarbital and phenytoin in combination. *J. Pharmacol. Exp. Ther.*, 200:570–575.

LeQuesne, P. M., Goldberg, V., and Vajda, F. (1976): Acute conduction velocity changes in guinea-pigs after administration of diphenylhydantoin. *J. Neurol. Neurosurg. Psychiatry*, 39:995–1000.

Letteri, J. M., Mellk, H., Louis, S., Durante, P., and Glazko, A. (1971): Diphenylhydantoin metabolism in uremia. *N. Engl. J. Med.*, 285:648–652.

Levin, S. R., Booker, J., Jr., Smith, D. F., and Grodsky, G. M. (1970): Inhibition of insulin secretion by diphenylhydantoin in the isolated perfused pancreas. *J. Clin. Endocrinol.*, 30:400–401.

Levine, R. R. (1978): Factors modifying the effects of drugs in individuals. Variability in response attributable to the biologic system. In: *Pharmacology: Drug Actions and Reactions*, 2nd edition, edited by R. R. Levine, pp. 241–266. Little, Brown and Company, Boston.

Levy, G. (1973): Pharmacokinetic control and clinical interpretation of steady-state blood levels of drugs. *Clin. Pharmacol. Ther.*, 16:130–134.

Levy, R. (1980): Phenytoin: Biopharmacology. In: *Antiepileptic Drugs: Mechanism of Action, Advances in Neurology, Vol. 27*, edited by G. H. Glaser, J. K. Penry, and D. M. Woodbury, pp. 315–322. Raven Press, New York.

Meldrum, B. S., and Nilsson, B. (1976): Cerebral blood flow and metabolic rate early and late in prolonged epileptic seizures induced in rats by bicuculline. *Brain*, 99:523–542.

Meldrum, B. S., Vigouroux, R. A., and Brierly, J. B. (1973): Systemic factors and epileptic brain damage: Prolonged seizures in paralyzed artificially ventilated baboons. *Arch. Neurol.*, 29:82–87.

Melikian, A. P., Straughn, A. B., Slywka, G. W. A., Whyatt, P. L., and Meyer, M. C. (1977): Bioavailability of 11 phenytoin products. *J. Pharmacokinet. Biopharmacol.*, 5:133–146.

Merlis, J. K. (1970): Proposal for an International Classification of the Epilepsies. *Epilepsia*, 11:114–119.

Merritt, H. H., and Putnam, T. J. (1938a): A new series of anticonvulsant drugs tested by experiments on animals. *Arch. Neurol. Psychiatry*, 39:1003–1015.

Merritt, H. H., and Putnam, T. J. (1938b): Sodium diphenylhydantoinate in treatment of convulsive disorders. *JAMA*, 111:1068–1973.

Mesdjian, E., Mesdjian, J. L., Bouyard, P., Dravet, C., and Roger, J., (1978): Effect of sodium valproate on phenobarbitone plasma levels in epileptic patients. In: *Advances in Epileptology*, edited by H. Meinardi and A. J. Rowan, pp. 266–268. Swets and Zeitlinger, Amsterdam.

Meunier, H., Carraz, G., Meunier, Y., Eymard, P., and Aimard, M. (1963): Proprietes pharmacodynamique de l'acide n-dipropylacetique. *Therapie*, 18:435–438.

Michael, J. R., and Mitch, W. E. (1976): Reversible renal failure and myositis caused by phenytoin hypersensitivity. *JAMA*, 236:2773–2775.

Michaux, L., Feld, M., and Labet, R. (1959): L'intoxication par les hydantoines: Manifestations neurologiques. *Presse Med.*, 67:210–212.

Miller, N. E., Forde, O. H., Thelle, D. S., and Mjos, O. D. (1977): The Tromso-heart-study. High density lipoprotein and coronary heart disease: A prospective case-control study. *Lancet*, 1:965–968.

Miller, C. A., and Long, L. M. (1951): Anticonvulsants. I. An investigation of N-R-alpha-R1-alpha-phenylsuccinimides. *J. Am. Chem. Soc.*, 73:4895–4898.

Miller, C. A., and Long, L. M. (1953a): Anticonvulsants. IV. An investigation of a (substituted phenyl) succinimide. *J. Am. Chem. Soc.*, 75:6256–6258.

Miller, C. A., and Long, L. M. (1953b): Anticonvulsants. III. An investigation of N-alpha-B-alkyl-succinimides. *J. Am. Chem. Soc.*, 75:373–375.

Miller, J. H. D., and Nevin, N. C. (1973): Congenital malformations and anticonvulsant drugs. *Lancet*, 1:328.

Miller, N. E., and Nestel, P. J. (1973): Altered bile acid metabolism during treatment with phenobarbital. *Clin. Sci. Mol. Med.*, 45:257–262.

Millichap, J. G. (1952): Milontin: A new drug in the treatment of petit mal. *Lancet*, 2:907–910.

Millichap, J. G. (1969): Systemic electrolyte and neuroendocrine mechanisms. In: *Basic Mechanisms of the Epilepsies*, edited by H. H. Jasper, A. A. Ward, Jr., and A. Pope, pp. 709–726. Little, Brown and Company, Boston.

Millichap, J. G. (1974): Metabolic and endocrine factors. In: *Handbook of Clinical Neurology: The Epilepsies*, edited by P. J. Vinken and G. W. Bruyn, pp. 311–324. North Holland, Amsterdam.

Millichap, J. G., Jones, J. D., and Ruchis, B. P. (1964): Mechanisms of anticonvulsive action of ketogenic diet. *Am. J. Dis. Child.*, 107:593–604.

Millichap, J. G., Woodbury, D. M., and Goodman, L. S. (1955): Mechanisms of the anticonvulsant action of acetazolamide, a carbonic anhydrase inhibitor. *J. Pharmacol. Exp. Ther.*, 115:251–258.

Miribel, J., and Poirier, F. (1961): Effects of ACTH and adrenocortical hormone in juvenile epilepsy. *Epilepsia*, 2:345–353.

Miyahara, J. T., Esplin, D. W., and Zablocka, B. (1966): Differential effects of depressant drugs on presynaptic inhibition. *J. Pharmacol. Exp. Ther.*, 154:118–127.

Mohler, H., and Okada, T. (1977): Benzodiazepine receptor: Demonstration in the central nervous system. *Science*, 198:849–851.

Monnet, P., Rosenberg, D., and Bovier-Lapierre, M. (1968): Thérapeutique anticomitiale administrée pendant la grossesse et maladie hémorrhagique du nouveau-né. *Rev. Fr. Gynecol.*, 63:695–702.

Monson, R. R., Rosenberg, L., Hartz, S. C., Shapiro, S., Heinonen, O. P., and Slone, D. (1973): Diphenylhydantoin and selected congenital malformations. *N. Engl. J. Med.*, 289:1049–1052.

Moore, M. T. (1959): Pulmonary changes in hydantoin therapy. *JAMA*, 171:1328–1333.

Morrell, F., Bradley, W., and Ptashne, M. (1959): Effects of drugs on discharge characteristics of chronic epileptogenic lesions. *Neurology*, 9:492–498.

Morris, H. H. (1979): Lidocaine: A neglected anticonvulsant. *South. Med. J.*, 72:1564–1566.

Morselli, P. L. (1975): Carbamazepine: Absorption, distribution and excretion. In: *Complex Partial Seizures and Their Treatment, Advances in Neurology, Vol. 11*, edited by J. K. Penry and D. D. Daly, pp. 279–293. Raven Press, New York.

Morselli, P. L., Cassano, G. B., Placidi, G. F., Muscettola, G. B., and Rizzo, M. (1973): Kinetics of the distribution of ^{14}C-diazepam and its metabolites in various areas of cat brain. In: *The Benzodiazepines*, edited by S. Garattini, E. Mussini, and L. O. Randall, pp. 129–143. Raven Press, New York.

Mosekilde, L., Hansen, H. H., Christensen, M. S., Lund, B., Sprensen, O. H., Melsen, F., and Norman, A. W. (1979): Fractional intestinal calcium absorption in epileptics on anticonvulsant therapy. *Acta Med. Scand.*, 205:405–409.

Mountain, K. R., Hirsh, J., and Gallus, A. S. (1970): Neonatal coagulation defect due to anticonvulsant drug treatment in pregnancy. *Lancet*, 1:265–268.

Muller, W., and Wollert, U. (1973): Characteristics of the binding of benzodiazepines to human serum albumin. *Arch. Pharmacol.*, 280:229–237.

Mutani, R., and Fariello, R. (1969): Effetti dell'acido n-dipropylacetico (Depakene) sull'attivita del focus epilettogenico corticale da cobalto. *Riv. Patol. Nerv. Ment.*, 90:40–49.

Myers, G. J. (1975): The therapy of myoclonus. In: *Myoclonic Seizures*, edited by M. H. Carlton, pp. 121–160. Excerpta Medica, New York.

Naestoft, J., and Larsen, N. E. (1974): Quantitative determination of clonazepam and its metabolites in human plasma by gas chromatography. *J. Chromatogr.*, 93:113–122.

Nanda, R. N., Johnson, R. H., Keogh, H. J., Lambie, D. G., and Melville, I. D. (1977a): Treatment of epilepsy with clonazepam and its effect on other anticonvulsants. *J. Neurol. Neurosurg. Psychiatry*, 40:538–543.

Nanda, R. N., Johnson, R. H., Keogh, H. J., Lambie, D. G., Melville, I. D., and Shakir, R. A. (1977b): Treatment of chronic epilepsy for 1 to 2 years with clonazepam. In: *Epilepsy: The Eighth International Symposium*, edited by J. K. Penry, pp. 163–168. Raven Press, New York.

Nandedkar, A. K. N., Kutt, H., and Fairclough, G. F., Jr. (1978): Correlation of the "EMIT" with a gas-liquid chromatographic method for determination of antiepileptic drugs in plasma. *Clin. Toxicol.*, 12:483–494.

National Institutes of Health (1980): Febrile Seizures: NIH Consensus Development Conference Summary, Vol. 3, No. 2. National Institutes of Health, Bethesda, Maryland.

Nelson, K. B., and Ellenberg, J. H. (1978): Prognosis in children with febrile seizures. *Pediatrics*, 61:720–727.

Neophytides, A. N., Nutt, J. G., and Lodish, J. R. (1979): Thrombocytopenia associated with sodium valproate. *Ann. Neurol.*, 5:389–390.

Ney, R. L. (1969): Effects of dibutyryl cyclic AMP on adrenal growth and steroidogenic capacity. *Endocrinology*, 84:168–170.

Nicol, C. F., Tutton, J. C., and Smith, B. H. (1969): Parenteral diazepam in status epilepticus. *Neurology*, 19:332–343.

Nicoll, R. A., and Iwamoto, E. T. (1978): Action of pentobarbital on sympathetic ganglion cells. *J. Neurophysiol.*, 41:977–986.

Niebyl, J. R., Blake, D. A., and Freeman, J. M. (1979): Carbamazepine levels in pregnancy and lactation. *Obstet. Gynecol.*, 53:139–140.

Nikkilä, E. A., Kaste, M., Ehnholm, C., and Viikari, J. (1978): Elevation of high-density lipoprotein in epileptic patients treated with phenytoin. *Acta Med. Scand.*, 204:517–520.

Nishihari, K., Uchino, K., Saitoh, Y., Honda, Y., Nakagawa, F., and Tamura, Z. (1979): Estimation of plasma unbound phenobarbital concentration by using mixed saliva. *Epilepsia*, 20:37–45.

Noble, E. P., Gillies, R., Vigran, R., and Mandel, P. (1976): The modification of the ethanol withdrawal syndrome in rats by Di-n-propylacetate. *Psychopharmacology*, 46:127–131.

Nogen, A. G. (1978): The utility of clonazepam in epilepsy of various types. Observations with 22 childhood cases. *Clin. Pediatr.*, 17:71–74.

Norris, F. H., Jr., Colella, J. A. B., and McFarlin, D. (1964): Effect of diphenylhydantoin on neuromuscular synapse. *Neurology*, 14:869–876.

Nowack, W. J., Johnson, R. N., Englander, R. N., and Hanna, G. (1979): Effects of valproate and ethosuximide on thalamocortical excitability. *Neurology*, 29:96–99.

Nutt, J. G., Neophytides, A. N., and Lodish, J. R. (1978): Lowered erythrocyte-sedimentation rate with sodium valproate. *Lancet*, 2:636.

Nutt, J., Williams, A., Plotkin, C., Eng, N., Ziegler, M., and Calne, D. B. (1979): Treatment of Parkinson's disease with sodium valproate: Clinical, pharmacological, and biochemical observations. *Can. J. Neurol. Sci.*, 6:337–343.

Oder-Cederlof, I., and Borga, O. (1974): Kinetics of diphenylhydantoin in uremic patients—consequences of decreased plasma protein binding. *Eur. J. Clin. Pharmacol.*, 7:31–37.

O'Donohoe, N. V. (1964): Treatment of petit mal with ethosuximide. *Dev. Med. Child Neurol.*, 6:498–501.

Olah, K., Szoke, A., and Vojta, Z. S. (1979): On the mechanisms of Kolb's N-P selective detector. *J. Chromatogr. Sci.*, 17:497–502.

Oliver, A. P., Hoffer, B. J., and Wyatt, R. J. (1977): The hippocampal slice: A system for studying the pharmacology of seizures and for screening anticonvulsant drugs. *Epilepsia*, 18:543–548.

Ooi, B. S., Kant, K. S., Hanenson, I. B., Pesce, A. J., and Pollack, V. E. (1977): Lymphocytotoxins in epileptic patients receiving phenytoin. *Clin. Exp. Immunol.*, 30:56–61.

Osiewicz, R., Aggarwal, V., Young, R. M., and Sunshine, I. (1974): The quantitative analysis of phenobarbital with trimethylanilinium hydroxide. *J. Chromatogr.*, 88:157–164.

Ottoson, J. O. (1955): The effect of Xylocaine in electric convulsive treatment. *Experientia*, 11:453–454.

Ounsted, C. (1978): Preventing febrile convulsions. *Dev. Med. Child Neurol.*, 20:799–800.

Oxbury, J. M., and Whitty, C. W. M. (1971): Causes and consequences of status epilepticus in adults. *Brain*, 94:733–744.

Painter, M. J., Pippenger, C. E., MacDonald, H., and Pitlick, W. (1978): Phenobarbital and diphenylhydantoin levels in neonates with seizures. *J. Pediatr.*, 92:315–319.

Palmer, L., Bertilsson, L., Collste, P., and Rawlins, M. (1973): Quantitative determination of carbamazepine in plasma by mass fragmentography. *Clin. Pharmacol. Ther.*, 14:827–832.

Parker, W. A., and Shearer, C. A. (1979): Phenytoin in hepatotoxicity: A case report and review. *Neurology*, 29:175–178.

Parsonage, M. (1975): Treatment with carbamazepine. In: *Complex Partial Seizures and Their Treatment, Advances in Neurology, Vol. 11*, edited by J. K. Penry and D. D. Daly, pp. 221–236. Raven Press, New York.

Parsonage, M. J. (1967): Use of diazepam in the treatment of severe convulsive status epilepticus. *Br. J. Med.*, 3:85–88.

Patel, I. H., and Levy, R. H. (1979): Valproic acid binding to human serum albumin and determination of free fraction in the presence of anticonvulsants and free fatty acids. *Epilepsia*, 20:85–90.

Patsalos, P. N., and Lascelles, P. T. (1977): Effect of sodium valproate on plasma protein binding of diphenylhydantoin. *J. Neurol. Neurosurg. Psychiatry*, 40:570–574.

Patton, J. R., and Dudley, K. H. (1979): Synthesis of 2-methylcarbamazepine, a new internal standard for chromatographic assays of carbamazepine (Tegretol). *J. Heterocyclic Chem.*, 16:257–262.

Paxton, J. W., Rowell, F. J., and Ratcliffe, J. G. (1977): The evaluation of a radioimmunoassay for diphenylhydantoin using an iodinated tracer. *Clin. Chim. Acta*, 79:81–92.

Pearce, I., Heathfield, K. W. G., and Pearce, J. M. S. (1977): Valproate sodium in Huntington's Chorea. *Arch. Neurol.*, 34:308–309.

Pearce, J., and Ron, M. A. (1968): Thrombocytopenia after carbamazepine. *Lancet*, 2:223.

Pecci, J., and Giovanniello, T. J. (1975): Gas chromatographic studies of phenobarbital and diphenylhydantoin after flash heater alkylation. *J. Chromatogr.*, 109:163–167.

Pelkonen, R., Fogelholm, R., and Nikkila, E. A. (1975): Increase in serum cholesterol during phenytoin treatment. *Br. Med. J.*, 4:85.

Pellmar, T. C., and Wilson, W. A. (1977): Synaptic mechanism of pentylenetetrazole: Selectivity for chloride conductance. *Science*, 197:912–914.

Penny, J. L. (1963): Megaloblastic anemia during anticonvulsant drug therapy. *Arch. Int. Med.*, 111:744–749.

Penry, J. K. (1979): The use of antiepileptic drugs. *Ann. Int. Med.*, 90:207–218.

Pentikainen, P. J., Neuvonen, P. J., and Elfving, S. M. (1975): Bioavailability of four brands of phenytoin tablets. *Eur. J. Clin. Pharmacol.*, 9:213–218.

Perchalski, R. J., Andresen, B. D., and Wilder, B. J. (1976): Reaction of carbamazepine with dimethylformamide dimethylacetal. *Clin. Chem.*, 22:1229–1230.

Perchalski, R. J., Bruni, J., Wilder, B. J., and Willmore, L. J. (1979): Simultaneous determination of the anticonvulsants, cinromide (3-bromo-n-ethyl-cinnamamide)3-bromo-cinnamamide and carbamazepine in plasma by high performance liquid chromatography. *J. Chromatogr.*, 163:187–193.

Perchalski, R. J., Scott, K. N., Wilder, B. J., and Hammer, R. H. (1973): Rapid, simultaneous GLC determination of phenobarbital, primidone and diphenylhydantoin. *J. Pharmacol. Sci.*, 62:1735–1736.

Perchalski, R. J., and Wilder, B. J. (1974a): Rapid gas liquid chromatographic determination of carbamazepine in plasma. *Clin. Chem.*, 20:492–493.

Perchalski, R. J., and Wilder, B. J. (1974b): GLC microdetermination of plasma anticonvulsant levels. *J. Pharmacol. Sci.*, 63:806–807.

Perchalski, R. J., and Wilder, B. J. (1978a): Gas liquid chromatographic determination of carbamazepine and phenylethylmalonamide in plasma after reaction with dimethylformamide dimethylacetal. *J. Chromatogr.*, 145:97–103.

Perchalski, R. J., and Wilder, B. J. (1978b): Evaluation of on-column methylation in gas-liquid chromatographic quantitation of antiepileptic drugs. In: *Antiepileptic Drugs: Quantitative Analysis and Interpretation*, edited by C. E. Pippenger, J. K. Penry, and H. Kutt, pp. 75–85. Raven Press, New York.

Perchalski, R. J., and Wilder, B. J. (1978c): Determination of benzodiazepine anticonvulsant in plasma by high performance liquid chromatography. *Anal. Chem.*, 50:554–557.

Perchalski, R. J., and Wilder, B. J. (1979): Reverse phase liquid chromatography at increased temperature. *Anal. Chem.*, 51:774–776.

Perlstein, M. A., and Andelman, M. B. (1946): Tridione: Its use in convulsive and related disorders. *J. Pediatr.*, 29:20–40.

Permin, H., and Sestoft, L. (1977): Deposits of plasma proteins in the skin during treatment with carbamazepine and diphenylhydantoin. *Acta Med. Scand.*, 202:113–117.

Perrier, D., Rapp, R., Young, B., Kostenbauder, H., Cady, W., Pancorbo, S., and Hackman, J. (1976): Maintenance of therapeutic plasma levels via intramuscular administration. *Ann. Int. Med.*, 85:318–321.

Perucca, E. (1976): A study of intoxication with antiepileptic drugs among a large in-patient population. *Seventh International Symposium on Clinical Pharmacology*, Pavia, Italy.

Perucca, E., Garratt, A., Hebdige, S., and Richens, A. (1978): Water intoxication in epileptic patients receiving carbamazepine. *J. Neurol. Neurosurg. Psychiatry*, 41:713–718.

Peters, B. H., and Samaan, N. A. (1969): Hyperglycemia with relative hypoinsulinemia in diphenylhydantoin toxicity. *N. Engl. J. Med.*, 281:91–92.

Peterson, H. D. (1966): Association of trimethadione therapy and myasthenia gravis. *N. Engl. J. Med.*, 274:506–507.

Pfeifer, H. J., Greenblatt, D. J., and Koch-Weser, J. (1976): Clinical use and toxicity of intravenous lidocaine, a report from the Boston Collaborative Drug Surveillance Program. *Am. Heart J.*, 92:168–173.

Pincus, J. H., Yaari, Y., and Argov, Z. (1980): Phenytoin: Electrophysiological effects at the neuromuscular junction. In: *Antiepileptic Drugs: Mechanisms of Action, Advances in Neurology, Vol. 27*, edited by G. H. Glaser, J. K. Penry, and D. M. Woodbury, pp. 363–376. Raven Press, New York.

Pinder, R. M., Brogden, R. N., Speight, T. M., and Avery, G. S. (1976): Clonazepam: A review of its pharmacological properties and therapeutic efficacy in epilepsy. *Drugs*, 12:321–361.

Pinder, R. M., Brogden, R. N., Speight, T. M., and Avery, G. S. (1977): Sodium valproate: A review of its pharmacological properties and therapeutic efficacy in epilepsy. *Drugs*, 13:81–123.

Pippenger, C. E. (1976): Homogenous enzyme immunoassays for the quantitation of diphenylhydantoin, phenobarbital, and primidone in serum or plasma. An overview. In: *Quantitative Analytic Studies in Epilepsy*, edited by P. Kellaway and I. Petersen, pp. 59–69. Raven Press, New York.

Pippenger, C. E. (1979): High pressure liquid chromatography therapeutic drug monitoring: An overview. *J. Chromatogr. Sci.*, 10:495–506.

Pippenger, C. E., and Gillen, H. W. (1969): Gas chromatographic analysis for anticonvulsant drugs in biological fluids. *Clin. Chem.*, 15:582–590.

Pippenger, C. E., and Kutt, H. (1978): Common errors in the analysis of antiepileptic drugs. In: *Antiepileptic Drugs: Quantitative Analysis and Interpretation*, edited by C. E. Pippenger, J. K. Penry, and H. Kutt, pp. 199–208. Raven Press, New York.

Pippenger, C. E., Kutt, H. P., Penry, J. K., and Daly, D. (1977): Proficiency testing in determinations of antiepileptic drugs. *J. Anal. Toxicol.*, 1:118–122.

Pippenger, C. E., Penry, J. K., and Kutt, H., editors (1978): *Antiepileptic Drugs: Quantitative Analysis and Interpretation*. Raven Press, New York.

Pippenger, C. E., Penry, J. K., White, B. G., Daly, D. D., and Buddington, R. (1976): Interlaboratory variability in determination of plasma antiepileptic drug concentrations. *Arch. Neurol.*, 33:351–355.

Pippenger, C. E., Scott, J. E., and Gillen, H. W. (1969): Thin layer chromatography of anticonvulsant drugs. *Clin. Chem.*, 15:255.

Pisciotta, A. V. (1975): Hematologic toxicity of carbamazepine. In: *Complex Partial Seizures and Their Treatment, Advances in Neurology, Vol. 11*, edited by J. K. Penry and D. D. Daly, pp. 355–368. Raven Press, New York.

Pitlick, W., Painter, M., and Pippenger, C. E. (1978): Phenobarbital pharmacokinetics in neonates. *Biochem. Pharmacol. Ther.*, 23:346–350.

Plaa, G. L. (1975): Acute toxicity of antiepileptic drugs. *Epilepsia*, 16:183–191.

Pojer, J., Radivojevic, M., and Williams, T. F. (1972): Dupuytren's disease. Its association with abnormal liver function in alcoholism and epilepsy. *Arch. Int. Med.*, 129:561–566.

Polc, R., and Haefely, W. (1976): Effects of two benzodiazepines, phenobarbitone, and baclofen on synaptic transmission in the cat cuneate nucleus. *Naunyn Schmiedebergs Arch. Pharmacol.*, 294:121–132.

Polypchuk, G., Oreopoulos, D. G., Wilson, D. R., Harrison, J. E., McNeill, K. G., Meema, H. E., Ogilvie, R., Sturtridge, W. C., and Murray, T. M. (1978): Calcium metabolism in adult outpatients with epilepsy receiving long-term anticonvulsant therapy. *Can. Med. Assoc. J.*, 118:635–638.

Porter, R. J., and Penry, J. K. (1980): Phenobarbital: Biopharmacology. In: *Antiepileptic Drugs: Mechanisms of Action, Advances in Neurology, Vol. 27*, edited by G. H. Glaser, J. K. Penry, and D. M. Woodbury, pp. 493–500. Raven Press, New York.

Porter, R. J., Penry, J. K., Lacy, J. R., Newmark, M. E., and Kupferberg, H. J. (1979): Plasma concentrations of phensuximide, methsuximide and their metabolites in relation to clinical efficacy. Neurology, 29:1509–1513.

Poser, C. M. (1974): Modification of therapy for exacerbation of seizures during menstruation. Letter to the editor. *J. Pediatr.*, 84:779–780.

Prensky, A. L., Raff, M. C., Moore, M. J., and Schwab, R. S. (1967): Intravenous diazepam in the treatment of prolonged seizure activity. *N. Engl. J. Med.*, 276:779–784.

Prescott, L. F. (1975): Pathological and physiological factors affecting drug absorption, distribution, elimination and response in man. In: *Handbook of Clinical Pharmacology, Vol. 28, Part 3*, edited by J. R. Gillette and J. R. Mitchell, pp. 234–257. Springer-Verlag, New York.

Preskorn, S. H., and Denner, L. J. (1977): Benzodiazepines and withdrawal psychosis. *JAMA*, 237:36–38.

Prichard, J. W. (1980a): Phenobarbital: Proposed mechanism of antiepileptic action. In: *Antiepileptic Drugs: Mechanisms of Action, Advances in Neurology, Vol. 27*, edited by G. H. Glaser, J. K. Penry, and D. M. Woodbury, pp. 553–562. Raven Press, New York.

Prichard, J. W. (1980b): Phenobarbital: Introduction. In: *Antiepileptic Drugs: Mechanisms of Action, Advances in Neurology, Vol. 27*, edited by G. H. Glaser, J. K. Penry, and D. M. Woodbury, pp. 473–492. Raven Press, New York.

Prieur, A. M., LeBovar, Y., Griscelli, C., and Mozziconacci, P. (1973): Carbamazepine agranulocytosis. (French.) *Sem. Hop. Paris*, 49:3275–3278.

Prince, D. A., and Farrel, D. (1969): Centroencephalic spike and wave discharges following parenteral penicillin injection in the cat. *Neurology*, 19:309–310.

Puro, D. G., and Woodward, D. J. (1973): Effects of diphenylhydantoin on activity of rat cerebellar Purkinje cell. *Neuropharmacology*, 12:433–440.

Putnam, T. J., and Merritt, H. H. (1937): Experimental determination of anticonvulsant properties of some phenyl derivatives. *Science*, 85:525–526.

Pynnönnen, S., Sillanpää, M., Frey, H., and Iisalo, E. (1977): Carbamazepine and its 10,11-epoxide in children and adults with epilepsy. *Eur. J. Clin. Pharmacol.*, 11:129–133.

Raabe, W., and Gumnit, R. J. (1977): Anticonvulsant action of diazepam: Increase of cortical postsynaptic inhibition. *Epilepsia*, 18:117–120.

Rambeck, B. (1979): Pharmacological interactions of methsuximide with phenobarbital and phenytoin in hospitalized epileptic patients. *Epilepsia*, 20:147–156.

Ramsay, R. E., Hammond, E. J., Perchalski, R. J., and Wilder, B. J. (1979): Brain uptake of phenytoin, phenobarbital, and diazepam. *Arch. Neurol.*, 36:535–539.

Rane, A., Bertilsson, L., and Palmer, L. (1975): Disposition of placentally transferred carbamazepine (Tegretol) in the newborn. *Eur. J. Clin. Pharmacol.*, 8:283–284.

Rane, A., and Wilson, J. T. (1976): Clinical pharmacokinetics in infants and children. *Clin. Pharmacokinet.*, 1:2–24.

Rapport, R. L., and Shaw, C. M. (1977): Phenytoin related cerebellar degeneration without seizures. *Ann. Neurol.*, 2:437–439.

Rauh, C. E., and Gray, W. D. (1968): The anticonvulsant potency of inhibitors of carbonic anhydrase in young and adult rats and mice. *J. Pharmacol. Exp. Ther.*, 161:329–334.

Rawlings, M. M., Collste, P., Bertilsson, L., and Palmer, L. (1975): Distribution and elimination kinetics of carbamazepine in man. *Eur. J. Clin. Pharmacol.*, 8:91–96.

Rawson, M. D. (1968): Diphenylhydantoin intoxication and cerebrospinal fluid protein. *Neurology*, 18:1009–1011.

Record, K. E., Rapp, R. P., Young, B. A., and Kostenbauder, H. B. (1979): Oral phenytoin loading in adults: Rapid achievement of therapeutic plasma levels. *Ann. Neurol.*, 5:268–270.

Rey, E., d'Athis, P., de Lauture, D., Dulac, O. Aicardi, J., and Olive, G. (1979): Pharmacokinetics of carbamazepine in the neonate and in the child. *Int. J. Clin. Pharmacol. Biopharm.*, 17:90–96.

Reynolds, E. H. (1972): Diphenylhydantoin: Hematological aspects of toxicity. In: *Antiepileptic Drugs*, edited by D. M. Woodbury, J. K. Penry, and R. P. Schmidt, pp. 247–262. Raven Press, New York.

Reynolds, E. H. (1975a): Neurotoxicity of carbamazepine. In: *Complex Partial Seizures and Their Treatment, Advances in Neurology, Vol. 11*, edited by J. K. Penry and D. D. Daly, pp. 345–353. Raven Press, New York.

Reynolds, E. H. (1975b): Chronic antiepileptic toxicity: A review. *Epilepsia*, 16:319–352.

Reynolds, E. H., Chanarin, I., and Matthews, D. M. (1968): Neuropsychiatric aspects of anticonvulsant megaloblastic anemia. *Lancet*, 1:394–397.

Reynolds, E. H., and Travers, R. (1974): Serum anticonvulsant concentrations in epileptic patients with mental symptoms. *Br. J. Psychiatry*, 124:440–445.

Richards, R. K., Taylor, J. D., and Asher, D. T. (1954): Experimental studies on the physiological distribution and metabolism of phenacemide (Phenurone). *Epilepsia*, 3:120–121.

Richardson, S. G. N., Fletcher, D. J., and Jeavons, P. M. (1976): Sodium valproate and platelet function. In: *Clinical and Pharmacological Aspects of Sodium Valproate (Epilim) in the Treatment of Epilepsy*, edited by N. J. Legg, pp. 119–122. MCS Consultants, Tunbridge Wells.

Richens, A. (1977*a*): Interactions with antiepileptic drugs. *Drugs*, 13:266–275.

Richens, A. (1977*b*): Drug interactions in epilepsy. In: *Drug Interactions*, edited by D. G. Grahame-Smith, pp. 239–249. University Park Press, Baltimore, Maryland.

Richens, A. (1979): Clinical pharmacokinetics of phenytoin. *Clin. Pharmacokinet.*, 4:153–169.

Richens, A., and Ahmad, S. (1975): Controlled trial of sodium valproate in severe epilepsy. *Br. Med. J.*, 4:255–256.

Richens, A., Scoular, I. T., Ahmad, S., and Jorden, B. J. (1976): Pharmacokinetics and efficacy of Epilim in patients receiving long-term therapy with other antiepileptic drugs. In: *Clinical and Pharmacological Aspects of Sodium Valproate (Epilim) in the Treatment of Epilepsy*, edited by N. J. Legg, pp. 78–88. MCS Consultants, Tunbridge Wells.

Richens, A., and Warrington, S. (1979): When should plasma drug levels be monitored? *Drugs*, 17:488–500.

Richens, A., and Woodford, F. P. (1976): *Anticonvulsant Drugs and Enzyme Induction*. Elsevier, Amsterdam.

Richie, M. J., and Cohen, P. J. (1975): Local anesthetics. In: *The Pharmacological Basis of Therapeutics*, edited by L. S. Goodman and A. Gilman, pp. 379–403. MacMillan, New York.

Rigelman, S., Rowland, M., and Epstein, W. L. (1970): Griseofulvin-phenobarbital interaction in man. *JAMA*, 213:426–431.

Robb, E. W., and Westbrook, J. J., III (1963): Preparation of methyl esters for gas liquid chromatography of acids by pyrolysis of tetramethylammonium salts. *Anal. Chem.*, 35:1644–1647.

Rodbard, D., Bridson, W., and Rayford, P. L. (1969): Rapid calculation of radioimmunoassay results. *J. Lab. Clin. Med.*, 74:770–781.

Rodin, E. A., Rim, C. S., Kitano, H., Lewis, R., and Rennick, P. M. (1976): A comparison of the effectiveness of primidone versus carbamazepine in epileptic outpatients. *J. Nerv. Ment. Dis.*, 163:41–46.

Roger, J. C., Rodgers, G., and Soo, A. (1973): Simultaneous determination of carbamazepine (Tegretol) and other anticonvulsants in human plasma by gas liquid chromatography. *Clin. Chem.*, 19:590–592.

Rollinson, R. D., and Gilligan, B. S. (1979): Postanoxic action myoclonus (Lance-Adams Syndrome) responding to valproate. *Arch. Neurol.*, 36:44–45.

Rosen, J. A. (1968): Dilantin dementia. *Trans. Am. Neurol. Assoc.*, 93:273.

Rosenberg, I. H., Streiff, R. R., Godwin, H. A., and Castle, W. B. (1968): Impairment of intestinal deconjugation of dietary folate. A possible explanation of megaloblastic anemia associated with phenytoin therapy. *Lancet*, 2:530–532.

Roussounis, S. H., and de Rudolf, N. (1977): Clonazepam in the treatment of children with intractable seizures. *Dev. Med. Child Neurol.*, 19:326–334.

Rowan, A. J., Binnie, C. D., Warfield, C. A., Meinardi, H., and Miejer, J. W. A. (1979): The delayed effect of sodium valproate on the photoconvulsive response in man. *Epilepsia*, 20:61–68.

Rubenstein, K. K., Schneider, R. S., and Ullman, E. F. (1972): Homogeneous enzyme immunoassay. A new immunochemical technique. *Biochem. Biophys. Res. Commun.*, 47:846.

Ruf, R., and Sauter, R. (1977): Influence of phenobarbital on the serum level of phenytoin and effect of phenytoin on primidone metabolism. In: *Epilepsy: The Eighth International Symposium*, edited by J. K. Penry, pp. 147–150. Raven Press, New York.

Salcman, M., Defendini, R., Correll, J., and Gilman, S. (1978): Neuropathological changes in cerebellar biopsies of epileptic patients. *Ann. Neurol.*, 3:10–19.

Saleh, A. E. C., and Mendes de Leon, D. E. (1968): Fatal pancytopenia in the course of treatment with carbamazepine. (Dutch.) *Ned. Tijdschr. Geneeskd.*, 112:2089–2090.

Salem, R. B. Yost, R. L., Torosian, G., Davis, F. T., and Wilder, B. J. (1980): Investigation of the crystallization of phenytoin in normal saline. *Drug Intelligence and Clinical Pharmacy*, 14:605–608.

Salem, R. B., Wilder, B. J., Yost, R. L., Doering, P. L., Lee, C. C. (1981): Rapid phenytoin infusion for administration of loading doses. *Am. J. Hosp. Pharm.* 38:354–357.

Sapirstein, V. S., Lees, M. B., and Trachtenberg, M. C. (1978): Soluble and membrane bound carbonic anhydrases from rat CNS: Regional development. *J. Neurochem.*, 31:283–287.

Sawaya, M. C. B., Horton, R. W., and Meldrum, B. S. (1975): Effects of anticonvulsant drugs on the cerebral enzymes metabolizing GABA. *Epilepsia*, 16:649–655.

Schain, R. J., and Watanabe, K. (1976): Origin of brain growth retardation in young rats treated with phenobarbital. *Exp. Neurol.*, 50:806–809.

Schallek, W., Schlosser, W., and Randall, L. O. (1972): Recent developments in the pharmacology of the benzodiazepines. *Adv. Pharmacol. Chemother.*, 10:119–183.

Schauf, C. L., David, F. A., and Marder, J. (1974): Effects of carbamazepine on the ionic conductances of myxicola giant axons. *J. Pharmacol. Exp. Ther.*, 189:538–543.

Schettini, A., and Wilder, B. J. (1974): Effects of anticonvulsant drugs on enflurane induced cortical dysrhythmias. *Anesth. Analg. (Cleve.)*, 53:951–962.

Schier, G. M., Gan, I. E. T., Halpern, B., and Korth, J. (1980): Measurement of sodium valproate by direct-insertion chemical ionization/mass spectrometry. *Clin. Chem.*, 26:147–149.

Schmidt, D. (1976): Measurement of diphenylhydantoin and phenobarbital by enzyme immunoassay and gas liquid chromatography. *J. Neurol.*, 213:41.

Schmidt, D., and Kupferberg, H. J. (1975): Diphenylhydantoin, phenobarbital, and primidone in saliva, plasma and cerebrospinal fluid. *Epilepsia*, 16:735–741.

Schmidt, D., Goldberg, V., Guelen, P. J. M., Johanessen, S., Van der Kleijn, E., Meijer, J. W. A., Meinardi, H., Richens, A., Schneider, H., Stein-Lavie, Y., and Symann-Louette, N. (1977): Evaluation of a new immunoassay for determination of phenytoin and phenobarbital: Results of a European collaborative control study. *Epilepsia*, 18:367–374.

Schmidt, D., Kupferberg, H. J., Porter, R. J., and Penry, J. K. (1980): Primidone withdrawal in patients with intractable epilepsy (abstract). In: *Epilepsy: Xth International Symposium, Vancouver, Canada*, edited by J. A. Wada and J. K. Penry, p. 132. Raven Press, New York.

Schmidt, R. F., Vogel, M. E., and Zimmerman, G. (1967): Die Wirkung von Diazepam auf die praesynaptische Hemung und andere Rueckenmarksreflexe. *Naunyn Schmiedebergs Arch. Exp. Pathol. Pharmakol.*, 258:69–82.

Schmidt, R. P., and Wilder, B. J. (1968): *Epilepsy*. F. A. Davis, Philadelphia.

Schneider, H. (1975): Carbamazepine: The influence of other antiepileptic drugs on its serum level. In: *Clinical Pharmacology of Antiepileptic Drugs*, edited by H. Schneider, D. Janz, C. Gardner-Thorpe, H. Meinardi, and A. L. Sherwin, pp. 189–196. Springer-Verlag, New York.

Schneider, H. (1977): Long-term treatment in severe epilepsy (institutionalized patients). II. Retrospective evaluation of carbamazepine. In: *Epilepsy: The Eighth International Symposium*, edited by J. K. Penry, pp. 57–62. Raven Press, New York.

Schneider, J. (1961): Urinary excretion of electrolytes in centrencephalic epileptics. *Epilepsia*, 2:358–366.

Schnell, R. C., and Miya, T. S. (1970): Altered absorption of drugs from the rat small intestine by carbonic anhydrase inhibition. *J. Pharmacol. Exp. Ther.*, 174:177–184.

Schobben, F., and Van der Kleijn, E. (1974a): Determination of sodium di-n-propylacetate in plasma by gas-liquid chromatography. *Pharmaceutisch Weekblad*, 109:30–33.

Schobben, F., and Van der Kleijn, E. (1974b): Pharmacokinetics of distribution and elimination of sodium di-n-propylacetate in mouse and dog. *Pharmaceutisch Weekblad*, 109:33–41.

Schobben, F., Van der Kleijn, E., and Gabreels, E. J. M. (1975): Pharmacokinetics of di-n-propylacetate in epileptic patients. *Eur. J. Clin. Pharmacol.*, 8:97–105.

Schobben, F., Vree, T. B., and Van der Kleijn, E. (1977): Pharmacokinetics, metabolism and distribution of 2-n-propyl-pentanoate (sodium valproate) and the influence of salicylate comedication. In: *Advances in Epileptology*, edited by H. Meinardi and A. J. Rowan, pp. 271–277. Swets and Zeitlinger, Amsterdam.

Schoffeniels, E., Franck, G., Hertz, L., and Tower, D. B., editors (1978): *Dynamic Properties of Glia Cells*. Pergamon Press, Oxford.

Scholfield, C. N. (1978): A barbiturate induced intensification of the inhibitory potential in slices of guinea pig olfactory cortex. *J. Physiol.*, 275:559–566.

Scholl, M. L., and Schwab, R. S. (1971): The triggering of grand mal and psychomotor spells by spike and wave discharge. *Electroencephalogr. Clin. Neurophysiol.*, 31:419.

Scholtz, W. (1959): The contribution of patho-anatomical research to the problem of epilepsy. *Epilepsia*, 1:36–55.

Schottelius, D. D., and Fincham, R. W. (1978): Clinical application of serum primidone levels. In: *Antiepileptic Drugs: Quantitative Analysis and Interpretation*, edited by C. E. Pippenger, J. K. Penry, and H. Kutt, pp. 273–282. Raven Press, New York.

Schulte, C. J. A., and Good, T. A. (1966): Acute intoxication due to methsuximide and diphenylhydantoin. *J. Pediatr.*, 68:635–637.

Schwade, E. D., Richards, R. K., and Everett, G. M. (1956): Peganone®, a new anticonvulsant drug. *Dis. Nerv. Syst.*, 17:155–158.

Schwartz, J. R., and Vogel, W. (1977): Diphenylhydantoin: Excitability reducing action in single myelinated nerve fibers. *Eur. J. Pharmacol.*, 44:241–249.

Sellers, E. M., and Kalant, H. (1976): Alcohol intoxication and withdrawal. *N. Engl. J. Med.*, 294:757–762.

Serrano, E. E., Roye, D. B., Hammer, R. H., and Wilder, B. J. (1973): Plasma diphenylhydantoin values after oral and intramuscular administration of diphenylhydantoin. *Neurology*, 23:311–317.

Serrano, E. E., and Wilder, B. J. (1974): Intramuscular administration of diphenylhydantoin. *Arch. Neurol.*, 31:276–278.

Shakir, R. A., Behan, P. O., Dick, H., and Lambie, D. G. (1978): Metabolism of immunoglobulin A_1 lymphocyte function and histocompatibility antigens in patients on anticonvulsants. *J. Neurol. Neurosurg. Psychiatry*, 41:307–311.

Shakir, R. A., Nanda, R. N., Lambie, D. G., and Johnson, R. H. (1979): Comparative trial of valproate sodium and clonazepam in chronic epilepsy. *Arch. Neurol.*, 36:301–304.

Shand, D. G., Mitchell, J. R., and Oates, J. A. (1975): Pharmacokinetic drug interactions. In: *Handbook of Experimental Pharmacology, Vol. 28, Part 3*, edited by J. R. Gillette and J. R. Mitchell, pp. 272–314. Springer-Verlag, New York.

Shapiro, M. (1958): Acceleration of gingival wound healing in non-epileptic patients receiving DPH sodium. *Exp. Med. Surg.*, 16:41–53.

Sharpe, S. L., Cooreman, W. M., Bloomme, W. J., and Lakeman, G. M. (1976): Quantitative enzyme immunoassay: Current status. *Clin. Chem.*, 22:733–738.

Sherwin, A. W. (1978): Clinical pharmacology of ethosuximide. In: *Antiepileptic Drugs: Quantitative Analysis and Interpretation*, edited by C. E. Pippenger, J. K. Penry, and H. Kutt, pp. 283–295. Raven Press, New York.

Sherwin, A. L., and Robb, J. P. (1972): Ethosuximide: Relation of plasma levels to clinical control. In: *Antiepileptic Drugs*, edited by D. M. Woodbury, J. K. Penry, and R. P. Schmidt, pp. 443–448. Raven Press, New York.

Sherwin, A. L., Robb, J. P., and Lechter, M. (1973): Improved control of epilepsy by monitoring plasma ethosuximide. *Arch. Neurol.*, 28:178–181.

Shorvon, S. D., Chadwick, D., Galbraith, A. W., and Reynolds, E. H. (1978): One drug for epilepsy. *Br. Med. J.*, 1:474–476.

Shorvon, S. D., and Reynolds, E. H. (1977): Unnecessary poly pharmacy for epilepsy. *Br. Med. J.*, 2:1635–1637.

Shouldon, I., Kartzinal, R., and Chase, T. N. (1976): Huntington's disease: Treatment with dipropylacetic acid and gamma-aminobutyric acid. *Neurology*, 26:61–63.

Similä, S., von Wendt, L., Linna, S. L., Saukkonen, A. L., and Huhtaniemi, I. (1979): Dipropylacetate and hyperglycinemia. *Neuropädiatrie*, 10:158–160.

Simler, S., Ciesielski, L., Maitre, M., Randrianarisoa, H., and Mandel, P. (1973): Effect of sodium n-dipropylacetate on audiogenic seizures and brain gamma-aminobutyric acid level. *Biochem. Pharmacol.*, 22:1701–1708.

Simon, D., and Penry, J. K. (1975): Sodium di-n-propylacetate (DPA) in the treatment of epilepsy: A review. *Epilepsia*, 16:549–573.

Simonsen, N., Olsen, P. Z., Kuehl, V., Lund, M., and Wendelboe, J. (1976): A comparative controlled study between carbamazepine and diphenylhydantoin in psychomotor epilepsy. *Epilepsia*, 17:169–176.

Simpson, G., Kunz, E., and Slafta, J. (1965): Use of sodium Dilantin in the treatment of leg ulcers. *NY State J. Med.*, 65:886–888.

Singh, A. N., Saxena, B. M., and Germain, M. (1977): Anticonvulsive psychotropic effects of carbamazepine in hospitalized epileptic patients: A long-term study. In: *Epilepsy: The Eighth International Symposium*, edited by J. K. Penry, pp. 47–56. Raven Press,New York.

Sjö, O., Hvidberg, E. F., Naestoft, J., and Lund, M. (1975): Pharmacokinetics and side-effects of clonazepam and its 7-aminometabolite in man. *Eur. J. Clin. Pharmacol.*, 8:249–254.

Slater, G. E., and Johnston, D. (1978): Sodium valproate increases potassium conductance in aplysia neurons. *Epilepsia*, 19:379–384.

Slavin, B. N., Fenton, G. M., Laundy, M., and Reynolds, E. H. (1974): Serum immuno-globulin in epilepsy. *J. Neurol. Sci.*, 23:353–357.

Sloan, L. L., and Gilger, A. P. (1947): Visual effects of tridione. *Am. J. Ophthalmol.*, 30:1387–1405.

Smith, B. T., and Masotti, R. E. (1971): Intravenous diazepam in the treatment of prolonged seizure activity in neonates and infants. *Dev. Med. Child Neurol.*, 13:630–634.

Smith, G. A., McKauge, L., Dubetz, J. H., Tyrer, J. H., and Eadie, M. J. (1979*a*): Factors influencing plasma concentrations of ethosuximide. *Clin. Pharmacokinet.*, 4:38–52.

Smith, Q. T., Hamilton, M. J., Biros, M. H., and Pihlstrom, B. L. (1979*b*): Salivary and plasma IgA of seizure subjects receiving phenytoin. *Epilepsia*, 20:17–23.

Snider, R. S., and Del Cerro, M. (1967): Drug-induced dendrite sprouts on Purkinje cells in the adult cerebellum. *Exp. Neurol.*, 17:466–480.

Snider, R. S., and Del Cerro, M. (1972): Diphenylhydantoin: Proliferating membranes in cerebellum resulting from intoxication. In: *Antiepileptic Drugs*, edited by D. M. Wood-bury, J. K. Penry, and R. P. Schmidt, pp. 237–245. Raven Press, New York.

Snyder, L. R., and Kirkland, J. J. (1979): *Introduction to Modern Liquid Chromatography*, 2nd edition. Wiley, New York.

Sohn, R. S., and Ferrendelli, J. A. (1976): Anticonvulsant drug mechanism: Phenytoin, phenobarbital and ethosuximide and calcium flux in isolate presynaptic endings. *Arch. Neurol.*, 33:626–629.

Solomon, G. E., Hilgartner, M. W., and Kutt, H. (1972): Coagulation defects caused by diphenylhydantoin. *Neurology*, 22:1165–1171.

Solomon, G. E., Hilgartner, M. W., and Kutt, H. (1974): Phenobarbital-induced coagulation defects in cats. *Neurology*, 24:920–924.

Solow, E. B., and Green, J. B. (1971): The determination of ethosuximide in serum by gas chromatography. Preliminary results of clinical application. *Clin. Chim. Acta*, 33:87–90.

Solow, E. B., and Green, J. B. (1972): The simultaneous determination of multiple anti-convulsant drug levels by gas-liquid chromatography. Method and clinical application. *Neurology*, 22:540–555.

Solow, E. B., and Kenfield, C. P. (1977): A micro method for the determination of clon-azepam in serum by electron-capture gas-liquid chromatography. *J. Anal. Toxicol.*, 1:155–157.

Solow, E. B., Metaxas, J. M., and Summers, T. R. (1974): Antiepileptic drugs: A current assessment of simultaneous determination of multiple drug therapy by gas-liquid chro-matography on-column methylation. *J. Chromatogr. Sci.*, 12:256–260.

Sommerbeck, K. W., Theilgaard, A., Rasmussen, K. E., Løhren, V., Gram, L., and Wulff, K. (1977): Valproate sodium: Evaluation of so-called psychotropic effect. A controlled study. *Epilepsia*, 18:159–167.

Sorel, L. (1972): 196 Cases of infantile myoclonic encephalopathy with hypsarrhythmia (IMEH: West syndrome) treated with ACTH: danger of synthetic ACTH. *Electroence-phalogr. Clin. Neurophysiol.*, 32:576.

Sorel, L., and Dusaucy-Bauloye, A. (1958): A propos de ce cas d'hypsarythmia de Gibbs. Son traitement spectaculair par l'ACTH. *Acta Neurol. Belg.*, 58:130.

Sorrell, T. C., Forbes, I. J., Burness, F. R., and Rischbieth, R. H. C. (1971): Depression of immunologic function in patients treated with phenytoin sodium (sodium diphenylhy-dantoin). *Lancet*, 2:1233–1235.

Soulayrol, R., and Roger, J. (1970): Effects psychiatriques defavorables des medications anti-epileptiques. *Rev. Neuropsychiatr. Infant*, 18:591–598.

South, T. (1972): Teratogenic effect of anticonvulsants. *Lancet*, 2:1154.

Speidel, B. D., and Meadow, S. R. (1972): Maternal epilepsy and abnormalities of the fetus and newborn. *Lancet*, 2:839–843.

Spiehler, V., Sun, L., Miyada, D. S., Sarandis, S. G., Walwick, E. R., Klein, M. W., Jordan, D. B., and Jessen, B. (1976): Radioimmunoassay, enzyme immunoassay, spec-trophotometry and gas-liquid chromatography compared for determination of phenobar-bital and diphenylhydantoin. *Clin. Chem.*, 22:749–753.

Stambaugh, R. V., Morgan, A. F., and Enwonwa, C. O. (1973): Ascorbic acid deficiency associated with Dilantin hyperplasia. *J. Periodont.*, 44:244–247.

Stamp, T. C. B., Round, J. M., Rowe, D. J. F., and Haddad, J. G. (1972): Plasma levels and therapeutic effect of 25-hydroxycholecalciferol in epileptic patients taking anticon-vulsant drugs. *Br. Med. J.*, 4:9–12.

Stephens, W. P., Coe, J. Y., and Baylis, P. H. (1978): Plasma arginine vasopressin con-centrations and antidiuretic action of carbamazepine. *Br. Med. J.*, 1:1445–1447.

Stephenson, J. B. P., House, F. M., and Stromberg, P. (1977): Medium-chain triglycerides in a ketogenic diet. *Dev. Med. Child Neurol.*, 19:693–694.

Sterman, M. B. (1977): Clinical implications of EEG biofeedback training: A critical appraisal. In: *Biofeedback: Theory and Research*, edited by G. E. Schwartz and J. Beatty, pp. 389–411. Academic Press, New York.

Sterman, M. B., and Friar, L. (1972): Suppression of seizures in an epileptic following sensorimotor EEG feedback training. *Electroencephalogr. Clin. Neurophysiol.*, 33:89–95.

Sternbach, L. H. (1973): Chemistry of 1,4-benzodiazepines and some aspects of the structure-activity relationship. In: *The Benzodiazepines*, edited by S. Garattini, E. Mussini, and L. O. Randall, pp. 1–26. Raven Press, New York.

Stevenson, G. W. (1966): On column methylation of barbituric acid. *Anal. Chem.*, 38:1948–1949.

Stores, G. (1975): Behavioral effects of anticonvulsant drugs. *Dev. Med. Child Neurol.*, 17:647–658.

Strain, G. M., VanMeter, W. G., and Brockman, W. H. (1978): Elevation of seizure thresholds: A comparison of cerebellar stimulation, phenobarbital, and diphenylhydantoin. *Epilepsia*, 19:493–504.

Strong, J. M., Abe, T., Gibbs, E. L., and Atkinson, A. J. (1974): Plasma levels of methsuximide and n-desmethylmethsuximide during methsuximide therapy. *Neurology*, 24:250–255.

Suchy, F. J., Balistreri, F. J., Buchino, J. J., Sondheimer, J. M., Bates, S. R., Kearns, G. L., Stull, J. D., and Bove, K. E. (1979): Acute hepatic failure associated with the use of sodium valproate. *N. Engl. J. Med.*, 300:962–966.

Sutor, A. H., and Jesdinsky-Buscher, C. (1974): Coagulation changes caused by dipropylacetic acid. *Med. Welt*, 25:447–449.

Suzuki, M., Maruyama, H., Ishibashi, Y., Seki, T., Hoshino, M., Maekawa, K., Yogo, T., and Sato, Y. (1972): A double-blind comparative trial of sodium dipropylacetate and ethosuximide in epilepsy in children: With special emphasis on pure petit mal seizures. (Japanese.) *Med. Prog.*, 82:470–488.

Swinyard, E. A. (1949): Laboratory assay of clinically effective antiepileptic drugs. *J. Am. Pharm. Assoc. Sci. Ed.*, 38:201–204.

Swinyard, E. A., and Castellion, A. W. (1966): Anticonvulsant properties of some benzodiazepines. *J. Pharmacol. Exp. Ther.*, 151:369–375.

Swinyard, E. A., and Toman, J. E. P. (1950): A comparison of the anticonvulsant actions of some phenylhydantoins and their corresponding phenylacetylureas. *J. Pharmacol. Exp. Ther.*, 100:151–157.

Symmington, G. R., Leonard, D. P., Shannon, P. J., and Vajda, F. J. E. (1978): Sodium valproate in Huntington's disease. *Am. J. Psychiatry*, 135:352–354.

Syversen, G. B., Morgan, J. P., Weinbtraub, M., and Myers, G. J. (1977): Acetazolamide-induced interference with primidone absorption. *Arch. Neurol.*, 34:80–84.

Taburet, M., Aymard, P., and Richardet, J. M. (1975): Influences of joint therapy on phenobarbital blood levels. *Ann. Biol. Clin.*, 33:231.

Tallman, J. F., Thomas, J. W., and Gallagher, D. W. (1978): GABAergic modulations of benzodiazepine binding site sensitivity. *Nature*, 247:383–385.

Tan, B. K., Leijnse-Ybema, H. J., and Zee, M. F. H. (1976): Sodium valproate in Huntington's chorea. *Clin. Neurol. Neurosurg.*, 79:62–65.

Tassinari, C. A., Dravet, C., Roger, J., Cano, J. P., and Gastaut, H. (1972): Tonic status epilepticus precipitated by intravenous benzodiazepine in five patients with Lennox-Gastaut syndrome. *Epilepsia*, 13:421–435.

Taverner, D., and Bain, W. A. (1958): Intravenous lignocaine as an anticonvulsant in status epilepticus and serial epilepsy. *Lancet*, 2:1145–1147.

Taylor, J., editor (1958): *Selected Writings of John Hughlings Jackson. Vol. 1. On Epilepsy and Epileptiform Convulsions.* Basic Books, New York.

Tchicaloff, M., and Gaillard, F. (1970): Quelques effects indesirables des medicaments antiepileptiques sur les rendements intellectuals. *Rev. Neuropsychiatr. Infant*, 18:599–602.

Tenckhoff, H., Sherrard, D. J., Hickman, R. O., and Ladda, R. L. (1968): Acute diphenylhydantoin intoxication. *Am. J. Dis. Child.*, 116:422–425.

Theobald, W., and Kunz, H. A. (1963): Zur Pharmakologie des Antiepilepticums 5-carbamul-5H-dibenzo (b,f)azepin. *Arzneim. Forsch.*, 13:122–125.

Thoma, J. J., Ewald, T., and McCoy, M. (1978): Simultaneous analysis of underivatized phenobarbital, carbamazepine, primidone, and phenytoin by isothermal gas-liquid chromatography. *J. Anal. Toxicol.*, 2:219–225.

Tigelaar, R. E., Rapport, R. L., II, Inman, J. K., and Kupferberg, H. J. (1973): A radioimmunoassay for diphenylhydantoin. *Clin. Chim. Acta*, 43:231–241.

Todorov, A. B., Lenn, N. J., and Gabor, A. J. (1978): Exacerbation of generalized nonconvulsive seizures with ethosuximide therapy. *Arch. Neurol.*, 35:389–391.

Toman, J. E. P. (1952): Neuropharmacology of peripheral nerve. *Pharmacol. Rev.*, 4:168–218.

Toman, J. E. P. (1965): Drugs effective in convulsive disorders. In: *The Pharmacological Basis of Therapeutics*, edited by L. S. Goodman and A. Gilman, pp. 215–236. MacMillan, New York.

Touchstone, J. C., and Dobbins, M. F. (1978): *Practice of Thin-Layer Chromatography.* Wiley, New York.

Tower, D. B., and Young, G. M. (1973): The activities of butyrylcholinesterase and carbonic anhydrase, the rate of anaerobic glycolysis, and the question of a constant density of glial cells in cerebral cortices of various mammalian species from mouse to whale. *J. Neurochem.*, 20:269–278.

Treasure, R., and Toseland, P. A. (1971): Hyperglycemia due to phenytoin toxicity. *Arch. Dis. Child.*, 46:563–564.

Treiman, D. M., and Delgado-Escueta, A. V. (1980): Status epilepticus. In: *Critical Care of Neurologic and Neurosurgical Emergencies*, edited by R. A. Thompson and J. R. Green, pp. 53–99. Raven Press, New York.

Trimble, M. (1979): The effect of anticonvulsant drugs on cognitive abilities. *Pharmacol. Ther.*, 4:677–685.

Trimble, M. R., and Reynolds, E. H. (1976): Anticonvulsant drugs and mental symptoms: A review. *Psychol. Med.*, 6:169–178.

Troupin, A. S., and Friel, P. (1975): Anticonvulsant levels in saliva, serum and cerebrospinal fluid. *Epilepsia*, 16:223–227.

Troupin, A. S., Friel, P., Wilensky, A. J., Morretti-Ojemann, L., Levy, R. H., and Fiegl, P. (1979): Evaluation of clorazepate (Tranxene) as an anticonvulsant—a pilot study. *Neurology*, 29:458–466.

Troupin, A. S., Green, J. R., and Halpern, L. M. (1975): Carbamazepine (Tegretol) as an anticonvulsant. A controlled double-blind comparison with diphenylhydantoin (Dilantin). *Acta Neurol. Scand.*, 60:13–26.

Troupin, A., Ojemann, L. M., Halpern, L., Dodrill, C., Wilkus, R., Friel, P., and Feigl, P. (1977): Carbamazepine—a double-blind comparison with phenytoin. *Neurology*, 27:511–519.

Tunnicliff, G., Smith, J. A., and Ngo, T. T. (1979): Competition for diazepam receptor binding by diphenylhydantoin and its enhancement by gamma aminobutyric acid. *Biochem. Biophys. Res. Commun.*,

Uges, D. R. A., and Bouma, I. P. (1978): An improved determination of clonazepam in serum by high performance liquid chromatography. *Pharmaceutisch Weekblad*, 113:1156–1158.

Uhlemann, E. R., and Neims, A. H. (1972): Anticonvulsant properties of the ketogenic diet in mice. *J. Pharmacol. Exp. Ther.*, 180:231–238.

Urechia, C. I., and Lichter, C. (1958): Histopathologic examination of the diencephalon in status epilepticus. *Neurobiologia*, 3:299–305.

Urquhart, N., Godolphin, W., and Campbell, D. J. (1979): Evaluation of automated enzyme immunoassay for five anticonvulsants and theophylline adapted to a centifugal analyzer. *Clin. Chem.*, 25:785–787.

Utterback. R. A. (1958): Parynchymatous cerebellar degeneration complicating diphenylhydantoin (Dilantin) therapy. *Arch. Neurol.*, 80:180–181.

Vajda, F. J. E., Mihaly, G. W., Miles, J. L., Donnan, G. A., and Bladin, P. F. (1978): Rectal administration of sodium valproate in status epilepticus. *Neurology*, 28:897–899.

Vakil, S. D., Critchley, E. M.R., Philips, J. C., Fokim, Y., Haydock, C., Cocks, A., and Dyer, T. (1976): The effect of sodium valproate (Epilim) on phenytoin and phenobarbitone blood levels. In: *Clinical and Pharmacological Aspects of Sodium Valproate (Epilim) in the Treatment of Epilepsy*, edited by N. J. Legg, pp. 75–77. MCS Consultants, Tunbridge Wells.

Vallarta, J. M., Bell, D. B., and Reichert, A. (1974): Progressive encephalopathy due to chronic hydantoin intoxication. *Am. J. Dis. Child.*, 128:27–34.

Van Creveld, S. (1958): Nouveaux aspects de la maladie hémorrhagique du nouveau-né. *Arch. Fr. Pediatr.*, 15:721–735.

Vandemark, F. L., and Adams, R. F. (1976):Ultramicro gas chromatographic analysis for anticonvulsants with use of a nitrogen selective detector. *Clin. Chem.*, 22:1062–1065.

Van der Kleijn, E., Collste, P., Norlander, B., Agurell, S., and Sjoqvist, F. (1973): Gas chromatographic determination of ethosuximide and phensuximide in plasma and urine of man. *J. Pharm. Pharmacol.*, 25:324–327.

Van der Kleijn, E., Van Rossum, J. M., Muskens, E. T. J. M., and Rijntjes, N. V. M. (1971): Pharmacokinetics of diazepam in dogs, mice and humans. *Acta Pharmacol. Toxicol.* [*Suppl. 3*], 29:109–127.

Van der Korst, J. K., Colenbrander, H., and Cats, A. (1966): Phenobarbital and the shoulder-hand syndrome. *Ann. Rheum. Dis.*, 25:553–555.

Varma, R., and Hishino, A. Y. (1979): Simple gas chromatographic measurement of valproic acid in psychiatric patients. Effect of levels on other simultaneous administered anticonvulsants. *Neurosci. Lett.*, 11:353.

Vassella, F., Pavlincova, E., Schneider, H. J., Rudin, H. J., and Karbowski, K. (1973): Treatment of infantile spasms and Lennox-Gastaut syndrome with clonazepam (Rivotril). *Epilepsia*, 14:165–175.

Vazquez, A. J., Diamond, B. I., and Sabelli, H. C. (1975): Differential effects of phenobarbital and pentobarbital on isolated nervous tissue. *Epilepsia*, 16:601–608.

Veall, R. M., and Hogarth, H. C. (1975): Thrombocytopenia during treatment with clonazepam. *Br. Med. J.*, 4:462.

Vessell, E. S. (1972): Pharmacogenetics. *N. Engl. J. Med.*, 287:904–909.

Vessell, E. S. (1973): Factors causing interindividual variations of drug concentrations in blood. *Clin. Pharmacol. Ther.*, 16:135–148.

Victor, M., and Adams, R. D. (1953): The effect of alcohol on the nervous system. *Res. Publ. Assoc. Res. Nerv. Ment. Dis.*, 32:526–573.

Victor, M., and Brausch, C. (1967): The role of abstinence in the genesis of alcoholic epilepsy. *Epilepsia*, 8:1–20.

Victor, A., Lundberg, P. O., and Johansson, E. D. B. (1977): Induction of sex hormone binding globulin by phenytoin. *Br. Med. J.*, 2:934–935.

Villarreal, H. J., Wilder, B. J., Willmore, L. J., Bauman, A. W., Hammond, E. J., and Bruni, J. (1978): Effect of valproic acid on spike and wave discharges in patients with absence seizures. *Neurology*, 28:886–891.

Viswanathan, C. T., Booker, H. E., and Welling, P. G. (1978): Bioavailability of oral and intramuscular phenobarbital. *J. Clin. Pharmacol.*, 18:100–105.

Volpe, J. J. (1977): Neonatal seizures. *Clin. Perinatol.*, 4:43–63.

Volzke, E., Doose, H., and Stephen, E. (1967): The treatment of infantile spasms and hypsarrhythmia with Mogadon®. *Epilepsia*, 8:64–70.

Von Krebs, A. (1964): Chloasenartige Hyperpigmentierungen nach Behandlung mit Hydantoinpraparaten. *Schweiz. Med. Wochenschr.*, 94:748–757.

Vrai, P. V. (1978): Acute intoxication during a combined treatment of sodium valproate and phenobarbitone. In: *Advances in Epileptology*, edited by H. Meinardi and A. J. Rowan, pp. 366–369. Swets and Zeitlinger, Amsterdam.

Vyas, I., and Carney, M. W. P. (1975): Diazepam withdrawal fits. *Br. Med. J.*, 2:44.

Wad, N. T., and Hanifl, E. J. (1977): Simplified thin-layer chromatographic method for simultaneous determination of clonazepam, diazepam, and their metabolites in serum. *J. Chromatogr.*, 143:214–218.

Wad, N. T., Hanifl, E., and Rosenmund, H. (1977): Rapid thin-layer chromatographic method for the simultaneous determination of carbamazepine, diphenylhydantoin, mephenytoin, phenobarbital and primidone in serum. *J. Chromatogr.*, 143:89–93.

Wad, N., T., and Rosenmund, H. (1978): Rapid quantitative method for the simultaneous determination of carbamazepine, carbamazepine-10,11-epoxide, diphenylhydantoin, mephenytoin, phenobarbital and primidone in serum by thin-layer chromatography. *J. Chromatogr.*, 146:167–168.

Wad, N., Rosenmund, H., and Hanifl, E. (1976): A simplified quantitative method for the simultaneous determination of diazepam and its metabolite in serum by thin-layer chromatography. *J. Chromatogr.*, 128:231–234.

Wada, J. A. (1977): Pharmacological prophylaxis in the kindling model of epilepsy. *Arch. Neurol.*, 34:389–395.

Wahlström, G., and Nordberg, A. (1978): Decreased brain weights in rats after long-term barbital treatments. *Life Sci.*, 23:1583–1590.

Walker, J. E., Homan, R. W., Vasko, M. R., Crawford, I. L., Bell, R. D., and Tasker, W. G. (1979): Lorazepam in status epilepticus. *Ann. Neurol.*, 6:207–213.

Wallace, J. E., Biggs, J., and Dahl, E. V. (1965): Determination of diphenylhydantoin by ultraviolet spectrophotometry. *Anal. Chem.*, 37:410–413.

Wallace, J. E., and Hamilton, H. E. (1974): Diphenylhydantoin microdetermination in serum and plasma by ultraviolet spectrophotometry. *J. Pharmacol. Sci.*, 63:1795–1798.

Wallis, W., Kutt, H., and McDowell, F. (1968): Intravenous diphenylhydantoin in treatment of acute repetitive seizures. *Neurology*, 18:513–525.

Waltregny, A., and Dargent, J. (1975): Preliminary study of parenteral lorazepam in status epilepticus. *Acta Neurol. Belg.*, 75:219–229.

Wang, L. K., Costello, C. E., and Biemann, K. (1976): Methylation artifacts in gas chromatography of serum extracts. *J. Chromatogr.*, 116:321–331.

Wasterlain, C. G. (1972a): Breakdown of brain polysomes in status epilepticus. *Brain Res.*, 39:278–284.

Wasterlain, C. G. (1972b): Inhibition of cerebral protein synthesis in status epilepticus. *Neurology*, 22:427 *(Abstr.)*.

Wasterlain, C. G., and Plum, F. (1973): Vulnerability of developing rat brain to electroconvulsive seizures. *Arch. Neurol.*, 29:38–45.

Weinstein, A. W., and Allen, R. J. (1966): Ethosuximide treatment of petit mal seizures. *Am. J. Dis. Child.*, 111:63–73.

Wells, C. E. (1957): Trimethadione: Its dosage and toxicity. *Arch. Neurol. Psychiatry*, 77:140–155.

Welton, D. G. (1950): Exfoliative dermatitis and hepatitis due to phenobarbital. *JAMA*, 143:232–234.

Westenberg, H. G. M., and DeZeeuw, R. A. (1976): Rapid and sensitive liquid chromatographic determination of carbamazepine, suitable for use in monitoring drug anticonvulsant therapy. *J. Chromatogr.*, 118:217–224.

Westenberg, H. G. M., Van der Kleijn, E., Oei, T. T., and DeZeeuw, R. A. (1978): Kinetics of carbamazepine and carbamazepine-epoxide determined by use of plasma and saliva. *Clin. Pharmacol. Ther.*, 23:320–328.

Westreich, G., and Kneller, W. (1972): Intravenous lidocaine for status epilepticus. *Minerva Med.*, 55:807–809.

Whittle, B. A. (1976): Pre-clinical teratological studies on sodium valproate (Epilim) and other anticonvulsants. In: *Clinical and Pharmacological Aspects of Sodium Valproate (Epilim) in the Treatment of Epilepsy*, edited by N. J. Legg, pp. 105–111. MCS Consultants, Tunbridge Wells.

Whittle, S. R., and Turner, A. J. (1978): Effects of the anticonvulsant sodium valproate on α-aminobutyrate and aldehyde metabolism in ox brain. *J. Neurochem.*, 31:1453–1459.

Wilder, B. J. (1981): Experimental studies, models and phylogenetic aspects of secondary epileptogenesis. In: *Secondary Epileptogenesis*, edited by A. Mayersdorf and R. P. Schmidt. Raven Press, New York. *(In press.)*

Wilder, B. J., and Buchanan, R. A. (1981): Methsuximide for refractory complex partial seizures. *Neurology (In press.)*

Wilder, B. J., Buchanan, R. A., and Serrano, E. E. (1973*a*): Correlation of acute diphenylhydantoin intoxication with plasma levels and metabolic excretion. *Neurology*, 23:1329–1332.

Wilder, B. J., and Ramsay, R. E. (1976): Oral and intramuscular phenytoin. *Clin. Pharmacol. Ther.*, 19:360–364.

Wilder, B. J., Ramsay, R. E., Willmore, L. J., Feussner, G. G., Perchalski, R. J., and Shumate, J. B. (1977): Efficacy of intravenous phenytoin in the treatment of status epilepticus. *Ann. Neurol.*, 1:511–518.

Wilder, B. J., Serrano, E. E., and Ramsay, R. E. (1973*b*): Plasma diphenylhydantoin levels after loading and maintenance doses. *Clin. Pharmacol. Ther.*, 14:798–801.

Wilder, B. J., Serrano, E. E., Ramsay, R. E., and Buchanan, R. A. (1974*a*): A method for shifting from oral to intramuscular diphenylhydantoin administration. *Clin. Pharmacol. Ther.*, 16:507–513.

Wilder, B. J., Willmore, L. J., Bruni, J., and Villarreal, H. J. (1978): Valproic acid: Interaction with other anticonvulsant drugs. *Neurology*, 28:892–896.

Wilder, B. J., Streiff, R. R., and Hammer, R. H. (1972): Diphenylhydantoin: Absorption, distribution and excretion. In: *Antiepileptic Drugs*, edited by D. M. Woodbury, J. K. Penry, and R. P. Schmidt, pp. 137–148. Raven Press, New York.

Wilder, R. M. (1921): The effect of ketonemia on the course of epilepsy. *Mayo Clin. Bull.*, 2:307–308.

Wilensky, A. J., Levy, R. H., and Troupin, A. S. (1978): Clorazepate kinetics in treated epileptics. *Clin. Pharmacol. Ther.*, 24:22–30.

Wilensky, A. J., and Lowden, A. J. (1973): Inadequate serum levels after intramuscular administration of diphenylhydantoin. *Neurology*, 23:318–324.

Wilkus, R. J., Dodrill, C. B., and Troupin, A. S. (1978): Carbamazepine and the electroencephalogram of epileptics: A double blind study in comparison to phenytoin. *Epilepsia*, 19:283–291.

Willmore, L. J., Wilder, B. J., Bruni, J., and Villarreal, H. J. (1978): Effect of valproic acid on hepatic function. *Neurology*, 28:961–964.

Wilson, J. T., Hojer, B., Tomson, G., Rane, A., and Störqvist, F. (1978): High incidence of a concentration-dependent skin reaction in children treated with phenytoin. *Br. Med. J.*, 1:1583–1586.

Winfield, D. A., Benton, P., Espir, M. L. E., and Arthur, L. J. H. (1976): Sodium valproate and thrombocytopenia. *Br. Med. J.*, 2:981.

Wisdom, G. B. (1976): Enzyme immunoassay. *Clin. Chem.*, 22:1243–1255.

Withrow, C. D. (1980*a*): Oxazolidinediones. In: *Antiepileptic Drugs: Mechanisms of Action, Advances in Neurology, Vol. 27*, edited by G. H. Glaser, J. K. Penry, and D. M.. Woodbury, pp. 577–586. Raven Press, New York.

Withrow, C. D. (1980*b*): The ketogenic diet: Mechanism of anticonvulsant action. In: *Antiepileptic Drugs: Mechanisms of Action, Advances in Neurology, Vol. 27*, edited by G. H. Glaser, J. K. Penry, and D. M. Woodbury, pp. 635–642. Raven Press, New York.

Withrow, C. D., and Woodbury, D. M. (1972*a*): Trimethadione and other oxazolidine-diones: Absorption, distribution, and excretion. In: *Antiepileptic Drugs*, edited by D. M. Woodbury, J. K. Penry, and R. P. Schmidt, pp. 389–394. Raven Press, New York.

Withrow, C. D., and Woodbury, D. M. (1972*b*): Trimethadione and other oxazolidine-diones: Biotransformation. In: *Antiepileptic Drugs*, edited by D. M. Woodbury, J. K. Penry, and R. P. Schmidt, pp. 395–398. Raven Press, New York.

Withrow, C. D., and Woodbury, D. M. (1972*c*): Trimethadione and other oxazolidine-diones: Interactions with other drugs. In: *Antiepileptic Drugs*, edited by D. M. Woodbury, J. K. Penry, and R. P. Schmidt, pp. 399–402. Raven Press, New York.

Wolf, B. (1978): Dipropylacetate and propionyl CoA carboxylate. *Lancet*, 2:369.

Wolf, P., and Haas, H. L. (1977): Effects of diazepines and barbiturates on hippocampal recurrent inhibition. *Naunyn Schmiedebergs Arch. Pharmacol.*, 299:211–218.

Wolf, S. M. (1977): Effectiveness of daily phenobarbital in the prevention of febrile seizure recurrences in "simple" febrile convulsions and "epilepsy triggered by fever." *Epilepsia*, 18:95–99.

Wolf, S. M. (1979): Controversies in the treatment of febrile seizures. *Neurology*, 29:287–290.

Wolf, S. M., Carr, A., Davis, D. C., Davidson, S., Dale, E. P., Forsythe, A., Goldenberg, E. D., Hanson, R., Lulejian, G. A., Nelson, M. A., Treitman, P., and Weinstein, A. (1977): The value of phenobarbital in the child who has had a single febrile seizure: A controlled prospective study. *Pediatrics*, 59:378–385.

Wood, M. H., Sampson, D. C., and Hensley, W. J. (1977): The estimation of plasma valproate by gas liquid chromatography. *Clin. Chim. Acta*, 77:343.

Woodbury, D. M. (1952): Effects of chronic administration of anticonvulsant drugs, alone and in combination with desoxycorticosterone, on electroshock seizure threshold and tissue electrolytes. *J. Pharmacol. Exp. Ther.*, 105:46–57.

Woodbury, D. M. (1972): Sulfonamides and derivatives: Acetazolamide. In: *Antiepileptic Drugs*, edited by D. M. Woodbury, J. K. Penry, and R. P. Schmidt, pp. 465–475. Raven Press, New York.

Woodbury, D. M. (1977): Pharmacology and mechanisms of action of antiepileptic drugs. In: *Scientific Approaches to Clinical Neurology*, edited by E. S. Goldensohn and S. H. Appel, pp. 693–726. Lea and Febiger, Philadelphia.

Woodbury, D. M. (1980a): Phenytoin: Proposed mechanisms of anticonvulsant action. In: *Antiepileptic Drugs: Mechanisms of Action, Advances in Neurology, Vol. 27*, edited by G. H. Glaser, J. K. Penry, and D. M. Woodbury, pp. 447–472. Raven Press, New York.

Woodbury, D. M. (1980b): Convulsant drugs: Mechanisms of action. In: *Antiepileptic Drugs: Mechanisms of Action, Advances in Neurology, Vol. 27*, edited by G. H. Glaser, J. K. Penry, and D. M. Woodbury, pp. 249–304. Raven Press, New York.

Woodbury, D. M. (1980c): Antiepileptic drugs: Carbonic anhydrase inhibitors. In: *Antiepileptic Drugs: Mechanisms of Action, Advances in Neurology, Vol. 27*, edited by G. H. Glaser, J. K. Penry, and D. M. Woodbury, pp. 617–634. Raven Press, New York.

Woodbury, D. M. (1980d): Phenytoin: Introduction and history. In: *Antiepileptic Drugs: Mechanisms of Action, Advances in Neurology, Vol. 27*, edited by G. H. Glaser, J. K. Penry, and D. M. Woodbury, pp. 305–315. Raven Press, New York.

Woodbury, D. M., and Kemp, J. W. (1977): Basic mechanisms of seizures: Neurophysiological and biochemical etiology. In: *Psychopathology and Brain Dysfunction*, edited by C. Shagass, S. Gerson, and A. J. Friedhoff, pp. 149–182. Raven Press, New York.

Woodbury, D. M., Penry, J. K., Schmidt, R. P., editors (1972): *Antiepileptic Drugs*. Raven Press, New York.

Wu, A. (1974): Concerning on column methylation of phenobarbital. A letter. *Clin. Chem.*, 20:630.

Yanai, J., Roselli-Austin, L., and Tabakoff, B. (1979): Neuronal deficits in mice following prenatal exposure to phenobarbital. *Exp. Neurol.*, 64:237–244.

Yeo, P. P. B., Bates, D., Howe, J. G., Ratcliffe, W. A., Schardt, C. W., Heath, A., and Evered, D. C. (1978): Anticonvulsants and thyroid function. *Br. Med. J.*, 1:1581–1583.

Young, A. B., Zukin, S. R., and Snyder, S. H. (1974): Interaction of benzodiazepines with central nervous system glycine receptors: Possible mechanism of action. *Proc. Natl. Acad. Sci. USA*, 71:2246–2250.

Young, R. S. K., Bergman, I., Gang, D. L., and Richardson, E. P. (1980): Fatal Reye-like syndrome associated with valproic acid. *Ann. Neurol.*, 7:389.

Yunis, A. A., Arimura, B. K., Lutcher, C. L., Blasquez, J., and Halloran, M. (1967): Biochemical lesion in Dilantin-induced erythroid aplasia. *Blood*, 30:587–600.

Zakusov, V. V., Ostrovskaya, R. U., Markovitch, V. V., Molodavken, G. M., and Bulayev, V. M. (1975): Electrophysiological evidence for an inhibitory action of diazepam upon brain cortex. *Arch. Int. Pharmacodyn. Ther.*, 214:188–205.

Zimmerman, F. T., and Burgemeister, B. B. (1954): Use of N-methyl-α,α-methylphenyl-succinimide in treatment of petit mal epilepsy. *Arch. Neurol. Psychiatry*, 72:720–725.

Zingales, I. A. (1973): Diazepam metabolism during chronic medication. Unbound fraction in plasma, erythrocytes, and urine. *J. Chromatogr.*, 75:55–78.

Zucker, P., Daum, F., and Cohen, M. I. (1977): Fatal carbamazepine hepatitis. *J. Pediatr.*, 91:667–668.

Subject Index